中华传统医学文化教育与普及丛书

中 医 理 论

Basic Theory of Traditional Chinese Medicine

（汉英对照）

郑湘瑞　著

李晓婧　孙俊芳　主　译

许二平　中文主审

张加民　英文主审

U0254625

东南大学出版社
SOUTHEAST UNIVERSITY PRESS
·南京·

内 容 提 要

《中医理论》在论述中国传统文化体系中系列相对的概念，如天与地、上与下、昼与夜、明与暗、阴与阳、虚与实以及五行相生相克等的基础上，阐述了系列概念在中医中的体现和运用，解释了中医如何将这些概念上升到哲学高度，并从藏象学说、气血津液、十四经络、病因病机、望闻问切、中药理论、中医养生等方面介绍、论述了中医的基础理论，以帮助读者初步认识、了解中医，体会其辩证体系和思辨方式，为进一步深入学习奠定基础。

本书适用于从事中医学习、研究及对中医或中国传统文化有兴趣的人员，也可作为汉语国际教育、来华外国留学生及中国传统文化推广的教材使用。

图书在版编目（CIP）数据

中医理论：汉英对照 / 郑湘瑞著；李晓婧，孙俊芳

主译 . —南京：东南大学出版社，2018.6

ISBN 978-7-5641-7716-4

Ⅰ.①中… Ⅱ.①郑… ②李… ③孙 Ⅲ.①中医医学基础－汉、英 Ⅳ.① R22

中国版本图书馆 CIP 数据核字（2018）第 070988 号

中 医 理 论（汉 英 对 照）

著 者	郑湘瑞		**责任编辑**	刘 坚
主 译	李晓婧 孙俊芳			
电 话	（025）83793329 **QQ**：635353748		**邮 箱**	liu-jian@seu.edu.cn
出版发行	东南大学出版社		**出 版 人**	江建中
社 址	南京市四牌楼 2 号（210096）		**邮 编**	210096
销售电话	（025）83794561/83794121/83794174/83795801/83795802/83792174/57711295（传真）			
网 址	http://www. seupress. com		**电子邮箱**	press@seupress.com
经 销	全国各地新华书店		**印 刷**	虎彩印艺股份有限公司
开 本	787mm×1092mm 1/16		**印 张**	14.25 **字 数** 370 千
版 次	2018 年 6 月第 1 版		**印 次**	2018 年 6 月第 1 次印刷
书 号	ISBN 978-7-5641-7716-4			
定 价	45.00 元			

* 本书内所有文字、图片均不得转载、演绎、违者必究。

* 本书若有印装质量问题，可随时向我社营销部调换，电话（025-83891830）

总序

　　人类在漫长的发展进程中创造了丰富多彩的文明，中华文明是世界文明多样性、多元化的重要组成部分，对世界文明进步产生了积极影响。中医药是中华优秀传统文化的典型代表，强调道法自然、天人合一、阴阳平衡、调和致中，体现了中华文化的内核。中医药还提倡"辨证论治"，"仁心仁术"，更丰富了中华文化内涵，为中华民族认识和改造世界提供了有益启迪。

　　中医药的文化内涵和学术价值也越来越为世人接纳和认可。目前已有130个中医药类项目列入国家级非物质文化遗产代表性项目名录，"中医针灸"列入联合国教科文组织人类非物质文化遗产代表作名录，《黄帝内经》和《本草纲目》入选世界记忆名录。屠呦呦因发现"青蒿素——一种用于治疗疟疾的药物"，荣获2011年美国拉斯克临床医学奖和2015年诺贝尔生理学或医学奖。因将传统中药的砷剂与西药结合而显著提高急性早幼粒细胞白血病的疗效，王振义、陈竺获得第七届圣捷尔吉癌症研究创新成就奖。

　　在"一带一路"背景下的今天，中医药文化的国际发展尤其引人瞩目。然而这套丛书的目的不在于把中医药文化拿出去给世人看，乃是邀请世人走进中医药的世界，一起来领略天覆地载、万物悉备中的春生夏长、秋收冬藏、君臣佐使、浮沉升降，体味在这个古老的东方国度里某些生活态度和思维方式何以形成，人们与自然如何彼此相应。

　　这套丛书共分四册：《中医理论》将带你进入中医药独特的思维方式和理论体系中。在这里，你将认识一对对概念，如天与地、上与下、内与外、昼与夜、明与暗、寒与热、虚与实、散与聚，既相互对立，又在此消彼长中获得动态的平衡。你也将领略金木水火土之间的运动变化、相生相克，以及五行如何从五种具体物质中抽象出来，上升为哲学的理性概念。在这里，心为君主，肺为相傅，肝为将军，脾胃为仓廪之官；在这里，你会看到有形的五脏和无形的经络；你将看到中医如何"视其外应，测知其内"，并学会如何"顺时摄养"，保持机体内外环境的协调统一。

　　《中医名言》是历代名家名言的集锦，许多隽永的句子今天依然闪烁着智慧的光芒。这里有丰富的医学人文思想："医，仁术也。仁人君子，必笃于情。""无恒德者，不可以作医。也有对生命的尊重："人命至重，有贵千金，一方济之，德逾于此。"许多名言简洁而练达，言有尽而意无穷，有种不可言说的美感：坚者削之、客者除之、劳者温之、结者散之、留者攻之、燥者濡之、散者收之、损者温之、逸者行之、惊者平之、微者逆之、甚者从之……

　　《中医名家》对历代名医进行了介绍，包括生平简介、医学贡献、学术思想以及趣闻轶事等等，使读者从更加直观具体的角度来了解中医学的思想，而且每个医家各有所长，如清朝叶桂所言"内伤必取法乎东垣"（《叶氏医案存真》）。你在这里会深入了解很多名医，如孙思邈、华佗、扁鹊、张仲景、王叔和、葛洪等，也会结识一些普通人不太熟悉但是有过突出贡献的医生：薛己、缪希雍、喻昌等。有些是宫廷御医，有些却游走于民间市井街巷，有些出身名门，有些家境贫寒，他们以高尚的医德和精湛的医术使他们的影响超越了时代和国界。

　　《中医名著》对有代表性的历代中医典籍的主要内容、学术思想做了整理。其中，《黄帝内经》是中医理论体系的奠基之作，被奉为"医家之宗"；《伤寒杂病论》是我国医学在临床方

中医名著

Masterpieces of Traditional Chinese Medicine

面获得迅速发展的一个重要标志。你还将看到我国第一部医学百科全书——《千金方》，中医第一部临床急救手册——《肘后备急方》，最早的针灸学专著——《针灸甲乙经》，我国现存最早的药物学专著——《神农本草经》，中医关于药物炮制的第一部专书——《雷公炮炙论》，以及几百年来令医学界争论不休的《医林改错》……

没有任何一门学科的语言像中医语言一样有如此丰富的修辞：逆水行舟、闭门留寇、滋水涵木、提壶揭盖、釜底抽薪；治上焦如羽，非轻不举；治下焦如权，非重不沉。

也没有哪门学科的术语具备如此和谐的音节和对仗的词语：盛者责之，虚者责之；郁火宜发，实火宜泻；发表不远热，攻里不远寒；攻不可以收缓功，补不可以求速效。

中医哲学的深邃思想也体现在字里行间，在望闻问切、理法方药中，往往有更多哲理的意蕴：天地之理，有开必有合；用药之机，有补必有泻；见病医病，医家大忌；急则治其标，缓则治其本。

在这个世界里，万物是彼此关联的：寒极生热，热极生寒；乙癸同源，肝肾同治；有诸内者，必形诸外。

在这个世界中，人与天地自然的关系是和谐的，人们日出而作，日落而息。阴阳自和者，必自愈。

在这个世界里，医生不只是医生，可以是统帅千军的将领，因为"用药如用兵"。善用兵者，必先屯粮；善治邪者，必先养正。其高者，因而越之；其下者，引而竭之；其在皮者，汗而发之；其慓悍者，按而收之；其实者，散而泻之。用补之法，贵乎先轻后重，务在成功；用攻之法，必须先缓后峻，及病则已。

在这个世界里，并非有病的人才需要医生，也并非能治病的人就是最好的医生，因为圣人"不治已病治未病，不治已乱治未乱"。病也远不仅仅出于风、寒、暑、湿、燥、火，还有喜、怒、忧、思、悲、恐、惊。

虽然中医是崇尚经典的：医之为书，非《素问》无以立论，非《本草》无以主方。然而这套丛书的目的绝不在于怀旧或尚古，而在于启发我们今天的生活，因为"善言天者，必有验于人；善言古者，必有合于今；善言人者，必有厌于己。"

"未医彼病，先医我心。"今天的社会充满了浮躁和喧哗，亲爱的读者，在走近这套丛书的时候，请先预备一颗安静的心。有医术，更要有医道。术可暂行一时，道则永远流传。这套丛书未必要培养高明的医者，但其中蕴含的生命哲理或能伴你一生。

李照国
于 2017 年 8 月

Preface

Humanity has created a colorful civilization in the long course of development, and the civilization of China is an important component of the diverse world civilization, producing a positive impact on the progress of human civilization. TCM is the epitome of traditional Chinese culture. Applying such principles as "man should observe the law of nature and seek for the unity of the heaven and humanity", "yin and yang should be balanced to obtain the golden mean". TCM embodies the core value of Chinese civilization. TCM also advocates "syndrome differentiation and treatment", and "mastership of medicine lying in proficient medical skills and lofty medical ethics", which enriches Chinese culture and provides an enlightened base for Chinese to study and transform the world.

TCM's cultural connotation and academic value are increasingly gaining acceptance around the world. Up till now, 130 TCM elements have been incorporated into the Representative List of National Intangible Cultural Heritage, with TCM acupuncture and moxibustion been included in the Representative List of the Intangible Cultural Heritage of Humanity by UNESCO, and *Huangdi's Internal Classic* and *Compendium of Materia Medica* are listed in the Memory of the World Register. Tu Youyou won the 2011 Lasker Award in clinical medicine and the 2015 Nobel Prize in Physiology or Medicine for discovering qinghaosu (artemisinin) to cure malaria. Wang Zhenyi and Chen Zhu were awarded the Seventh Annual Szent-Gyorgyi Prize for Progress in Cancer Research for combining the Western medicine ATRA and the TCM compound arsenic trioxide to treat acute promyelocytic leukemia (APL).

Under the background of "One Belt One Road Initiative", the global development of TCM has been put under the spotlight. Yet the motivation of the series is not to show TCM to the world, but to bring people to get into the world of TCM, to explore the realm with the covering of the heavens in the upper and the support of the earth in the lower, with the generating spring, growing summer, harvesting autumn and storing winter; and to comprehend the monarch, minister, assistant and guide (metaphors of medicines based on their functions) and the floating, sinking, ascending and descending of Chinese herbs; to have a taste of the way that styles of life and ways of thinking are formed, and how they adjust themselves to achieve the harmony with the environment in this ancient oriental kingdom.

The series include four books: *Basic Theory of TCM* will bring you into a unique way of thinking and the system of TCM theory. Here you will get to know a set of opposite concepts, such as the heaven and the earth, up and down, inside and outside, day and night, light and dark, cold and heat, deficiency and excess, the scattered and the gathered, yet are in dynamic balance through constant waxing and waning. You will also get to know the movement and change, promotion and restriction of wood, fire, earth, metal and water and see how the five elements are abstracted from the five materials and sublimated into philosophical rational concept. Here the

中医名著

Masterpieces of Traditional Chinese Medicine

heart is like a monarch, the lung is an assistant, the liver is a general, and the spleen and stomach are barn officials; here you will see the tangible five zang-organs and feel the intangible meridian system. You will know how the TCM doctors know the inside by observing the outside and how to regulate the spirit according to the changes of the four seasons to harmonize the internal and external environments of the body.

TCM Mottos is a collection of the famous sayings in TCM history, many of which are still glittering with the light of wisdom. Here you will read rich thoughts of medical humanities, "Medicine is a kind of compassionate skill. Benevolent gentlemen should be affectionate. Without solid morality, a person cannot become a doctor." It also shows the respect for human lives, "Human life is topmost and valuable, while a treatable formula is much more valuable." With their simplicity and expressiveness, the sayings here are inexpressibly beautiful with few words but infinite meanings: Diseases caused by hardness of qi should be treated with reducing therapy; invasion of evil should be treated with eliminating therapy. Overstrain should be treated with warming therapy; stagnation should be treated with dispersing therapy. Retention disease should be treated with attacking therapy. Dryness disease should be treated with moistening therapy. Flaccidity disease should be treated with astringing therapy. Impairment disease should be treated with warming therapy. Stagnancy disease should be treated with dredging therapy. Fright should be treated with calming therapy. Mild disease should be treated with contrary therapy; severe disease should be treated with conforming therapy. . .

Masters of TCM is an introduction of the famous doctors in Chinese history, including their lives, medical contribution, academic thoughts and anecdotes. You will learn about the TCM thinking from a more concrete and personal perspective. Each doctor has his own specialty, just as Ye Gui says, "To find treatment methods of internal diseases, all doctors refer to Li Dongyuan." (*Yeshi Yi'an Cunzhen*, written by Ye Gui of the Qing Dynasty) Here you will learn about some not so familiar names like Xue Ji, Miao Xiyong, Yu Chang, as well as some famous ones like Sun Simiao, Hua Tuo, Bian Que, Zhang Zhongjing, Wang Shuhe, and Ge Hong. Some of them were court physicians, yet others worked in villages and towns; some were born to the purple, yet some were of very humble-birth, whose influence all go beyond time and borders owing to their noble morality and outstanding medical skills.

Masterpieces of TCM introduces the content and academic value of some important TCM works in the history of Chinese medicine. *Huangdi's Internal Classic* lays the foundation of TCM theoretical system, thus it is called "the source of medical thoughts". *Treatise on Cold Damage and Miscellaneous Diseases* is a symbol of China's rapid development in clinical medicine. You will also read about the first medical encyclopedia in China——*Thousand Golden Prescriptions*, the first clinical first-aid manual of traditional Chinese medicine—*Handbook of Prescriptions for Emergency*, the earliest extant book on acupuncture and moxibustion *A—B Classic of Acupuncture and Moxibustion*, the earliest classic on materia medica extant in China——*Shennong's Classic of*

Masterpieces of Traditional Chinese Medicine

中医名著

Materia Medica, the first monograph on processing of drugs——*Master Lei's Discourse on Medicine Processing*, and the book with endless arguments for hundreds of years in the medical world——*Correction on Errors in Medical Works*...

No other discipline has the language like TCM with so rich rhetorical expressions: sailing against the current, closing the door to keep the intruders, replenishing water to nourish wood, raising the kettle and opening the lid, taking away the firewood from under the cauldron; the disease of the upper energizer should be treated by drugs with light, clear, ascending and float natures, while the disease of the lower energizer should be treated by heavy, suppressing, greasy, nourishing and subduing drugs, which can affect the lower part of the body.

No other discipline has the terms with such melody in sound and symmetry in words: Diseases, be there symptoms excessive or deficient, should be explored from the root cause. Stagnant fire should be dispersed; excessive fire should be treated by clearing heat and reducing fire. When relieving pathogenic factors from the exterior, the use of drugs hot in nature should not be avoided; when attacking the interior, the use of drugs cold in nature should not be avoided. Attacking the pathogen should not be too slow, while nourishing should not be too rapid and effective.

The profound philosophical wisdom is often embodied in the simple TCM expressions. In the four examinations, the theories, treatments, formulas and drugs, you can draw deeper lessons: change in the world including opening and closing process; the mechanism of prescription including tonifying and purifying. Doctors should abstain from treating the exterior symptoms of the disease, but relieving the secondary in an urgent case and removing the primary in a chronic case.

In this world, everything is closely related with each other: Extreme cold generates heat and extreme heat produces cold. Yi (the second heavenly stem) and Gui (the tenth heavenly stem) have the same origin, which means that the liver and the kidney should be treated together. Every change inside the body is certainly manifested outside correspondingly.

In this world, human beings have a harmonious relationship with the nature: People get up to work when the sun rises and have rest when the sun sets. If yin and yang become harmonized by themselves, the disease will be cured.

In this world, doctors are more than doctors, but also commanders of the army since "treatment and prescription are similar to the command of military forces in the war". A general good at leading army will certainly store enough provisions to conserve energy and build up strength. A skillful doctor will certainly support and protect the vital qi when he is treating the disease and eliminating the pathogens. If the pathogenic factors have accumulated in the upper, vomiting therapy should be used. If the pathogenic factors have accumulated in the lower, dredging therapy should be used. If the pathogenic factors are in the skin, sweating therapy can be used. If the pathogenic conditions are acute, measures should be taken to control them. For excess or sthenia syndrome, dispersing therapy and purging therapy can be used. The treatment of invigoration should be light first and heavy then. The purgative method should be moderate first and fierce then.

In this world, not only the patients need doctors, and the best doctor is not the one who can treat diseases, since sages usually pay less attention to the treatment of a disease, but more to the prevention of it. They deal with problems before they appear, instead of dealing with them after they have appeared. Diseases are not only caused by wind, cold, heat, dampness, dryness and fire, but also joy, anger, worry, thinking, sorrow, fear and fright.

Although TCM greatly honors classic works: medical books are rooted in theories of *Su Wen* and based on formulas of *Compendium of Material Medica*, the purpose of the series is far from nostalgia or archaism, because "Those who are good at explaining the heavens must be able to prove it with human affairs, those who are good at discussing history must be able to relate it to the present situation and those who are good at talking about others must be able to delineate themselves."

Before curing diseases, doctors should keep their own mind correct first. Anyone who is going to open the series should bear a peaceful mind although today's society is filled with restlessness and noise. Medical doctrines always go before medical skills. Medical skills are used only for a time, while medical doctrines last through ages. This series of books will not necessarily equip you to be a qualified doctor, but the philosophy of life in them may benefit you for the rest of your life.

Li Zhaoguo

August, 8,2017

目 录
CONTENTS

绪言　理论体系
Introduction　Theoretical System

中国是医药文化发祥最早的国家之一,有文字可考的医学史长达数千年。在已出土的殷商时期甲骨文中,便有大量关于疾病的名称,在卜筮史料中记载了大量医药卫生的内容,形成了医学的雏形。西周《周礼·天官》记载了我国最早的医学分科,把医生分为食医(营养师)、疾医(内科)、疡医(外科)和兽医。

《黄帝内经》吸收了秦汉以前的天文、历法、气象、数学、生物、地理等多学科的重要成果,在阴阳、五行等学说指导下,总结了春秋战国以前的医疗成就和治疗经验,确定了中医学的理论框架,系统地阐述了脏腑、经络、气血津液、诊断、治疗、预防等问题,建立了独特的理论体系,成为中医学发展的基础和理论源泉。它与张仲景的《伤寒杂病论》分别是中医学基本理论和辨证论治的奠基之作。二者与《神农本草经》《难经》一起,被历代医家奉为经典,由

China, as one of the earliest countries of medical culture, has a recorded history of medical science for several thousand years. In the inscriptions on bones or tortoise shells of the Shang dynasty, there are a lot of disease names. Under the situation of coexistence of doctors and witch doctors, a large amount of information about medicine and health is found in the historical materials of divination, forming the medical prototype. The earliest medical division of China is recorded in *Rites of the Zhou* in which doctors are divided into dietitians (nutritionists), physicians (internal medicine), surgeons (surgery) and veterinarians.

Under the guidance of the theory of yin and yang and the five elements, *Huangdi's Inernal Classic (Huangdi Neijing)* absorbs the significant achievements of astronomy, calendar, meteorology, mathematics, biology, geography, and other subjects and summarizes the medical achievements and treatment experience before the Spring and Autumn period and the Warring States period. It builds up the theoretical framework of TCM and systematically expounds viscera, meridians, qi-blood and body fluid, diagnosis, treatment and prevention and other issues. It establishes a unique theoretical system which becomes the basis and theoretical source of the development of TCM. The Canon and Zhang Zhongjing's *Treatise on Cold Damage and Miscellaneous Diseases (Shanghan Zabing Lun)* are respectively the foundation works of the basic theory of TCM and "treatment based on syndrome differentiation". The two books, together with *Shennong's classic of Materia Medica (Shennong Bencao Jing)* and Classic *of Difficult*

此确立了中医学独特的理论体系，给后世医学的发展以深远的影响。

中医学理论体系是包括理、法、方、药在内的一个整体，主要阐明中医学的基本理论、基本规律和基本方法。它是以整体观念为主导思想，以阴阳、五行学说等为论理方法，以脏腑、经络、精气血津液为生理病理基础，以辨证论治为诊治特点的独特的医学理论体系。

理、法、方、药是中医药学关于诊断与治疗操作规范的整体性概括。中医临床诊疗的焦点集中体现在"方"或"方剂"上，俗称"药方"。药方自然由药物组成，其组成绝不是药物简单的堆积和罗列，它一定是药物之间君、臣、佐、使的配伍关系及其剂量的最佳选择，是对特定疾病病变所确定的相应的治疗原则和治疗方法的体现，即所谓的"法"；方剂有效与否取决于其是否符合中医药学理论对疾病病变机理作出的准确的解释和判断，即所谓的"理"。

辨证论治就是理、法、方、药具体运用于临床的过程。

辨证是指分析、辨识疾病的证候，即诊断的过程。中医诊断，主要采用望、闻、问、切四种诊察疾病的方法，简称四诊。望诊是对患者的神色、形态、五官、舌象

Issues (*Nan Jing*) are regarded as classics by doctors in the past dynasties, which establish the unique theoretical system of TCM and give a far-reaching impact on the development of medicine in later generations.

The theoretical system of TCM is a wholeness including the theory, method, prescription and medicine, which mainly expounds the basic theory, rules and methods of TCM. It is a unique theoretical system of medicine which takes the concept of holism as the guiding ideology, the theory of yin and yang and five elements as the logical method, the viscera, meridians, essence, qi, blood and body fluid as the physiological and pathological basis, and, is characterized by syndrome differentiation in diagnosis and treatment.

The theory, method, prescription and medicine are the general summary of the clinical standard of diagnosis and treatment in TCM. The focus of clinical diagnosis and treatment of TCM is reflected in "prescription" which is composed of medicines but far more than a simple mixture of medicines; it is supposed to be the optimal combination of the compatibility relations among monarch, minister, assistant and guide (metaphors of medicines based on their functions) and their doses; it is also the embodiment of the corresponding treatment principle and treatment methods for certain lesions, which is called the "method"; effective prescriptions depend on whether they conform to the accurate interpretation and judgment for the lesion mechanism made according to the theory of TCM, which is called "the theory".

Treatment based on syndrome differentiation is a process in which the theory, method, prescription and medicine are applied to the clinical practice.

Syndrome differentiation means analyzing and identifying the syndrome of the disease, which is the process of diagnosis. The diagnosis in TCM is mainly based on four ways—observing, listening, inquiring and pulse-taking. By the way of observing, the doctor purposefully observes

以及分泌物、排出物等进行有目的地观察,以了解病情,测知脏腑病变。闻诊是从患者语言、呼吸等声音以及由患者体内排出的气味来辨别内在的病情。问诊是通过对患者及知情者的询问,以了解患者平时的健康状态、发病原因、病情经过和患者的自觉症状等。切诊是诊察病人的脉象和身体其他部位,以测知体内变化的情况。四诊各有其特定的诊察内容,不能互相取代,必须四诊合参,才能系统而全面地获得临床资料,为辨证提供可靠依据。

辨证需要以脏腑、气血津液、经络、病因、病机等基础理论为依据,对四诊所收集的症状、体征,以及其他临床资料进行分析、综合,辨清疾病的原因、性质、部位,以及邪正之间的关系,进而概括、判断为何种证候,为论治提供依据。

论治是在辨证基础上拟定出相应的治疗方法和措施。如果说辨证侧重的是"理",那么论治就是"法"、是"方"、是"药"。辨证是论治的前提,论治是辨证的延续,也是辨证的检验和补充。辨证与论治在诊治疾病过程中,相互联系,密不可分,是理、法、方、药在临床上的具体应用。

总之,中医理论体系主要由"理"、"法"、"方"、"药"构成。"理"包括生理(脏腑、气血津液、经络)

the patient's complexion, shape, facial features, tongue image, secretion and discharge to know the illness and the pathological changes of viscera. By the way of listening the doctor identifies the internal disease according to the patient's voice, breath and smell. By the way of inquiring the doctor inquires the patient and the related persons for his or her state of health, the cause and process of the disease and his or her physical condition and symptoms. By pulse-taking the doctor examines the patient's pulse and other parts of the body to know the change of the body. Each of the four ways of diagnosis has its specific content, and cannot be replaced by each other. The combination of the four ways can obtain systematical and comprehensive clinical data to provide a reliable basis for syndrome differentiation.

Syndrome differentiation needs the theory of viscera, essence, qi, blood and body fluid, meridians, etiology and pathogenesis as the basis to analyze and summarize the symptoms, signs, and other clinical data collected through four ways of examination; then it needs to distinguish the cause, nature, location and relationship between the good and the evil; it further needs to summarize and judge the syndromes to provide the basis for treatment determination.

Treatment determination is the corresponding treatment method and measure worked out on the basis of syndrome differentiation. Syndrome differentiation is focused on "theory" while treatment determination, on "method", "prescription" and "medicine". Syndrome differentiation is the premise of treatment determination which is a continuation, a test and supplement of syndrome differentiation. In the process of diagnosis and treatment of disease, they are mutually contacted as the specific clinical application of the theory, method, prescription and medicine.

In a word, the theoretical system of TCM is mainly composed of the "theory", "method", "prescription" and "medicine". "Theory" includes physiology (viscera,

中医理论

Basic Theory of Traditional Chinese Medicine

和病理(病因病机);"法"即诊法,包括辨证、治疗原则和方法。"方"即处方、方剂;"药"即药物学。理法方药又在阴阳、五行等哲学理论指导下统一于中医的整体观念中,成为完整的理论与实践的统一体。

qi, blood, body fluid and meridians) and pathology (etiology and pathogenesis); "method" includes syndrome differentiation, treating principles and clinical methods; "prescription" means the formula and combination of medicines in prescription; "medicine" is pharmacology. In the light of the philosophy of yin and yang, five elements, etc., these four are unified in the concept of holism of TCM as a unity of theory and practice.

中医理论

Basic Theory of Traditional Chinese Medicine

第一章　阴阳五行

Chapter 1　Theories of Yin-Yang and the Five Elements

阴阳五行是中国古代用以认识自然和解释自然的世界观和方法论，是中医学理论的重要组成部分。阴阳、五行各自有其系统的理论并且贯穿中医理论体系的各个方面：从生命起源到人体的组织结构、从生理功能到病理变化、从分析归纳疾病的证候类型到诊断和治疗疾病乃至养生保健，无不与阴阳五行理论相关。

The theories of yin-yang and the five elements, as the important component of the theory of TCM, are the perspective and methodology that people used to understand and expound the nature in ancient China. Respectively, yin-yang and the five elements have their own systematical theory permeated throughout all aspects of TCM theory: the origin of life, the organic structures, physiological functions, pathological changes of the human body, diagnosis, treatment and health care.

1　阴阳学说

阴阳学说是关于对立统一规律的认识，物质世界在阴阳二气的相互作用下，不断运动变化。阴阳学说渗透到医学领域，促进了中医学理论体系的形成和发展，逐渐与中医学融为一体，形成了中医学的阴阳学说。中医学用阴阳的运动规律来解释说明生命的起源，人体的生理功能、病理变化，指导疾病的诊断和防治，贯穿于中医的理、法、方、药。

1　The Theory of Yin-Yang

The theory of yin-yang is about the understanding of the law of opposition and unity, and about movements and changes of material world by the interaction of yin and yang. It permeates into the medical field, facilitating the formation and development of TCM and shaping the theory of yin-yang in TCM when it is gradually integrated with TCM. It is applied to explain the origin of life, physiological functions and pathological changes of the human body, to guide the diagnosis and prevention of diseases, and to set the basis of theory, method, prescription and medicine of TCM.

1.1　阴阳的基本含义

阴阳是对自然界相互关联的事物和现象对立双方属性的概括和总结。它既可以表示相互对

1.1　The Basic Meaning of Yin-yang

Yin-yang is the summary of two opposite aspects of interrelated things or phenomena in the nature. It not only refers to the things and phenomena that are opposite to

中医理论

Basic Theory of Traditional Chinese Medicine

立的事物或现象,如天与地、日与月、水与火等;又可以表示同一事物或现象内部对立的两个方面,如寒与热、升与降、明与暗等。

阴阳最初指日光的向背,如山之南、水之北为阳;山之北、水之南为阴。后来用以概括自然界相互关联而又相互对立的事物和现象。一般而言,凡属于运动的、外向的、上升的、温热的、明亮的、功能的皆属于阳的范畴;而相对静止的、内在的、下降的、寒凉的、晦暗的、物质的属于阴的范畴。

事物的阴阳属性不是绝对的,而是相对的。阴阳这种相对性表现为:一方面,在一定条件下,阴和阳之间可以发生相互转化,阴可以转化为阳,阳也可以转化为阴。如寒证可以转化为热证,热证也可以转化成寒证。病变的寒热性质变了,其阴阳属性也随之改变。另一方面表现为阴阳的无限可分性,即阴中有阳,阳中有阴,阴阳之中复有阴阳,不断地一分为二,以至无穷。如,昼为阳,夜为阴。而上午为阳中之阳,下午则为阳中之阴;前半夜为阴中之阴,后半夜则为阴中之阳。随着对立面的改变,阴阳之中又可以再分阴阳。

也就是说,随着时间的推移或所运用范围的不同,事物的性质或对立面改变了,则其阴阳属性也随之而改变。这种阴阳属性的相对性,不但说明了事物或现象阴阳属性的规律性、复杂性,同

each other, such as the heaven and the earth, the sun and the moon, water and fire and so on, but also refers to two aspects inside the same thing or phenomenon, such as cold and heat, rise and fall, brightness and darkness, etc.

Originally, yin and yang refer to the two sides of the mountain: the side facing the sun is yang and the reverse side is yin. Therefore the south of a mountain and the north of a river is yang; the north of a mountain and the south of a river is yin. Then, everything in the natural world with opposition and interdependence can be attributed to either yin or yang respectively. Generally speaking, things that are movable, exterior, ascending, warm, bright and those bear functional activities are yang, while those relatively still, interior, descending, cold, dark and materialistic are yin.

Things' yin-yang attributes are relative rather than absolute. The relativity of yin-yang manifests as follows: in certain circumstances, on the one hand, either yin or yang may transform into its opposite aspect. For instance, cold syndrome can transform into heat syndrome and vice versa. The change in the cold or warm nature of pathology may promote the change of yin and yang. On the other hand, the relativity can be manifested by the infinite divisibility of yin and yang, namely there is yang in the yin and yin in the yang. Furthermore, any aspect of yin or yang can be sub-divided into yin and yang into infinity. For example, the day belongs to yang, and the night pertains to yin. Morning is the yang aspect of yang, while afternoon is the yin aspect of yang. The first half of the night is the yin aspect of yin, while the second half of the night is the yang aspect of yin. As the change of opposition, sub-division of yin and yang would occur.

With the passage of time or difference of application scope, the nature and opposition change will trigger the change of yin and yang. The relative degree of yin and yang not only shows the regularity, complexity of yin and yang on things or phenomena, but also the comprehensive properties of them. In a word, all things or phenomena

时也说明了阴阳概括事物或现象的广泛性，即每一事物或现象都包含着阴阳两个方面，都是可以一分为二的。

1.2 阴阳学说的基本内容

阴阳之间的关系极其复杂，但也有规律可循。概括起来，主要包括以下几个方面：

1.2.1 阴阳对立制约

阴阳的对立制约主要表现于阴阳之间的相互制约、相互斗争。阴阳双方的对立是绝对的，如天与地、上与下、内与外、动与静、升与降、出与入、昼与夜、明与暗、寒与热、虚与实、散与聚等。阴与阳在相互制约和相互斗争中取得了统一，即取得了动态平衡。万事万物都是阴阳对立的统一。

在中医学中，阴阳对立制约有广泛的应用：

用以说明人体的组织结构：体表为阳，体内为阴；体表的背部属阳，腹部属阴；上半身为阳，下半身属阴；四肢外侧为阳，内侧为阴。五脏为阴，六腑为阳。五脏之中，心肺为阳，肝脾肾为阴；心肺之中，心为阳中之阳，肺为阳中之阴；肝脾肾之间，肝为阳，脾肾为阴等。人的一切组织结构，既是有机联系的，又可以划分为相互对立的阴、阳两部分。所以说："人生有形，不离阴阳。"（《素

include yin and yang, and can be sub-divided.

1.2 The Basic Content of Yin-Yang Theory

The relationship between yin and yang is complex, but there are still rules to follow. To sum up, there are several aspects as the following:

1.2.1 The opposition and restriction of yin and yang

The opposition between yin and yang is mainly manifested in their restriction and combat with each other. The opposition between yin and yang is absolute, such as the heaven and the earth, up and the down, inside and outside, being dynamic and static, rise and fall, out and in, day and night, light and dark, cold and heat, deficiency and excess, the scattered and the gathered and so on. Yin and yang get unity during the process of struggle and restraint with each other, acquiring dynamic balance. The opposition and interdependence of yin and yang lie in all kinds of things and phenomena.

In TCM, the opposition and restriction of yin and yang has a wide range of applications:

It is applied to explain organic structures of human body: the exterior pertains to yang while the interior to yin; the back pertains to yang while the chest and abdomen to yin; the upper part of body pertains to yang while the lower part to yin; the outer side of the limbs pertains to yang while the inner side to yin; the five zang-organs pertain to yin while the six fu-organs to yang. Among the five zang-organs, the heart and lung pertain to yang while the liver, spleen and kidney, to yin; between the heart and lung, the heart is considered as the yang aspect of yang while the lung, the yin aspect of yang; among the liver, spleen and kidney, the liver pertains to yang while spleen and kidney to yin. All the tissues and structures of mankind have organic links, but also can be divided into yin and yang. So it is said: "Human beings have a physical shape which is inseparable from yin and yang". (*Plain Questions: Discussion on*

中医理论 Basic Theory of Traditional Chinese Medicine

问·宝命全形论》)

用以阐释生命活动：就生命物质的结构和功能而言，用阴阳来表述则生命物质为阴（精），生命机能为阳（气）。其运动转化过程则是阳化气，阴成形，即阴阳的对立统一。就生命现象而言，无非气的升降出入，升降和出入的平衡，同样是阴阳双方在对立制约中，取得了统一，维持着动态平衡状态，即所谓"阴平阳秘"，机体才能进行正常的生命活动。如果阴阳的动态平衡被打破，出现阴阳失调，就会导致疾病的发生。

在诊断方面症状分阴阳：如色泽鲜明者属阳，晦暗者属阴；语声高亢洪亮者属阳，低微无力者属阴；呼吸有力、声高气粗者属阳，呼吸微弱、声低气怯者属阴；口渴喜冷者属阳，口渴喜热者属阴；脉之浮、数、洪、滑等属阳，沉、迟、细、涩等属阴。

在临床辨证中，只有分清阴阳，才能抓住疾病的本质，做到执简驭繁。所以辨别阴证、阳证是诊断的基本原则。八纲辨证中，表证、热证、实证属阳；里证、寒证、虚证属阴，在临床上具有重要意义。在脏腑辨证中，脏腑气血阴阳失调可表现出许多复杂的证候，但不外阴阳两大类。

根据阴阳对立制定其相应的治疗原则：损其有余，补其不足，或实者泻之，虚者补之。如

Preserving Health and Protecting Life) (*Suwen*)

It is applied to explain life activities: the vital substance pertains to yin(essence) while the vital functions pertain to yang(qi) so far as the structure and function of life and material are concerned. The transformation process is that yang transforms to qi, and yin takes shape. That is the unity and opposition of yin and yang. Phenomenon of life is nothing more than ascending and descending of qi. The balance of ascending and descending is the same with the opposition and restriction of yin and yang, achieving unity and maintaining a state of dynamic equilibrium, so that the normal state of life can be maintained. If dynamic equilibrium of yin and yang is broken, the imbalance of yin and yang will occur, and so causes diseases.

In the process of diagnosis, the symptoms can be categorized into yin and yang: bright complexion pertains to yang, while grayish complexion, to yin; sonorous voice pertains to yang, while low and weak voice, to yin; high voice and rough breath pertains to yang, while weak breath and low sound, to yin; preference of cold and being thirsty pertains to yang, while preference for heat and being thirsty, to yin; floating, rapid, large and slippery pulses pertain to yang while deep, slow, fine and unsmooth pulses, to yin.

In syndrome differentiation, only by distinguishing between yin and yang can the doctor understand the nature of the diseases. So distinguishing yin syndrome from yang syndrome is the basic principle of diagnosis. In the eight principles of syndrome differentiation, the external syndrome, excess syndrome and heat syndrome pertain to yang syndrome, while the internal syndrome, cold syndrome and deficiency syndrome, to yin. It has important clinical significance. The imbalance of yin and yang of blood and viscera may exhibit many complex syndromes, but they all belong to two categories of yin and yang.

Therapeutic treatment principles should be adhered to according to the opposition and restriction of yin and yang: excess should be reduced and deficiency should be

中医理论

Basic Theory of Traditional Chinese Medicine

阳盛则热属实热证,宜用寒凉药以制其阳,治热以寒,即"热者寒之"。阴盛则寒属寒实证,宜用温热药以制其阴,治寒以热,即"寒者热之"。阴虚不能制阳而致阳亢者,属虚热证,治当滋阴以抑阳。若阳虚不能制阴而造成阴盛者,属虚寒证,治当扶阳制阴。

1.2.2　阴阳互根互用

互根指相互对立的事物之间的相互依存、相互依赖,任何一方都不能脱离另一方而单独存在。阴阳所代表的性质或状态,如天与地、上与下、动与静、寒与热、虚与实、散与聚等等,不仅互相排斥,而且互为存在的条件。如上属阳,下属阴,没有上也就无所谓下;没有下也就无所谓上;昼属阳,夜属阴,没有昼就无所谓夜;没有夜也就没有昼。热属阳,寒属阴,没有热也就无所谓寒;没有寒也就没有热。

互用是指阴阳不仅相互依存,还可以表现为阴阳之间相互促进、相互助长。如物质属阴,功能属阳,物质是生命的基础,功能是生命的体现。物质是功能的基础,功能则是物质的反映。脏腑功能活动健全,就会不断地促进营养物质的化生;而营养物质的充足,则能保护脏腑活动功能的平衡。

阴阳两个方面,任何一方都不能脱离另一方而单独存在。如果双方失去了互为存在的条件,有阳无阴谓之"孤阳",有阴无阳

supplemented. To be more specific, excess-heat syndrome due to the exuberance of pathogenic factors of yang nature should be treated by clearing away the heat while excess-cold syndrome due to the exuberance of pathogenic factors of yin nature should be treated by eliminating the cold. Deficiency-cold syndrome causing excess-heat should be treated by nourishing yin while deficiency-heat syndrome causing excess-cold should be treated by nourishing yang.

1.2.2　Interdependence and interaction between yin and yang

Interdependence means the mutual dependence between opposite things and the fact that any party cannot exist alone without the opposite one. The quality and state which yin and yang represent, like heaven and earth, the upper and the lower, dynamic and static, cold and heat, deficiency and excess, scattering and gathering and so on, are not only mutually exclusive, but also are the prerequisites of each other's existence. For example, the upper belongs to yang, the lower belongs to yin. There will be no lower part without upper part and vice versa. The day pertains to yang and night to yin. There is no day without night and vice versa. Heat pertains to yang while cold to yin. There is no heat without cold and vice versa.

Interaction means that yin and yang are not only interdependent, but also promote and support each other. For example, substance pertains to yin, and function pertains to yang. The substance is the basis of life and the function reflects life. Substance is the basis of function while function is the reflection of the substance. If the function of organs is normal, it will continuously promote the transformation of nutrient substance, and adequate nutrients can protect the balance of the functions of organs.

Yin and yang must exist in pair and no side can be isolated. If they lose the existence prerequisite of each other, there is "solitary yang" without yin and "solitary yin" without yang. Solitary yin cannot grow, solitary yang

中医理论　Basic Theory of Traditional Chinese Medicine

谓之"孤阴"。孤阴不生,独阳不长,一切生物也就不能存在,不能生化和滋长了。如脾气(阳)虚弱的病人,因为脾胃为后天之本,气血生化之源,脾气(阳)虚弱,化源不足,会导致阴(血)亏损,这可称之为阳损及阴的气血两虚证。又如失血病人,由于血液(阴)的大量丢失,气随血脱,往往会出现形寒肢冷的阳虚之候,这可称之为阴损及阳的气血两虚证。

如果人体内阳气与阴液、物质与功能等阴阳互根关系遭到严重破坏,以至一方趋于消失,另一方也就失去了存在的前提,呈现孤阳或孤阴状态。这种阴阳的相离,意味着阴阳矛盾的消失,那么生命也就即将结束了。

所以阳根于阴,阴根于阳,无阳则阴无以生,无阴则阳无以化。阳蕴含于阴之中,阴蕴含于阳之中。

中医学用阴阳互根的观点,阐述人体脏与腑、气与血、功能与物质等在生理病理上的关系。

1.2.3　阴阳消长

消长:增减、盛衰之谓。阴阳对立双方不是处于静止不变的状态,而是始终处于动态的运动变化之中。运动变化是中医学对自然和人体生命活动认识的根本出发点,这是中医学的宇宙恒动观。阴阳消长是一个量变的过程。

四时季节气候的变化,寒暑的更替,就是阴阳消长的过程。从冬至春及夏,寒气渐减,温热日

cannot exist, which means all creatures will not exist, grow up or develop. For example, deficiency in qi can lead to deficiency of yin (blood), as the spleen and stomach are the acquired root and the source of transformation of qi and blood, which is known as dual-deficiency syndrome of qi and blood caused by yang damage affecting yin. Take another example, the patient with blood deficiency can have limbs cooling syndrome, because loss of blood damages qi, which is dual-deficiency syndrome of qi and blood caused by yin damage affecting yang.

If the interdependent relationship between yang-qi and yin-fluid, substance and function in the human body is severely damaged so that one side tends to disappear, and then the other loses premise of existence, and so solitary yin or yang will occur. Yin separating from yang means the contradiction between them disappears, and life will soon come to an end.

So yin and yang are rooted in each other. In other words, without yin there would be no yang; without yang there would be no yin. They rely on each other for existence.

According to the interdependence and interaction between yin and yang, TCM expounds the physiological and pathological relationships between the zang-organs and fu-organs, qi and blood, function and substance.

1.2.3　Waxing and waning between yin and yang

The opposition of yin and yang is not in a static state, but always in a dynamic change. In TCM, change is the fundamental starting point of awareness to nature and human life activities, which is the constantly dynamic concept about the universe. The waxing and waning between yin and yang is a quantitative process.

Seasonal climatic variation and passage of winter and summer is the process of waxing and waning of yin and yang. While the transition from winter cold through spring

增,气候则由寒逐渐变温变热,是"阴消阳长"的过程;由夏至秋及冬,热气渐消,寒气日增,气候则由热逐渐变凉变寒,则是"阳消阴长"的过程。

就人体生理活动而言,各种功能活动(阳)的产生,必然要消耗一定的营养物质(阴),这就是"阳长阴消"的过程;阳气能够促进阴精的化生,这是"阳生阴长";各种营养物质(阴)的化生,又必然消耗一定的能量(阳),这是"阳消阴长";阳气虚弱,化生能力减退,使阴精减少,称为"阳杀阴藏"。

1.2.4 阴阳转化

转化即转换、变化,是指阴阳对立的双方,在一定条件下可以相互转化,阴可以转化为阳,阳可以转化为阴。

阴阳转化是事物运动变化的基本规律。在阴阳消长过程中,发展到一定程度,超越了阴阳正常消长的阈值,事物必然向着相反的方面转化。阴阳的转化,必须具备一定的条件,这种条件中医学称之为"重"或"极",故曰:"重阴必阳,重阳必阴","寒极生热,热极生寒。"(《素问·阴阳应象大论》)

同样,在疾病发展的过程中,在一定条件下,阴证与阳证常常可以发生互相转化。如邪热壅肺的病人,表现为高热、面红、烦躁、脉数有力等,这是机体反应功

warmth into summer heat demonstrates the process of the waning of yin leading to waxing of yang, the transition from summer heat through autumn cool into winter cold is the waning of yang leading to waxing of yin.

For the physiological activities of human body, various functional activities (yang) will necessarily consume a certain amount of nutrient substance (yin), which is the process of "consumption of yin fosters yang". Yang qi can promote the production of yin essence, so it is "yin grows while yang is generating". The production of various nutrient substances (yin) will necessarily consume a certain amount of energy (yang), which is the process of "consumption of yang fosters yin". Deficient yang and declined production capacity leads to the decrease of yin essence, which is called "yin conceals when yang is restrained".

1.2.4 Transformation of yin and yang

Transformation means change. In certain circumstances, the opposite aspect of yin and yang can transform into each other; yin may transform into yang and yang, into yin.

Transformation of yin and yang is the basic law of how things move and change. When the waning and waxing movement of yin and yang develops to an "extreme" stage beyond the normal scope, undesirable results may turn up. Prerequisite conditions are needed for transformation of yin and yang, which can be called as "severe" or "extreme". So there is the saying, "yin in its extreme gives rise to yang while extreme yang gives rise to yin", "cold in its extreme generates heat while heat in its extreme generates cold" *(Plain Questions: Major Discussion on the Theory of Yin and Yang and the Corresponding Relationships among All the Things in Nature).*

Similarly, in the course of the development of the disease, under certain conditions, yin syndrome and yang syndrome may often transform into one another. For instance, a patient with pathogenic heat in the lung has high fever, flushing, irritability, forceful pulse and so on, which is

中医理论 Basic Theory of Traditional Chinese Medicine

能旺盛的表现，称之为阳证、热证、实证；但由于热毒极重，大量耗伤人体正气，在持续高热、面赤、烦躁、脉数有力的情况下，会突然出现面色苍白、四肢厥冷、精神萎靡、脉微欲绝等一派阴寒危象。这是机体反应能力衰竭的表现，称之为阴证、寒证、虚证。这种病症的变化属于由阳转阴。又如咳喘患者，当出现咳嗽喘促、痰液稀白、口不渴、舌淡苔白、脉弦等脉证时，其症属寒(阴证)，常因重感外邪、寒邪外束、阳气闭郁而化热，反而出现咳喘息粗、咳痰黄稠、口渴、舌红苔黄、脉数之候，其症又属于热(阳证)。这种病症的变化，是由寒证转化为热证，即由阴转为阳。明确这些转化，不仅有助于认识病症演变的规律，而且对于确定相应的治疗原则有着极为重要的指导意义。

总之，阴阳是中国古代哲学的基本范畴之一。中国古代哲学把阴阳当成事物的性质及其变化的根本法则，将许多具体事物都赋予了阴阳的含义。阴阳的对立、互根、消长、转化是阴阳学说的基本内容。这些内容不是孤立的，而是互相联系、互相影响、互为因果的。中医认为阴阳双方在动态的过程中保持相对的平衡，人体才能保持正常的运动规律。平衡是维持生命的手段，阴阳平衡是

a strong performance of the body's reaction function called yang syndrome, heat syndrome and excess syndrome; however, because of the intense toxic heat which greatly consumes vital qi, in the circumstance of a persistent fever, red face, irritability, rapid and forceful pulse, there can suddenly appear pale complexion, cold limbs, listlessness, faint pulse and other critical syndromes of yin cold. This is the failure of the body reaction ability called yin syndrome, cold syndrome and deficiency syndrome. This change of syndrome is the transformation of yang into yin. The patients with cough and asthma have cough and short breath, thin and white sputum, no thirst, pale tongue with white coating, wiry pulse and other pulse conditions, are indicated by cold syndrome (yin syndrome). Yet heat can be transformed from heavy exogenous evil, external cold pathogen and yang-qi obstruction, leading to cough, asthma and short breath, thick yellowish sputum, thirst, red tongue with yellowish coating and rapid pulse, which indicates heat syndrome (yang syndrome). The change of this kind of disease is from cold syndrome into heat syndrome, that is, from yin to yang. Knowing these changes is not only helpful to understand the law of the evolution of disease and syndrome, but also has a very important guiding significance to determine the corresponding treatment principles.

In short, theory of yin and yang is one of the basic categories of Chinese ancient philosophy in which yin and yang are considered as the nature of things and the fundamental law of their change, and many specific things have been given the meaning of yin and yang. The restriction, interdependence, waxing and waning, transformation between yin and yang are the basic contents of the theory of yin and yang. These contents are not isolated, but interrelated and mutually influenced, and in a cause-effect relationship. In TCM, it is believed that as long as yin and yang maintain the relative balance in the dynamic process, the human body can maintain normal law of movement. Balance is the means to sustain life, and the balance of yin and yang is a characteristic of health. The

健康的特征。阴阳双方在一定范围内的消长、转化，体现了人体动态平衡的生理活动过程。

growth and decline and transformation of yin and yang in a certain range reflect the process of physiological activity of the body's dynamic balance.

2 五行学说

五行学说以木、火、土、金、水五类特性及其生克制化规律来认识、解释自然的系统论、控制论和方法论。运用到中医学中，用以解释人体内脏之间的相互关系、脏腑组织器官的属性、运动变化及人体与外界环境的关系。

2.1 五行的基本概念

五行，是指木、火、土、金、水五种物质及其运动变化。"五"，是木、火、土、金、水五种物质；"行"，四通八达，流行和行用之谓，是行动、运动的古义，即运动变化，运行不息的意思。

古人运用抽象出来的五行特性，采用取象比类和推演络绎的方法，将自然界中的各种事物和现象分为五类，并以五行"相生"、"相克"的关系来解释各种事物和现象发生、发展、变化的规律。因此，五行学说是以木、火、土、金、水五种事物的特性及其相生、相克规律来认识世界、解释世界和探求宇宙变化规律的一种世界观和方法论。

五行最初的含义与"五材"有关，是指木、火、土、金、水五种基本物质或基本元素。木、火、土、金、水这五种物质是人类日常生产和生活中最为常见和不可缺少

2 Five Elements

The theory of five elements takes the characteristics of wood, fire, earth, metal and water and their cybernetics to understand and explain the system theory, cybernetics and methodology of the nature. It is applied to TCM to explain the relationship among the internal organs, the characteristics and change of viscera, tissues and organs, and the relationship between the body and the external environment.

2.1 The Basic Concept of Five Elements

Five elements (wu xing) refer to wood, fire, earth, metal and water and their movement and change. In Chinese, "wu" refers to the five materials; "xing" refers to extending and flowing in all directions, namely movement and change.

By abstracting the characteristics of five elements and through classification, manifestation and deduction, ancient Chinese divide things and phenomena in the nature into five categories and explain their law of occurrence, development and change through their relationship of promotion and restriction. Therefore, the theory of the five elements is a kind of world outlook and methodology to understand and explain the world and explore the change rule of the universe by their characteristics and law of promotion and restriction.

The original meaning of five elements is related to the "five materials" which refer to five kinds of basic substances or elements: wood, fire, earth, metal and water. They are the most common and indispensable basic materials in daily life. In the *Revelation to the Book of History (Shangshu*

中医理论 Basic Theory of Traditional Chinese Medicine

的基本物质,如《尚书·正义》说:
"水火者,百姓之所饮食也;金木
者,百姓之所兴作也;土者,万物
之所资生,是为人用。"由于人类
在生产和生活中经常接触这五种
物质,而且认识到这五种物质相
互作用,还可以产生出新的事物,
如《国语·郑语》说:"以土与金、
木、水、火杂,以成百物。"

2.2　五行的特性

五行一词,最早见于《尚
书》。该书对五行的特性从哲学
高度作了抽象概括,指出:"五行,
一曰水,二曰火,三曰木,四曰金,
五曰土。水曰润下,火曰炎上,木
曰曲直,金曰从革,土爱稼穑。"
此时的五行,已从木、火、土、金、
水五种具体物质中抽象出来,上
升为哲学的理性概念。五行的特
性是:

2.2.1　木曰曲直

曲直是"枝曲干直"的缩语,
是对树木生长形态的生动描述,
言其主干挺直向上,树枝曲折向
外,引申为木有生长、兴发、生机、
条达、舒展等特征。凡具有此类特
性的事物和现象,均可归属于木。

2.2.2　火曰炎上

炎,热也;上,向上,是指火具
有炎热、上升、光明的特性,引申为
凡具有炎热、上升、光明等性质或
作用的事物和现象,归属于火。

2.2.3　土爱稼穑

春种曰稼,秋收曰穑,指农

Zhengyi), there is the saying, "water and fire are related to people's diet; metal and wood are related to construction and manufacture; earth is related to growth of all things". Since human beings get into contact with five kinds of substances in their production and life, they recognize that the interaction among the five kinds of materials can also produce new things, as the saying goes in *History of Kingdoms* (Guo yu): *Kingdom of Zheng*: "Combining soil with metal, wood, water and fire makes hundreds of things."

2.2　Characteristics of Five Elements

The concept of the five elements originally appears in the *Book of History* (Shangshu) which abstractly concludes the characteristics of five elements from the view of philosophy by pointing out, "water moistens and flows downward; fire flares upward; wood bends and straightens; metal is for change; earth is for sowing and reaping." This explanation for the five elements is abstracted from the five materials and sublimated into philosophical rational concept. The characteristics of five elements are as the following:

2.2.1　Wood bends and straightens

It means the branches can bend and the stem is straight and grows upward, vividly depicting the tree's growth. It is extended that anything having the characteristics of growth, development, prosperity and vitality can be attributed to wood.

2.2.2　Fire flares upward

It means the fire has the characteristics of heat, ascending and bright. It is extended that anything having these characteristics can be attributed to fire.

2.2.3　Earth is for sowing and reaping

Sowing in spring and reaping in autumn refers to

中医理论

Basic Theory of Traditional Chinese Medicine

作物的播种和收获。土具有载物、生化的特性,五行以土为贵。凡具有生化、承载、受纳性能的事物或现象,皆归属于土。

2.2.4 金曰从革

从,顺从、服从;革,革除、改革、变革。金具有能柔能刚、变革、肃杀的特性。凡具有肃杀、潜能、收敛、清洁之意的事物或现象,均可归属于金。

2.2.5 水曰润下

润,湿润;下,向下。水具有滋润、就下、闭藏的特性。凡具有寒凉、滋润、就下、闭藏性能的事物或现象都可归属于水。

2.3 事物和现象的五行归类

五行学说根据五行特性,把自然界的各种事物或现象通过类比,运用归类和推演等方法,将其最终分成五大类。其具体方法是:

2.3.1 类比

类比是根据两个或两类事物在某些属性或关系上的相似或相同而推出它们在其他方面也可能相同或相似的一种逻辑方法。类比也是一种推理方法。类比法,中医学称之为"援物比类"或"取象比类"。中医学五行学说运用类比方法,将事物的形象(指事物的性质、作用、形态)与五行属性相类比,物象具有与某行相类似的特性,便将其归属于某行。

方位配五行:旭日东升,与木之升发特性相类,故东方归属于木;南方炎热,与火之炎上特

sowing and harvesting of crops. It is extended that anything having characteristics of generating, holding and receiving can be attributed to earth.

2.2.4 Metal is for change

Metal has the characteristics of flexibility, change and descending. It is extended that anything having characteristics of descending, astringing and clearing can be attributed to metal.

2.2.5 Water moistens and flows downward

Water has the characteristics of moistening, downward flowing and hiding. It is extended that anything having characteristics of cooling, moistening, downward flowing and hiding can be attributed to water.

2.3 Attribution of Things and Phenomena to the Five Elements

The theory of the five elements, based on their characteristics, divides various things or phenomena in the nature by analogy, classification and deduction and other methods into five categories. The specific methods are:

2.3.1 Analogy

Analogy is a logical method through which one can conclude the similarity or identity of two kinds of things in other aspects based on their similarity or identity in certain attributes. Analogy is a kind of reasoning method. The theory of the five elements by analogy method compares the image of things (the nature, function and shape) with the five elements. If the image has the similar characteristic with one of the five, it belongs to it.

Directions are compatible with the five elements: the feature of sunrise is similar to the feature of the wood's growth and flourishing, so the east pertains to wood; in the south, it is hot which is similar to the fire's flaring, so the

中医理论

Basic Theory of Traditional Chinese Medicine

中医理论

Basic Theory of Traditional Chinese Medicine

性相类,故南方归属于火。

五脏配五行:脾主运化而类于土之化物,故脾归属于土;肺主肃降而类于金之肃杀,故肺归属于金;心主血脉,温养全身,类于火之温煦,故心归属于火;肝主疏泄而类于木之升发条达,故肝归类于木;肾主封藏,主水而类于水之滋润,故肾归属于水。

2.3.2 推衍

推衍是根据已知的某些事物的属性,推衍至其他相关事物,以得知这些事物的属性的推理方法,有平行式推衍和包含式推衍两种类型。

平行式推衍:以木行推衍为例,根据木行的特性,在人体以肝为中心,推衍至胆、目、筋、怒、呼、握;在自然界以春为中心,推衍至东、风、生、青、酸、平旦、角等。肝与胆、目、筋、怒、呼、握,以及春与东、风、生、青、酸、平旦、角等之间并不存在包含关系,仅是在五脏之肝、五季之春的基础上发生了量的增加,其他四行均类此。

包含式推衍:五行学说按木、火、土、金、水五行之间生克制化规律,说明人体肝、心、脾、肺、肾五脏为中心的五脏系统,以及人体与自然环境各不同要素之间的统一性,便是五行推衍的具体应用。

总之,五行学说以天人相应为指导思想,以五行为中心,以空间结构的五方、时间结构的五季、

south pertains to fire.

Five zang-organs are compatible with the five elements. The spleen is similar to earth in transformation and generation, so it pertains to earth. The lung, similar to metal in descending, pertains to metal; the heart, similar to the fire in warming, so the heart pertains to fire; the liver, governing dredging and discharging, which is similar to the wood's growth and prosperity, so the liver pertains to wood; the kidney, dominating, sealing and hiding, which is similar to the water's moistening, so the kidney pertains to water.

2.3.2 Deduction

Deduction is a reasoning method referring to deducting the other related things and their properties based on the known attributes of certain things. It includes parallel and inclusive deduction.

Parallel deduction: take the deduction of wood as an example. The liver as the center of human body is related to the gallbladder, eye, tendon, anger, shouting and holding; spring as the center of the nature is related to east, wind, germination, green, sour, early morning and jue. There is no inclusive relationship between the liver and gallbladder, eye, tendon, anger, shouting and holding, spring and east, wind, germination, green, sour, early morning and jue, but there appears the increase in volume based on the liver and spring. The other four elements are the same.

Inclusive deduction: the theory of the five elements based on interdependence and restriction among them explains the five-zang system taking the liver, heart, spleen, lung and kidney as the center and the unity between the different elements of the human body and the natural environment. That is the specific application for the deduction of the five elements.

In a word, the theory of the five elements takes the correspondence between man and nature as the guiding ideology, the five elements as center, the five directions of spatial structure, the five seasons of the time structure, the

人体结构的五脏为基本框架,将自然界的各种事物和现象,以及人体的生理病理现象,按其属性进行归纳,即凡具有生发、柔和特性者统属于木;具有阳热、上炎特性者统属于火;具有长养、化育特性者统属于土;具有清静、肃杀特性者统属于金;具有寒冷、滋润、趋下、闭藏特性者统属于水,从而将人体的生命活动与自然界的事物和现象联系起来,形成了一个人体内外环境的五行结构系统,用以说明人体以及人与自然环境的统一性。

five zang-organs of human structure as the basic framework to induce all things and phenomena in the nature and physiological and pathological phenomena of human body according to their attributes. Things with the characteristics of generation and gentleness are attributed to wood; things with the characteristics of yang-heat, flaring, fire; things with the characteristics of growth and development, earth; things with the characteristics of clearing and descending, metal; things with the characteristics of cooling, moistening, downward flowing, hiding and sealing, water. Therefore, human life activities are linked with things and phenomena in the nature to form a structure system of the five elements inside and outside the human body, which is applied to illustrate the unity between the human body and the natural environment.

事物和现象的五行属性归类表

五行	五方	五季	五气	五化	五色	五味	五脏	五腑	五官	五体	五志	五声	五音
木	东	春	风	生	青	酸	肝	胆	目	筋	怒	呼	角
火	南	夏	暑	长	赤	苦	心	小肠	舌	脉	喜	笑	徵
土	中	长夏	湿	化	黄	甘	脾	胃	口	肉	思	歌	宫
金	西	秋	燥	收	白	辛	肺	大肠	鼻	皮毛	悲	哭	商
水	北	冬	寒	藏	黑	咸	肾	膀胱	耳	骨	恐	呻	羽

Attribution of things and phenomena to the five elements

five elements	five directions	five seasons	five climates	five changes	five colors	five flavors	five zang-organs	five fu-organs	five sense organs	five constituents	five emotions	five voices	five notes
wood	east	spring	wind	germination	green	sour	liver	gallbladder	eye	tendon	anger	shouting	jue
fire	south	summer	summer-heat	growth	red	bitter	heart	small intestine	tongue	vessel	joy	laughing	zhi
earth	center	long summer	dampness	transformation	yellow	sweet	spleen	stomach	mouth	muscle	thinking	singing	gong
metal	west	autumn	dryness	reaping	white	acrid	lung	large intestine	nose	skin and body hair	sorrow	crying	shang
water	north	winter	cold	storing	black	salty	kidney	bladder	ear	bone	fear	moaning	yu

中医理论 Basic Theory of Traditional Chinese Medicine

中国古代的科学方法具有勤于观察、善于推类、精于运数、重于应用和长于辨证的特点。在"仰观天象,俯察地理","近取诸身,远取诸物"的"观物取象"的基础上,"以类族辨物",并进一步"引而伸之,触类而长之",即触类旁通,由已知事物推广到其他未知的事物。五行学说的归类和推演的思维方法是:观物—取象—比类—运数(五行)—求道(规律),这是一种以直接观察为基础的综合类比的思维方法。

2.4 五行学说的基本内容

五行学说是解释宇宙自然运行变化的系统论、控制论和方法论。其基本内容主要包括:相生、相克、五行制化以及相乘相侮等。

2.4.1 相生

相生即递相资生、助长、促进之意。五行之间互相滋生和促进的关系称作五行相生。

五行相生的次序是:木生火,火生土,土生金,金生水,水生木。

在相生关系中,任何一行都有"生我"、"我生"两方面的关系,《难经》把它比喻为"母"与"子"的关系。"生我"者为母,"我生"者为"子"。所以五行相生关系又称"母子关系"。以火为例,生"我"者木,木能生火,则木为火之母;"我"生者土,火能生土,则土为火之子。余可类推。

The scientific method in ancient China is featured as observation, induction, calculation, application and syndrome differentiation. It is based on images abstracting from viewing, such as, observing the heavenly bodies and geography and taking objects from as close as the body and as far as the things around, to extend from the known to the unknown. The thinking method for classification and deduction of the five elements is as the following: observing—images abstracting—analogy—attribution (the five elements)—seeking Dao (law), which is a comprehensive analogy thinking method based on direct observation.

2.4 Essential Content of Theory of Five Elements

The theory of the five elements is the system theory, cybernetics and methodology explaining the move and change of the nature and the universe. Its basic content includes: promotion and restriction, subjugation and violation.

2.4.1 Promotion

Promotion means the mutual generation and interpromotion of five elements.

The order of promotion is: wood promotes fire, fire promotes earth, earth promotes metal, metal promotes water and water promotes wood.

In the promotion relationship, each element can be promoted and promote meanwhile. *Classic of Difficult Issues (Nanjing)* compared it to the relationship between "mother" and "child". To promote is alike maternity while to be promoted, child. The promotion relationship among the five elements is also known as "mother-child relationship". Take fire as an example, what to promote is wood which can generate fire, so wood is the mother of fire; what to be promoted is earth which can be generated by fire, so earth is the child of fire. The relationship among the other four elements can also be deduced likewise.

中医理论

Basic Theory of Traditional Chinese Medicine

2.4.2 相克

相克即相互制约、克制、抑制之意。五行之间相互制约的关系称之为五行相克。

五行相克的次序是：木克土，土克水，水克火，火克金，金克木，木克土。

在相克的关系中，任何一行都有"克我"、"我克"两方面的关系。《黄帝内经》称之为"所胜"与"所不胜"的关系。"克我"者为"所不胜"。"我克"者为"所胜"。所以，五行相克的关系，又叫"所胜"与"所不胜"的关系。以土为例，"克我"者木，则木为土之"所不胜"。"我克"者水，则水为土之"所胜"。余可类推。

在上述生克关系中，任何一行皆有"生我"和"我生"，"克我"和"我克"四个方面的关系。以木为例，"生我"者水，"我生"者火；"克我"者金，"我克"者土。

相生与相克是不可分割的两个方面。没有生，就没有事物的发生和成长；没有克，就不能维持正常协调关系下的变化与发展。因此，必须生中有克（化中有制），克中有生（制中有化），相反相成，才能维持和促进事物相对平衡协调和发展变化。五行之间这种生中有制、制中有生、相互生化、相互制约的生克关系，称之为制化。

2.4.3 母子相及

及，影响所及之意。母子相及是指五行生克制化遭到破坏

2.4.2 Restriction

It means one element of the five restricts and limits another one.

The sequence of restriction of the five elements is: wood restricts earth, earth restricts water, water restricts fire, fire restricts metal, metal restricts wood and wood restricts earth.

For restriction relationship, each element can be two sides of the "being restricted" and "restrict". *Huangdi's Internal Classic* describes it as the "dominator" and "subordinate". "The restricting" refers to "dominator" and the "being restricted" refers to "subordinate". Take earth as an example, the "restricted" is wood, so earth is called the "subordinate" of wood. "The restricting" is water, so earth is called the "dominator" of water. The others can be deduced like this.

In the above restriction relationship, each element of the five can promote or be promoted, restrict or be restricted. Take wood as an example, the "mother" is water and the "child" is fire; the "restricting" is metal and the "being restricted" is earth.

Promotion and restriction are two inseparable sides. Without promotion, there is no occurrence and growth of things; without restriction, the change and development under the normal coordinate relationship cannot be maintained. Therefore, there must be restriction in the generation (restriction in the change), and generation in the restriction (change in the restriction) in order to maintain and promote the relative balance and development. The relationship of restriction in the generation, generation in the restriction, mutual promotion and restriction is called promotion and restriction among the five elements.

2.4.3 Mutual involvement of the mother and the child

It means when the promotion and restriction of the five elements are damaged, abnormal phenomena of generation

中医理论

Basic Theory of Traditional Chinese Medicine

后所出现的不正常的相生现象，包括母病及子和子病及母两个方面。如木行，影响到火行，叫作母病及子；影响到水行，则叫作子病及母。

母病及子的一般规律是母行虚弱导致子行异常。如水不涵木，即肾阴虚不能滋养肝木，其临床表现在肾，则为肾阴不足，多见耳鸣、腰膝酸软、遗精等；在肝，则为肝之阴血不足，多见眩晕、消瘦、乏力、肢体麻木，或手足蠕动，甚则震颤抽搐等。

子病及母有三种情况：一是子行亢盛，引发母行亢盛，结果是子母两行皆亢盛，一般称为"子病犯母"；二是子行虚弱，上累母行，引起母行不足，终致子母两行俱虚；三是子行亢盛，损伤母行，导致子盛母衰，一般称为"子盗母气"。

疾病按相生规律传变，有轻重之分，"母病及子"为顺，其病轻；"子病犯母"为逆，病重。

根据相生规律确定治疗原则：临床上运用相生规律来治疗疾病，多属母病及子，其次为子盗母气。其基本治疗原则是补母和泻子，所谓"虚者补其母，实者泻其子"（《难经·六十九难》）。

will appear. It concerns two sides: the involvement of the child by its mother and the involvement of the mother by its child. For example, if wood affects fire, it is called the involvement of the child by its mother; if wood affects water, it is called the involvement of the mother by its child.

The general rule of the involvement of the child by its mother is that deficient mother gives birth to abnormal child. For example, if water is not sufficient to moisten wood, that's to say, deficient kidney-yin cannot nourish liver. If the clinical syndromes show in kidney, there will appear deficient kidney-yin, tinnitus, soreness and weakness of waist and knees and spermatorrhea and so on. If the clinical syndromes show in liver, there will appear deficient yin blood, leading to dizziness, emaciation, fatigue, numb limbs and wriggling of limbs, even quivering and jerking.

There are three conditions that the child may affect its mother. One is that if the child element becomes hyperactive, it will cause the excess of its mother resulting in both the mother and child becoming hyperactive, which is called "the child's disorder affects its mother"; the second one is that if the child element is deficient, it will affect its mother resulting in both the mother and child becoming deficient; the last one is that if the child element is excessive, it will result in hyperactive child and deficient mother, which is called "the child's disorder steals its mother's qi"

Diseases, serious or minor, might arise according to the promotion rules. The involvement of the child by its mother is normally minor disease while the involvement of the mother by its child tends to be serious.

Treatment principles should be determined according to the promotion rules. Clinical treatment according to the generation rules is mainly related to the involvement of the child by its mother, and then to the child's stealing its mother's qi. The basic treatment principles are tonifying the mother and reducing the child, which is known as "for the deficient tonifying the mother and for the excessive reducing the child" *(Classic of Difficult Issues: The Sixty-Nine Question)*.

依据五行相生规律确定的治法,常用的有滋水涵木法、益火补土法、培土生金法和金水相生法四种。

2.4.4　相乘

乘,即乘虚侵袭之意。相乘即相克太过,超过正常制约的程度,使事物之间失去了正常的协调关系。五行之间相乘的次序与相克同,但被克者更加虚弱,所以相乘又称为"倍克"或"过克"。

2.4.5　相侮

相侮是指五行中的任何一行本身太过,使原来克它的一行,不仅不能去制约它,反而被它所克制,即反克,又称反侮。

相乘相侮均为破坏相对协调统一的异常表现。相乘和相侮是一个问题的两个方面,发生的原因都在于:"太过"或"不及"。如木有余而金不能对木加以克制,木便过度克制其所胜之土,这叫作"乘",同时,木还恃己之强反去克制其"所不胜"的金,这叫作"侮"。反之,木不足,则不仅金来乘木,而且其所胜之土又乘其虚而侮之。所以说:"气有余,则制己所胜而侮所不胜,其不及,则己所不胜侮而乘之,己所胜轻而侮之"(《素问·五运行大论》)。

"太过"者属强,表现为机能亢进;"不及"者属弱,表现为机能衰退。因而治疗上须同时采取抑强扶弱的治疗原则,并侧重于

The therapies based on the promotion rules include the method of replenishing water to nourish wood, the method of assisting fire and strengthening earth, the method of reinforcing earth to strengthen metal and the method of mutual promotion of metal and water.

2.4.4　Subjugation

It means excessive restriction breaks the coordinate relations among things. The sequence of subjugation among the five elements is the same as the sequence of restriction, except that the restricted element becomes weaker. Therefore, subjugation is also called "double restriction" or "excessive restriction".

2.4.5　Violation

Violation means one element of the five elements is so powerful that its "restricting" element is reversely restricted by it.

Both subjugation and violation are the abnormal conditions due to breaking of the relative coordination. They are the two sides of one problem, the causes of which are being "excessive" or "deficient". Such as, if wood is so powerful that metal cannot restrict it, it will excessively restrict earth, which is called subjugation. The excessive wood will furthermore reversely restrict the weak metal, which is called violation. On the contrast, if wood is weak, metal will subjugate it and even the "being restricted" earth will reversely restrict it, which is called violation. So there is the saying, "the element with excessive qi subjugates its restricted element and violates its non-restricting element; the element with deficient qi is reversely restricted by its restricting element or subjugated by its restricted element." (*Plain Questions: Major Discussion on the Changes of Five Elements*).

The "excessive" are related to the powerful, appearing as hyperfunction; the "deficient" belongs to the weak appearing as hypofunction. Therefore, the therapeutic principles could be restraining the powerful and helping the

中医理论 Basic Theory of Traditional Chinese Medicine

制其强盛,使弱者易于恢复。若一方虽强盛而尚未发生克伐太过时,亦可利用这一治则,预先加强其所胜的力量,以阻止病情的发展。

依据五行相克规律确定的治法,常用的有抑木扶土法、培土制水法、佐金平木法和泻南补北法四种。

weak. If the powerful element has not restricted the other element excessively yet, the power of its "being restricted" element can still be reinforced to prevent the development of the disease. This can be used as a therapeutic method.

The therapeutic methods based on the restriction law of the five elements include: inhibiting wood to assist earth, banking up earth to treat water, assisting metal to subdue wood and reducing the south to tonify the north.

第二章　藏象学说

Chapter 2　Theory of Visceral Manifestation

中医学对脏腑生理、病理的认识,传统称为藏象学说。

脏古体是藏,而藏又通"藏"(cang),藏指隐藏于体内的脏腑。

象,其义有二,一指脏腑的生理病理表现于外的征象,二指人体和自然界相通应的事物和现象。象是脏的外在反映,脏是象的内在本质,两者结合起来就叫作"藏象"。

"藏象"一词,蕴含了中医学认识人体脏腑生理功能的独特思维方法,它是依据"有诸内必形诸外"的原理,运用"司外揣内"的法则,通过分析活的机体的外部表征,以表知里,来推导认识人体内部生理病理情况的。如,心开窍于舌,舌体红润光泽、转动灵活说明心的气血充足;舌尖红或糜烂疼痛可能是心火旺盛;舌质颜色淡红,说明心血不足;舌色紫暗或有瘀点可能是心血瘀阻。

藏象学说的特点是以五脏为中心的整体观:主要体现在以

In Traditional Chinese Medicine (TCM), the understanding of the physiology and pathology of the internal organs is called the Theory of Visceral Manifestation (Theory of Zangxiang).

Zang in ancient Chinese shares the same pronunciation and meaning with cang (hiding), so zang refers to the viscera hidden inside human body.

Xiang has two meanings: one is the external manifestation of physiological and pathological state; the other is the phenomenon of connection between human body and the nature. Xiang is the external reflection of zang, and at the same time, zang is the intrinsic nature of xiang. The combination of the two is called "zangxiang".

Zangxiang contains the special thinking method about the physiological function of human viscera in TCM. Based on the principle of "viscera inside the body are sure to manifest themselves externally", it applies the axiom of "operating the external to surmise the internal" and analyzes the external appearance of living body to know and investigate the internal physiological and pathological states. For example, the heart is linked to tongue in orifice. Red, moist, lustrous and flexible tongue manifests that qi and blood of the heart is sufficient; red tip of tongue, or erosion and pain of tongue manifests flaring of heart-fire; pale tongue manifests deficiency of heart-blood; purple, dark purple tongue or tongue with ecchymoses may manifest stagnation of heart-blood.

Zangxiang theory is characterized by the concept of holism with five internal organs as the centre, which

五脏为中心的人体自身的整体性及五脏与外界环境的统一性两个方面。

心、肝、脾、肺、肾合称五脏,属于实体性器官,作用是"化生和贮藏精气",即生化和贮藏气、血、津液等精微物质。精气是一种弥漫状态,而且是不断运动的,不能停滞,否则会引起气滞、血瘀、积水等症,所以中医描述五脏的状态是满而不能实。

胆、胃、小肠、大肠、膀胱、三焦合称六腑。腑通"府",有府库之意。从形象上看,六腑属于管腔性器官;从功能上看,六腑主"受盛和传化水谷",即接受和容纳食物,在向下传送的过程中,吸收食物中的营养成分(中医称"水谷精微"),排泄糟粕,主要是对饮食物起消化、吸收、输送、排泄的作用。由于六腑在消化吸收食物的过程中要保持虚实更替的状态,才能使得胃肠蠕动,促进消化物的下降,所以中医描述六腑的状态是实而不能满。

脑、髓、骨、脉、胆、女子胞六者合称奇恒之腑。奇者异也,恒者常也。奇恒之腑,形多中空,与腑相近;但内藏精气,又类于脏,似脏非脏,似腑非腑,而且不像脏腑之间有表里配伍的关系,故称之为"奇恒之腑"。

中医脏腑研究的对象重点是内脏的生理功能,但一定是通过形体、官窍等外在表现来反映的。

所谓形体,其广义者,泛指

is reflected in two aspects: the body's integrity with five internal organs as the center, and the unity of the external environment and internal organs.

The heart, lungs, spleen, liver and kidneys are collectively called the five zang-organs which are substantive organs with the function of transforming and storing qi, blood, body fluid and the other refined food nutrient. Essence-qi pervades inside the body and is in constant motion. If it stagnates, it will cause qi stagnation, blood stasis and edema and so on. So, the state of five zang-organs is described in TCM as fullness rather than solidness.

The gallbladder, stomach, large intestine, small intestine, bladder, tri-jiao form the six fu-organs which belong to luminal organs according to their appearance. As for function, the six fu-organs are to transport and transform food, namely to receive and digest food. In the process of transporting and transforming, nutrient is absorbed and waste is discharged. The main function of them are digesting, absorbing, transporting and discharging. The six fu-organs need to remain in excess and deficiency alternatively in the process of digesting and absorbing food, which can facilitate gastrointestinal peristalsis and the declining of digesta, so the state of the six fu-organs is described in TCM as solidness rather than fullness.

The brain, spinal cord, bone, pulse, gallbladder and womb form the extraordinary fu-organs. They are similar to the fu-organs because they are hollow inside; similar to the zang-organs in that they store essence-qi. They resemble the zang-organs and the fu-organs in some ways but are neither of them. Moreover, they do not have the exterior-interior and compatible relationships as the zang and fu-organs do. That's why they are called the extraordinary fu-organs.

The research focus of TCM is the physiological functions of internal organs which must be reflected on the outside performance of the body and orifices.

The so-called "body", in its broad sense, refers to the

中医理论 Basic Theory of Traditional Chinese Medicine

具有一定形态结构的组织,包括头、躯干和脏腑在内;其狭义者,指皮、肉、筋、骨、脉五种组织结构,又称五体。

关于官窍,官指机体有特定功能的器官,如耳、目、口、鼻、舌,又称五官,它们分属于五脏,为五脏的外候。窍,有孔穴、苗窍之意,是人体与外界相通连的窗口。官必有窍,窍多成官,故官窍并称。窍有七窍,七窍指头面部七个孔窍(眼二、耳二、鼻孔二、口)。五脏的精气分别通达于七窍。九窍又称九官,指七窍加前阴和后阴而言。

这些脏腑、组织、官窍,通过四通八达、无处不至的"经络"系统的沟通、连缀,形成了一个结构完全、统一的整体,形成了五个生理系统:

心系统:心、小肠、脉、舌。

肝系统:肝、胆、筋、目。

脾系统:脾、胃、肉、唇。

肺系统:肺、大肠、皮、鼻。

肾系统:肾、膀胱、骨、耳及二阴。

这五个系统各自有不同的功能。

心能推动和调控心脏的搏动而行血,反映在脉搏、舌头和面部。

肝主疏泄,能调畅气机,舒畅情绪,能贮藏血液,所以有"血海"之称,反映在筋脉、眼睛、爪甲上。

肺气宣发肃降以主持呼吸

tissues with certain shape and structure, including head, trunk, and internal organs; in its narrow sense, it refers to skin, muscles, tendons, bones and vessels. These five kinds of tissues are also known as the five body constituents.

The organs are apparatuses with specific functions, such as ears, eyes, mouth, nose and tongue, which are also known as facial features, the external reflection of the five internal organs. The orifice is the window connecting the body and the outside. The organs must have orifices and several orifices make up an organ, so they are always combined. There are seven orifices on a head-face (two eyes, two ears, two nostrils and one mouth). The energy-qi of the five zang-organs is connected with seven orifices. The nine orifices are also nine organs, including seven orifices and genitalia (front-yin) and anus (back-yin).

These organs, tissues, and the orifices, through the connection of meridian system spreading over the body, form a unity with five physiological systems:

the heart system: including the heart, small intestine, pulse and tongue;

the liver system: including the liver, gallbladder, tendons and eyes;

the spleen system: including the spleen, stomach, muscle and lips;

the lung system: including the lung, large intestine, skin and nose;

the kidney system: including the kidney, bladder, bone, ear, two yins (genitalia and anus).

These five systems function differently.

The heart can drive and regulate heart beat to propel blood circulation, which is reflected in the pulse, tongue and face.

The liver can balance the whole body's qi dynamic, smooth mood and store blood, so it is called the "Blood Sea" which is reflected in tendons, pulses, eyes, hands and nails.

The lung-qi, governing diffusion and descent, commands

并行水液,推动血液流动,反映在呼吸、皮毛和鼻部。

脾能运化水谷并控制、统领血液运行,反映在食物消化、肌肉和口唇色泽上。

肾藏精,主生长发育和生殖,水,反映在骨骼、牙齿、毛发、耳朵和二阴尤其是前阴(排尿及生殖)。

虽然五脏的功能不同,但也并非各行其是,只管发挥自己的功能而不顾整体,而是(包括六腑)在功能上密切配合、协调统一。单就血液循行而言,心主血,以推动血液的运行;肺主气,以辅助心而行血;肝藏血,以调解血液流量;脾统血,以规范血液运行不致溢出脉外。正是由于各脏密切配合,才能维持血液的正常循行。

由于脏与脏,腑与腑之间也是相互沟通联系的,所以,某一脏或腑的病变,还可以通过经络相互影响。例如,肝的疏泄功能失常,不仅肝脏本身出现病变,见有两肋胀满、腹胀的症状,还会影响脾的运化功能而出现食欲不振、腹痛腹泻的症状;也会影响到肺气的宣发肃降而见咳喘、肋痛;还会影响心神而见烦躁不安,失眠多梦。

脏与腑之间在生理、病理上也能相互影响。例如,肾是脏,膀胱是腑,肾与膀胱有表与里的关系。肾气虚就会影响膀胱的排尿

respiration, carries fluid and propels blood circulation, which is reflected in respiration, skin and body hair, fur and nose.

The spleen can transport and transform foodstuff, control and govern blood circulation, which is reflected in the digestion, muscle and lip color.

The kidney stores essence, governs growth and reproduction, and controls water, which is reflected in bones, teeth, hair, ears and two yins, especially the front yin (urination and reproduction).

Although the five zang-organs have different functions, they do not act separately. Instead, the five zang-organs (including six fu-organs) cooperate and coordinate with each other. As far as the blood circulation is concerned, the heart governs blood to propel blood circulation; the lung governs qi to assist the heart to propel blood; the liver stores blood to regulate the amount of blood; the spleen commands blood to regulate blood not to flow outside the pulse. Only when the five zang-organs coordinate closely, can the normal blood circulation be maintained.

Due to mutual affection among the zang- and fu-organs, lesions of certain zang-organ or fu-organ also interact with each other through the meridians. Take liver as an example: its dysfunction in regulating qi dynamic will not only show lesions in liver, developing symptoms of rib fullness and bloating, it will also affect the spleen's transportation and transformation, with the symptoms of anorexia, abdominal pain, and diarrhea; and it may also affect diffusion and descent of the lung-qi, causing cough and rib pain; and it may even affect mood, resulting in irritability, insomnia and dreaminess.

Zang-and fu-organs can affect each other physiologically and pathologically. For example, the kidney belongs to zang and the bladder, fu, and they have the exterior-interior relationship. Qi deficiency of the kidney will affect urinating

中医理论

Basic Theory of Traditional Chinese Medicine

功能,出现尿频或失禁,或者小便不利而水肿等症状。再如,肺与大肠相表里,大肠燥热,大便秘结,可以影响到肺气肃降而见咳喘。前者是脏影响腑,后者则是腑影响及脏。

所以,五脏之间既分工又合作,共同维持着人体复杂的生理活动。这种以五脏为中心,在组织结构及机能活动上相统一的观点,就称为"五脏一体观"。

人与自然界存在着密切的关系。人类生活在自然界中,自然界存在着人类赖以生存的必要条件。同时,自然界的变化,如季节气候、昼夜晨昏、地理环境等的不同,直接或间接地影响人体,而机体则相应地产生反应。

藏象学说把自然界的四时、五方、五气、五化等与人体五大系统密切联系,形成了"四时五脏"系统,构成了人体内外环境的统一体。

function of the bladder, causing frequent urination or incontinence or edema caused by urine negative. Another example is the lung and large intestine form an exterior-interior relationship. Dry and hot large intestine and constipation can affect the lung qi descending resulting in cough. In the former example, zang affects fu while the later, fu affects zang.

Therefore, the five-zang organs work separately while cooperate with each other, maintaining the complex physiological activities of the human body. The concept of unity in organizational structure and functional activities with the five-zang organs as the center is called "holism of five zang-organs".

Human beings and nature are closely related. Human beings live in nature and the nature provides the necessities for the survival of mankind. At the same time, the changes in nature, such as seasonal climate, day and night, dawn and dusk, different geographical environments directly or indirectly affect the human body, while the body acts correspondingly.

In the zangxiang theory, the four seasons, five regions, five qis and five stages have close relationship with human body's five systems, constituting "the four seasons and the five-organ system", forming the unity of internal and external environment of the human body.

五脏	心	肝	脾	肺	肾
五气	热(暑)	风	湿	燥	寒
五化	长	生	化	收	藏
五色	赤	青	黄	白	黑
五方	南	东	中	西	北
五季	夏	春	长夏	秋	冬

中医理论 Basic Theory of Traditional Chinese Medicine

five-zang organs	heart	liver	spleen	lung	kidney
five qis	heat	wind	dampness	dryness	coldness
five stages	growth	birth	transformation	restrain	storage
five colors	red	green	yellow	white	black
five regions	south	east	middle	west	north
five seasons	summer	spring	long summer	autumn	winter

如一年四季的气候各不相同：春温、夏热、秋凉、冬寒，形成了植物的生长规律：春生、夏长、秋收、冬藏；对应人体有春天多温病，夏天多热病，秋天多燥病，冬天多伤寒。所以有应春温之气以养肝，应夏热之气以养心，应长夏之气以养脾，应秋凉之气以养肺，应冬藏之气以养肾的养生原则。

心、肺、脾、肝、肾称为五脏，加上心包络又称六脏，但习惯上往往把心包络附属于心，所以五脏也包括了心包络。五脏的共同生理特点是化生和贮藏精气。同时五脏各有所司，而且与形体、官窍等有密切联系，构成了人体以五脏为中心的特殊系统。其中心的生理功能起着主宰作用。

Climate differ with the seasonal changes as warm spring, hot summer, cool autumn and cold winter, corresponding to the growth rules of plants: birth in spring, growth in summer, harvest in autumn and storage in winter. Accordingly, human body usually suffers from epidemic febrile disease in spring, fever in summer, dryness in autumn and typhoid in winter. So, there goes the principle of health preserving as nurturing the liver complying with spring's warmth, nurturing the heart complying with summer's heat, nurturing the spleen complying with long summer's qi, nurturing the lung complying with autumn's coolness, and nurturing the kidney complying with winter's storage.

The heart, lung, spleen, liver and kidney, known as the five-zang organs, are also called the six-zang organs together with pericardium. However, pericardium is often attached to the heart, so the five-zang organs also include pericardium. The common physiological characteristics of five-zang organs are to produce and store essence. At the same time, the five-zang organs, performing their own functions, have close contact with body and orifices, constituting the body's special system with the five-zang organs as the center. The physiological functions of the heart play a dominant role in the system.

1 心

心者，君主之官，神明出焉。

心的主要生理功能是心主血脉和心藏神，心脏系统包括心在体合脉、其华在面、在官窍为

1 Heart

The heart is like a monarch governing the five zang-organs from which the spirit comes out.

The main physiological functions of the heart system are to govern blood and store spirit. In the heart system it is

舌、在液为汗、在情志为喜，与夏气相通应，心与小肠相表里。

中医学认为，心脏在五脏中居于首要地位，起着主宰人体生命活动的作用。

1.1 生理功能

1.1.1 心主血脉

血指血液，脉指脉管，是血液运行的通道。心主血脉，是指心脏有推动血液循行于脉管之中、周流全身的作用。心脏的正常搏动，依赖于心气、心阳的推动和温煦作用，以及心血、心阴的营养和滋润作用。心脏有规律地跳动，与心脏相通的脉管亦随之产生有规律的搏动，即为"脉搏"。中医通过触摸脉搏的跳动，来了解心力、心率和心律，判断全身气血的盛衰，作为诊断疾病的依据之一，即为"脉诊"。心气充沛，血液充盈，脉道畅通，则面色红润而有光泽，脉象和缓均匀有力。如果心气不足，血液亏虚，则见面色淡白无华，脉象细弱无力等。若气血瘀滞，血脉受阻，而见面色灰暗，唇舌青紫，心前区憋闷和刺痛，脉象结、代、促、涩等。

心主血脉的功能与心气、心血、心阴、心阳密切联系，不可分割。心气是维持和促进心进行各项功能活动的动力；心血主要指

linked to vessels in body, gloss in the face, tongue in orifice, sweat in fluid and joy in emotion. The heart and summer-qi are interlinked. The heart and small intestine form an internal- external relationship.

In TCM, the heart occupies a leading position among the five zang-organs and dominates life activities.

1.1 Physiological Function

1.1.1 Heart governing blood vessels

Blood refers to blood fluid; vessels refer to blood vessels which are the passageway of blood circulation. The heart governing blood vessels means that the heart propels blood circulation within vessels of the whole body. The normal beating of the heart relies on the driving and warming functions of heart-qi and heart-yang, along with the nourishing and moistening effects of heart-blood and heart-yin. With regular beating of the heart, vessels interlinked with the heart beat rhythmically, which is called the pulse. Doctors of TCM feel the pulse to get the operating condition of heart vitality, heart rate and heart rhythm, even prosperity or decline of qi-blood throughout whole body. It is regarded as one of the base for diagnosis, which is called pulse-taking. If the heart-qi is sufficient, blood redundant, vessels smooth, complexion will be rosy and lustrous, and pulse will feel moderate, even and forceful. If the heart-qi is insufficient, blood deficient, complexion will be pale and illustrious, and pulse will feel thin, weak and forceless. If qi-blood gets stagnated, blood vessels are obstructed, complexion will take on grey and dark color, lips and tongue will become cyanotic, precordium will feel oppressed, stuffed and stabbingly painful, and pulse will feel knotted, intermittent, hasty and uneven.

The functions of the heart are closely connected with heart-qi, heart-blood, heart-yin and heart-yang. Heart-qi is an impetus to maintain and promote the functions and activities of the heart; heart-blood mainly refers to the blood which is passing through the heart and has the effects of

中医理论 Basic Theory of Traditional Chinese Medicine

流经心脏的血液,具有养心养神、敛藏、滋养心气、心阳等作用;心阴是心之阴液,具有滑利血脉、凉润、宁静、抑制等作用;心阳是心之阳气,具有温煦、推动、兴奋作用,与心阴相反相成。四者充盛协调,共同维持心脏进行功能活动。

1.1.2 心藏神

又称主神志,是指人的精神意识思维活动,主要归属于心,心为人体生命活动的主宰。五脏六腑必须在心的统一指挥下,才能进行统一协调的正常生命活动。中医学认为:血液是精神活动的物质基础。心主神明,主要依赖于心血与心阴的作用,血与阴都有滋养心神的功能。如心血不足,血不养心,会导致心神不安,出现心慌、失眠、多梦等病症;当然精神活动也能调节和影响血液循环。心神不安会引起血行不畅。由此可见,如果发生病变,两者之间可以相互影响。

1.2 心与体窍液时等的关系

1.2.1 心在体合脉,其华在面

心合脉,指全身血脉都归于心。脉搏及脉道的通利与心脏有直接的关联。面部血管丰富,最能够反映血液的情况,可以通过面部色泽变化来观察心主血脉及心藏神的功能。

supporting the heart and soul, storing and nourishing heart-qi and heart-yang and so on; as yin-fluid of the heart, heart-yin has the effects of smoothing blood vessels, cooling and lubricating, calming and restraining; as yang-qi of the heart, heart-yang has the effects of warming, promoting and exciting. Heart-yin and heart-yang are both opposite and complementary to each other. Heart-qi, heart-blood, heart-yin and heart-yang are connected with each other harmoniously, maintaining the functional activities of the heart.

1.1.2 Heart storing spirit

Heart storing spirit, or controlling mind, means human being's activities of mentality, consciousness and thinking pertain to the heart. The heart dominates life activities of the body. Under the unified command of the heart, five zang- and six fu-organs will harmoniously carry out normal life activities. In TCM, blood is the physical basis of all the mental activities. The heart controlling mind depends on the functions of heart-blood and heart-yin nourishing the heart and mind. If heart-blood is insufficient and blood can't nourish the heart, it will lead to restlessness of the heart and mind, even result in palpitation, insomnia and dreaminess. Oppositely, mental activities can also regulate and affect blood circulation. Restlessness of the heart will hinder blood circulation. Therefore the two (the heart and blood) will influence each other if any disease arises.

1.2 Relations of Heart with Body, Orifices, Fluid and Seasons

1.2.1 Linking to vessels in body and gloss in face

The heart is linked to vessels in body. The heart linking to vessels signifies that blood vessels of the whole body are controlled by the heart. The patency of vessel system has a direct correlation with the heart. Rich facial vessels can better reflect the situation of blood. The functions of the heart governing vessels and storing spirit can be observed by the changes of facial gloss.

中医理论

Basic Theory of Traditional Chinese Medicine

1.2.2　心在窍为舌

舌主司味觉和语言表达有赖于心主血脉和主神志的功能状态。心的生理功能正常，则舌体红润灵活、味觉灵敏、语言流利。如果心阳不足，可见舌质淡白胖嫩；心阴不足，则见舌头红绛色；心血不足，可见舌体瘦薄、舌色少华；心火上炎，可见舌边尖红，甚则生疮；心血瘀阻，可见舌质紫暗或有瘀斑；心藏神功能异常，可见舌头发硬、失语等。

1.2.3　心在液为汗

汗为津液所化生，是津液通过阳气的蒸腾气化后，从汗孔排出的液体。由于津液是血液的重要组成部分，而血又为心所主，且人在精神紧张或受惊时会出汗，与心神关系密切，故有"汗为心之液"的说法。

1.2.4　心在志为喜

是指心的生理功能和情志与"喜"有关。人有各种情绪。喜则气血通达有利于心功能的正常活动。但如果过度喜乐，就会耗散心神，所以有"喜伤心"的说法。

1.2.5　心与夏气相通应

自然界的四时阴阳消长变化，与人体五脏功能活动系统相通应。夏季气候炎热，人体阳气隆盛，心阳在夏季最旺盛。一般来说，阳气虚衰的病人，往往在夏季缓解(各类心脏病人以阳虚多

1.2.2　Linking to tongue in orifice

The tongue governing taste rests on the functional conditions of the heart governing blood vessels and storing spirit. When the physical function of the heart is normal, the tongue will be red, moist, flexible, and can taste acutely and speak fluently. If the heart-yang is deficient, the tongue will be pale and enlarged; if the heart-yin is inadequate, the tip of the tongue will become deep red; if the heart-blood falls short, the tongue will be thin and pale; flaring of the heart-fire may cause red margin and tip of tongue, even oral ulceration; stagnation of the heart-blood will make purple, dark tongue or tongue with ecchymoses; if the heart functions abnormally in storing spirit, there will be stiff tongue and aphasia.

1.2.3　Linking to sweat in secretion

Sweat is transformed from body fluid. It is the perspired secretion through sweat pores after the transpiration and gasification of body fluid by yang-qi. Body fluid is the major constituent of blood which is governed by the heart, and people will perspire when they are nervous and alarmed, which is closely connected with the heart-spirit, therefore sweat is regarded as "the secretion of the heart".

1.2.4　Linking to joy in emotion

The physical function of the heart is associated with "joy" in emotion. People have all kinds of emotions. Joy leads to sufficient qi-blood which is good for the normal functional activities of the heart. However, over-joy may cause the heart-spirit to be dissipative, just as the saying that "over-joy injures the heart".

1.2.5　Heart and the summer-qi interlinked

The four seasons, wax-wane and transformation of yin-yang are interlinked with the system of functions and activities of five zang-organs. Yang-qi increases in hot summer, and heart-yang gets the richest in this season. Generally speaking, symptoms of the patients with declined yang-qi tend to relieve in summer (patients

中医理论　Basic Theory of Traditional Chinese Medicine

见）。中医据此提出来"冬病夏治"的理论。在冬季发作或加重的病人，在夏天治疗，凭借内外阳气隆盛，可收到事半功倍的效果。

1.3　心与小肠相表里

小肠者，受盛之官，化物出焉。

小肠的主要生理功能是受盛化物、泌别清浊。

1.3.1　受盛化物

受盛，接受，以器盛物之意。化物，变化、消化、化生之谓。小肠的受盛化物功能主要表现在两个方面：一是小肠盛受了由胃腑下移而来的初步消化的饮食物，起到容器的作用，即受盛作用；二指经胃初步消化的饮食物，在小肠内必须停留一定的时间，由小肠对其进一步消化和吸收，将水谷化为可以被机体利用的营养物质，即"化物"作用。在病理上，小肠受盛功能失调，传化停止，则气机失于通调，滞而为痛，表现为腹部疼痛等。如化物功能失常，会导致消化、吸收障碍，表现为腹胀、腹泻、便溏等。

1.3.2　泌别清浊

泌，即分泌。别，即分别。清，即精微物质。浊，即代谢产物。所谓泌别清浊，是指小肠对承受胃初步消化的饮食物，在进一步消化的同时，进行分别水谷精微和代谢产物的过程。分清，就是将饮食物中的精华部分，包括饮料

with heart disease usually suffer from yang deficiency), which constitutes TCM's theory "winter disease cured in summer". Depending on sufficient yang-qi in and outside the body, curative effect on the patients who fall ill or get worse in winter will yield double effect with half the effort.

1.3　Heart and Small Intestine Forming an Internal– external Relationship

The small intestine is like an official of receiving and resolving food.

The small intestine has the main function of receiving and resolving food, separating the clear from the turbid.

1.3.1　Receiving and resolving food

The function of receiving and resolving food of the small intestine manifests in two aspects: firstly, the small intestine accepts the chyme sent down by the stomach, which is the receiving function; secondly, the small intestine further digests and absorbs the remaining chyme to transform it into nutrient essence which can be made use of by the body, which is the resolving function. In pathology, malfunction of receiving food causes stagnation manifested as abdominal pain; malfunction of resolving food causes digestive and absorptive disorder manifested as abdominal distension, diarrhea, loose stools, etc.

1.3.2　Separating the clear from the turbid

Separating the clear from the turbid is the metabolism process that the small intestine digests the chyme and separates them into foodstuff essence and waste. Separating the clear means the foodstuff essence is absorbed and conveyed up to the heart and lung through the ascending and distributing function of the spleen, and distributed all over

化生的津液和食物化生的精微，进行吸收，再通过脾之升清散精的作用，上输心肺，输布全身，供给营养。别浊，则体现为两个方面：其一，是将饮食物的残渣糟粕，传送到大肠，形成粪便，经肛门排出体外；其二，是将剩余的水分经肾脏气化作用渗入膀胱，形成尿液，经尿道排出体外。因为小肠在泌别清浊过程中，参与了人体的水液代谢，故有"小肠主液"之说。

小肠分清别浊的功能正常，则水液和糟粕各走其道而二便正常。若小肠功能失调，清浊不分，水液归于糟粕，即会出现水谷混杂、便溏泄泻等。因"小肠主液"，故小肠分清别浊功能失常不仅影响大便，也影响小便，表现为小便短少。所以泄泻初期常用"利小便即所以实大便"的方法治疗。

小肠的泌别清浊，实为脾之升清和胃之降浊功能的具体体现。

1.3.2 心与小肠相表里

手少阴经属心络小肠，手太阳经属小肠络心，心与小肠通过经脉相互络属构成了表里关系。

心与小肠生理上相互为用。心主血脉，心阳之温煦，心血之濡养，有助于小肠的化物功能；小

the body. Depriving the turbid falls on two parts: the turbid is sent to the large intestine in which stool is formed and through the anus exerted out of the body; the residual water infiltrating into the bladder through the kidney's gasification function transforms into urine which is discharged through the urethra. The small intestine is involved in the water metabolism of human body, as the saying goes, "the small intestine dominates thick fluid".

If the small intestine's function is normal, fluid and dreg go their respective ways, and urine and stool will be normal. If the small intestine's function is abnormal manifesting as fluid going into dreg and food and drink becoming mixed, there will be diarrhea. The dysfunction of the small intestine can lead to abnormal stool, and also abnormal urine as oliguria. So, in the early stages of diarrhea, the treatment of "promoting urine to make stool solid" is commonly practiced.

Separating the clear from the turbid is the specific manifestation of the spleen's function of ascending the clear and the stomach's function of descending the turbid.

1.3.2 Heart and small intestine forming an internal- external relationship

Hand-shaoyin belongs to the heart affiliated with the small intestine through the meridians and hand-taiyang belongs to the small intestine affiliated with the heart through the meridians. The heart and the small intestine form an internal-external relationship through mutual connection and affiliation of their meridians.

Heart and small intestine support each other physiologically. The heart governs blood vessels. Heart-yang's warming and heart-blood's nourishing functions help the small intestine resolving food. To resolve food, separate

肠主化物,泌别清浊,吸收水谷精微和水液,其中浓厚部分经脾气转输于心,化血以养其心脉。

心与小肠病理上相互影响。心经实火,可移热于小肠,引起尿少、尿涩赤刺痛、尿血等小肠实热的症状。反之,小肠有热,亦可循经脉上熏于心,可见心烦、舌赤糜烂等症状。此外,小肠虚寒,化物失职,水谷精微不生,日久可出现心血不足的病症。

附:心包络

心包络,简称心包,又称"膻中",是包在心脏外面的包膜,具有保护心脏的作用。心居包络之中,包络在心之外。手厥阴经属于心包络,故心包络可称为脏。

心是君主之官,五脏六腑之大主,自然不能随便被打扰,一般由心包代其行使功能,所以若外邪入侵,心包络当先受病,所谓"代心受邪"。温病学把外感热病中出现的神昏谵语等心功能失常的病理变化,称为"热入心包"或"痰热蒙蔽心包"。

2 肺

肺者,相傅之官,治节出焉。

肺经肺系(指气管、支气管

---

the clear from the turbid, the small intestine absorbs the essence and fluid from the food and transport the quintessence to the heart through the spleen-qi and transform it into blood to nourish heart vessel.

The heart and small intestine interact with each other pathologically. The excess fire in the heart meridian transfers to the small intestine, resulting in oliguria, urinary astringent, red urine, odynuria and hematuria and other excess heat symptoms of small intestine. On the contrary, the heat of the small intestine also can go up to the heart along meridians, resulting in upset mind, red tongue, erosion of tongue and other symptoms. In addition, if the small intestine is weak and cold neglecting its duty of dissolving food, foodstuff essence will not be absorbed and over time there will appear symptoms of insufficient blood.

Attachment: Pericardium

Pericardium (also called "shanzhong") is a tissue surrounding the heart to protect it. Pericardium meridian of hand-jueyin is a part of pericardium, so it is also called zang.

The heart, as the monarch governing five zang- and six fu-organs, could not be disturbed casually, so its functions are conducted by pericardium. When pathogenic factors invade the heart, they will attack pericardium first, which is called "replacing the heart to be attacked". In science of epidemic febrile disease of TCM, the pathogenic changes of coma, delirium and other malfunctions happen in exogenous febrile disease are described as "heat attacking pericardium" or "phlegm-heat fogging pericardium".

2 Lung

The lung is an assistance-organ in governing and regulating.

The lung through the lung system (of the trachea

等)与喉、鼻相连,故称喉为肺之门户,鼻为肺之外窍。

肺的主要生理功能是主气、司呼吸,主行水,朝百脉,主治节。肺在体合皮,其华在毛,在窍为鼻,在志为悲(忧),在液为涕,与秋气相通应。肺与大肠相表里。

肺在体腔中位居最高,具有覆盖诸脏、保护诸脏、抵御外邪的作用;肺通过气管、喉、鼻直接与外界相通,主一身之表,为脏腑之外卫。因此,肺的生理功能最易受外界环境的影响,如自然界的风、寒、暑、湿、燥、火"六淫"之邪侵袭人体,多首先入肺而导致肺卫失宣、肺窍不利等病变,多见发热恶寒、咳嗽、鼻塞等肺卫功能失调的症状,故称肺为华盖。

肺为清虚之体,且居高位,百脉之所朝,外合皮毛,开窍于鼻,与天气直接相通;六淫外邪侵犯人体,不论是从口鼻而入,还是侵犯皮毛,都容易犯肺而生病,内伤与其他脏腑病变,都可累及肺而生病,故又有肺为"娇脏"之说。

2.1 生理功能

2.1.1 肺主气、司呼吸

主,是主管,主持的意思。肺主气,包括主一身之气和呼吸之气两方面。

肺司呼吸,指肺是体内外气体交换的场所。人体通过呼吸进

and bronchi) is connected with the throat and nose, so the throat is known as a gateway of the lung and the nose as the outside orifice of the lung.

The main physiological function of the lung is that the lung controls respiratory qi, smoothens water passage, connects with vessels and governs the organs. The lung is linked to skin, reflecting its gloss in hair, to nose in offices, to sorrow and worry in emotion, to fluid in nose secretion, and corresponds to autumn-qi. The lung and the large intestine form an internal-external relationship.

The location of the lung is the highest among the internal organs. It plays the role of covering and protecting the other organs and resisting the evils. Through trachea, throat and nose, it directly communicates with the outside world, dominates qi throughout the body, and is the guard of zangfu. Therefore, the physiological function of the lung is most easily affected by the external environment. Such as, if wind, coldness, heat, dampness, dryness and fire (the "six evils") invade the body, they will first invade the lung leading to diseases of failure of dispersion and descending, such as, fever, coldness, cough and nasal obstruction. So, the lung is compared to "canopy".

The lobes of the lung are delicate and its location is the highest. It connects the vessels, associates with skin and body hair outside, with nose in orifice and interlinks directly with the weather. When the six evils invade the body, no matter they are through mouth and nose, or skin and body hair, they are apt to bring about lung diseases. All the injuries and other viscera lesions can cause lung diseases. Therefore, it has the name of "fragile organ".

2.1 Physiological Function

2.1.1 Lung governing qi and controlling respiration

The lung governs qi, which includes qi of the whole body and respiratory qi.

The lung controlling respiratory qi means it is the place of gas exchange inside and outside the body. The body

行气体交换,吸清呼浊,吐故纳新,将体内的浊气呼出,把自然界的清气吸入,使体内之气与自然界之气进行交换,以维持人体清浊之气的新陈代谢。

肺要保持其司呼吸功能的正常,主要依赖于肺气的宣发和肃降作用。宣发反映了肺气向上、向外的特点;肃降反映了肺气向下、向内的特点。因此,宣发的作用重在呼出体内的浊气,肃降的作用重在吸入自然界的清气。两者相反相成,相互协调,才能使气道畅通,呼吸自如,体内外气体得以正常交换。

肺主呼吸是一身之气的主要来源和体现,民间通过观察鼻部的气体出入,以"有气没气"来作为生命活动的重要现象。呼吸微弱,气生成不足,自然少气无力。肺有节律的呼吸(宣发和肃降),调节着全身气的向上、向外、向下、向内等升降出入运动。

2.1.2 肺通调水道

通,即疏通;调,即调节;水道,是水液运行和排泄的通道。肺的通调水道功能,是指肺的宣发和肃降运动对体内水液的输布、运行和排泄起着疏通和调节的作用。通过肺的宣发,水液向上、向外输布,布散全身,外达皮毛,代谢后以汗的形式由汗孔排泄;通过肺的肃降,将上部水津向下输送、下达于肾,并成为尿液生成之源,经肾的气化,将代谢后

exchanges gas through breath. Clear gas in nature is inhaled and turbid gas in body is exhaled. The exchange between gas in nature and in body maintains the metabolism of clear and turbid gases inside the human body.

Maintaining the lung's normal respiratory function mainly depends on the dispersing and descending of the lung qi. Dispersing reflects lung-qi's characteristic of going upward and outward; descending reflects lung-qi's characteristic of going downward and inward. Therefore, the function of dispersing is to exhale turbid gas out of the body and the function of descending, inhale clear gas into the body. They supplement while oppose and coordinate, to keep the airway open, breath free and gas exchange normal.

The lung governing respiratory qi is the main source and manifestation of qi of the whole body. Through observing gas coming into or out of nasal passage Chinese people usually consider "whether there is gas or not" as an important sign of life activities. Weak breathing and lack of gas generation can cause infirmity. Rhythmic breath (dispersing and descending) regulates the motion of the whole body's qi to go upward, outward, downward and inward.

2.1.2 Lung smoothing water passage

Smoothing means dredging and regulating. Water passage means the passage for circulation and excretion of water. That the lung smoothing water passage signifies the lung's dispersing and descending movement plays a role of dredging and regulating distribution, circulation and excretion of water in the body. Through the lung's dispersing, water is distributed upward and outward to skin and body hair and the whole body. Then it reaches the surface of the body, and is excreted through sweat pores as perspiration after it is metabolized. Through the lung's descending, the fluid of the upper part is distributed to the lower part—kidney as the source of urine formation.

的水液化为尿贮藏于膀胱,而排出体外。如果肺气的宣发肃降出现异常,会影响肺的通调水道功能,出现水液停滞,酿成痰饮,或水湿泛溢肌肤而成水肿等病变。

2.1.3 肺朝百脉、主治节

朝,有汇聚和朝向两种意思;百脉,许多经脉(此指血管)。肺朝百脉,是指全身的血液都通过经脉汇聚于肺,经肺的呼吸进行体内外清浊之气的交换,然后再将富含清气的血液通过经脉输送到全身。肺朝百脉的功能,是肺气的运动在血液循行中的具体体现,说明全身的血和脉虽统属于心,心气是血液在肺中循环运行的基本动力,但尚须肺的协助。因此,肺朝百脉的作用,是帮助心脏行血。

治节,就是治理调节,指肺具有治理调节全身脏腑及其功能的作用。肺的治节作用,主要体现在四个方面:一是肺主呼吸,人体的呼吸运动是有节奏地一呼一吸;二是随着肺的呼吸运动,治理和调节全身的气机,就是调节气的升降出入运动;三是通过调节气的升降出入运动而辅助心脏,推动和调节血液的运行;四是肺的宣发和肃降,治理和调节津液的输布、运行和排泄。

Through the kidney's gasification, the metabolized fluid was stored in bladder and excreted out of the body. The malfunction of the lung qi's dispersing and descending will influence lung's function in regulating water passage, leading to accumulation of water, manifesting as phlegm, or dampness over skin, manifesting as edema and other pathological changes.

2.1.3 Lung connecting with vessels and governing the organs

That the lung connecting with vessels means blood of the whole body converges in the lung through the vessels and operates the clear and turbid gas exchange through the lung's respiratory function, and then, blood with rich clear qi goes through the vessels to the whole body. The lung's function of connecting with vessels is the concrete embodiment of the movement of lung-qi in blood circulation, which signifies though blood and vessels are governed by the heart, the basic power of blood circulation in the lung, the heart-qi should be assisted by the lung. Hence, the function of the lung is to help promote blood circulation.

Governing means managing and regulating. It means the lung can manage and regulate all the organs and their functions in four aspects: the lung governs respiratory qi. Human respiratory movement is rhythmic breath; secondly, with respiratory movement, the lung governs and regulates the whole body's functional activity of qi, and adjusts the movement of qi in ascending, descending, exiting and entering; thirdly, it can promote and regulate blood circulation through adjusting the movement of qi in ascending, descending, exiting and entering; fourthly, dispersing and descending of the lung governs and regulates fluid distribution, running and excretion.

中医理论 Basic Theory of Traditional Chinese Medicine

2.2 肺与体窍液时等的关系

2.2.1 肺在体合皮，其华在毛

皮毛，包括皮肤、汗腺等组织，就是身体的表面。这些组织依赖于肺所宣发的卫气和津液的温养和润泽，是机体抵抗外邪的第一屏障。肺的生理功能正常，则皮肤致密，毫毛光泽，抵御外邪侵袭的能力就强；反之，肺气虚，宣发卫气和输精于皮毛的生理功能减弱，则卫表不固，抵抗外邪侵袭的能力低下，会出现多汗和容易感冒，或皮毛憔悴枯槁等现象。

2.2.2 肺在窍为鼻

鼻的嗅觉与喉部的发音都是肺气的作用，所以肺气和，呼吸利，则嗅觉灵敏，声音正常。由于肺开窍于鼻而与喉直接相通，所以外邪袭肺，多是从鼻喉而入；肺的病变也多见鼻塞、流涕、喷嚏、喉痒、音哑和失声等症状。

2.2.3 肺在液为涕

涕是鼻黏膜分泌的黏液，有润泽鼻窍的作用。鼻为肺窍，因此其分泌物亦属肺。肺的功能正常，鼻涕润泽鼻窍而不外流；如果肺寒，则鼻流清涕；肺热，则鼻流黄涕；肺燥，则鼻干。

2.2.4 肺在志为悲、忧

悲和忧对人体的主要影响是耗伤肺气。如悲忧过度，就会出现呼吸气短等肺气不足的现

2.2 Relations of Lung with Body, Orifices, Fluid and Seasons

2.2.1 Lung linking to skin, reflecting its gloss in hair

Skin and body hair, including skin, sweat glands and other tissues, is the surface of the body. Depending on the defensive qi dispersed by lung and the warm nourishing and moisture of secretion, these tissues are the first barrier of resisting exopathogens. If the lung's physiological function is normal, skin will be fine and close, hair will be lustrous and resistance against exopathogens will be strong. Conversely, if the lung-qi gets deficient and the physiological function of dispersing defensive qi and carrying essence to skin and hair weakens, there will appear weak resistance, excessive sweat, susceptible to cold or haggard skin and body hair.

2.2.2 Lung linking to nose in orifice

The nasal olfactory and larynx pronunciation depends on the function of the lung-qi. So, when the lung qi disperses smoothly, the nose will be keen with smell and voice will be normal. The nose is the orifice of lung, and the lung is linked with throat, therefore exopathogens attack the lung mainly through nose and throat. Pulmonary lesions will lead to symptoms such as stuffy nose. running nose, sneezing, itching throat, hoarseness and aphonia etc.

2.2.3 Lung associating with snivel in secretion

The secretion of nasal mucus can moisturize nasal orifice. The nose is the lung orifice, so its secretion also belongs to the lung. If the lung functions normally, the nasal secretion moisturizes nasal orifice and does not flow out of it. If the lung suffers from coldness, clear secretion runs out of nose. If the lung suffers from heat, yellow secretion runs out of nose.

2.2.4 Lung linking with sorrow and worry in emotion

The major influence of sorrow and worry is consumption of lung-qi. For example, over-sorrow will lead to short breath and deficiency of lung-qi. Conversely, if the lung

象。反之,在肺虚或肺宣降运动失调时,机体对外来的非良性刺激的耐受性就会下降,容易产生悲忧的情绪变化。

2.2.5 肺与秋气相应

时令至秋,暑去而凉生,草木皆凋。肺为清虚之体,性喜清润,与秋季气候清肃、空气明润相通应。同气相求,故肺与秋气相应。

秋金之时,燥气当令,此时燥邪极易侵入人体而耗伤肺的阴津,出现干咳、皮肤和口鼻干燥等肺的病变症状。

2.3 肺与大肠相表里

大肠者,传导之官,变化出焉。

大肠的主要生理功能是传化糟粕、吸收津液。

2.3.1 传化糟粕

大肠传导是指大肠接受由小肠下移的饮食残渣,再吸收完其中剩余的水分和养料后,使形成粪便,经肛门而排出体外,是整个消化过程的最后阶段,故有"传导之腑"、"传导之官"之称。大肠的传导功能,主要与肝之疏泄、胃之通降、脾之运化、肺之肃降以及肾之封藏有密切关系。

大肠有病,传导失常,主要表现为大便质和量的变化和排便次数的改变。如大肠传导失常,就会出现大便秘结或泄泻。若湿热蕴结于大肠,大肠气滞,又会出

qi gets deficient and the function of lung's dispersing and descending is abnormal, the tolerance of pessimistic stimulation by human body will decrease, and it is easy to lead to the emotional changes such as sorrow and worry.

2.2.5 Lung corresponding to autumn-qi

In autumn, summer-heat fades and coolness arises; grass and trees wither. The delicate lung which favors clearness and moisture corresponds to the clear, bright and moist weather in autumn. So, the lung corresponds to autumn-qi.

In dry autumn, dryness is apt to invade the human body and consume and injure the lung's yin-fluid, leading to dry cough, dry skin and nose and other pathological changes caused by dry lung.

2.3 Lung and the Large Intestine Forming an Internal–external Relationship

The large intestine is like an official governing transforming and changing.

The main physiological function of the large intestine is to transform and convey the waste, and absorb fluid.

2.3.1 Transforming and conveying the waste

Transforming and conveying of the large intestine means that the large intestine accepts the chyme sent down by the small intestine, absorbs the remained fluid and nourishment in the chyme, and makes the remains into stool which is exerted out of the body via anus. It is the last stage of digestion, so it is called "the fu or official of transforming and conveying the waste". Its function has the close relationship with the liver's function of regulating flow of qi, the stomach's dredging and descending, the spleen's transforming and transporting, the lung's descending and the kidney's sealing and storing.

Illness and disorder of the large intestine mainly manifest as the change in the quality and quantity of stool and frequency of defecation, such as constipation or diarrhea. If damp heat in the large intestine accumulates, there will appear qi stagnation in the large intestine, abdominal pain,

现腹痛、里急后重、下痢脓血等。

2.3.2　大肠主津

大肠重新吸收水分，参与调节体内水液代谢的功能，称之为"大肠主津"。大肠的病变也多与津液有关。如大肠虚寒，无力吸收水分，则水谷杂下，出现肠鸣、腹痛、泄泻等。大肠实热，消烁水分，肠液干枯，肠道失润，又会出现大便秘结不通之症。

大肠在脏腑功能活动中，积聚与输送并存，始终处于实而不能满的状态，故以降为顺，以通为用。大肠通降失常，以糟粕内结，壅塞不通为多，故有"肠道易实"之说。

2.3.3　肺与大肠相表里

手太阴经属于肺，络于大肠；手阳明经属于大肠，络于肺。通过经脉的相互络属，肺与大肠构成表里关系。

肺与大肠的生理联系，主要体现在肺气肃降与大肠传导功能之间的相互为用关系。肺气清肃下降，气机调畅，并布散津液，能促进大肠的传导，有利于糟粕的排出。大肠传导正常，糟粕下行，亦有利于肺气的肃降。两者配合协调，从而使肺主呼吸及大肠传导功能均归正常。

肺与大肠在病变时亦可相互影响。肺气壅塞，失于肃降，气

tenesmus and diarrhea sepsis etc.

2.3.2　Large intestine dominating thin fluid

The large intestine reabsorbs water and involves in regulating body fluid metabolism, which is known as the "the large intestine dominating thin fluid ". Its lesions are also always related to body fluid. Weak and cold large intestine is unable to absorb water, and so mixed food and drink will descend, resulting in borborygmus, abdominal pain and diarrhea. The real heat, however, consumes the fluid, bringing about the dry large intestine, even constipation.

The large intestine functions to accumulate and transport, and is always solid but not full, so its function of descent and smoothness plays an important role. The dysfunction of descent and smoothness causes waste blocked inside of the large intestine, so there is the saying "the large intestine is apt to be solid".

2.3.3　Lung and large intestine forming an internal-external relationship

The meridian of hand-taiyin belongs to the lung and connects with the large intestine through meridians; the meridian of hand-yangming belongs to the large intestine and connects with the lung through meridians. The lung and large intestine form an internal-external relationship, connected and affiliated with each other through meridians.

The physiological relationship of the lung and large intestine is mainly reflected in the interaction between the lung's descending and the large intestine's transforming. Purification and descent of the lung-qi smoothen qi and distribute the fluid, which is conducive to the large intestine's transformation and dross discharging. Conversely, if the large intestine functions normally and dross descends, it will be conducive to the lung-qi's descending. The coordination of the lung and the large intestine makes them function normally.

The pathological change of the lung and the large intestine can also affect each other. If the lung-qi is

不下行,津不下达,可引起腑气不通,肠燥便秘。若大肠实热,传导不畅,腑气阻滞,也可影响到肺的宣降,出现胸满咳喘。

blocked and lost in descending, qi and body fluid cannot descend, bringing about blocked fu-qi, dry large intestine and constipation. If there is real heat in the large intestine, there will appear unsmooth transformation and blocked fu-qi, which also affects the lung's dispersing and descending, resulting in full chest, cough and dyspnea.

3 脾

脾胃者,仓廪之官,五味出焉。

脾的生理功能是主运化,统摄血液。脾在体合肉而主四肢,在窍为口,其华在唇,在志为思,在液为涎,与长夏之气相通应,旺于四时。脾与胃相表里。

脾主管饮食物的消化以及营养物质的吸收和转输,对维持生命活动起着根本的作用,所以称"脾为后天之本,气血生化之源"。这一理论在养生防病方面非常重要,有指导意义。

3.1 生理功能

3.1.1 脾主运化

运,就是转运输送;化,就是消化吸收。脾主运化,指脾具有将水谷化为精微并将精微物质转运输送至全身各脏腑组织的功能,包括运化食物和运化水液两个方面。

饮食物消化,依赖于脾的运化功能将食物分解成水谷精微和糟粕。如果脾功能不足,会使消化功能减退,甚至出现吃什么排

3 Spleen

The spleen and stomach, barn organs, determine the five flavors.

The physiological function of the spleen is to govern transformation and transportation, dominating blood. The spleen is linked to muscles in body to dominate four limbs, to mouth in orifice to reflect its brilliance on lips, to saliva in secretion. The spleen interlinked with long summer-qi is vibrant in four seasons. The spleen and the stomach form an internal-external relationship.

The spleen is a general organ governing food digestion and nutrient absorption and having a fundamental effect of maintaining life activities. Therefore, the spleen is called the "acquired root" and the "origin of qi and blood". This theory has guiding significance for health preserving and disease prevention.

3.1 Physiological Function

3.1.1 Spleen governing transformation and transportation

The spleen governing transformation and transportation means the spleen can transform foodstuff, as well as drink into essence and transport it to all organs and tissues around the whole body.

Food digestion relies on the spleen's function of transforming and transporting food into essence and dregs. Malfunction of the spleen will make the digestive function decline, resulting in discharge of undigested food, which is called in TCM "complete grain in stool"; the spleen

中医理论　Basic Theory of Traditional Chinese Medicine

什么的现象,中医称之为"完谷不化";通过脾的运化,将水谷精微上输于心肺,经肺之宣发向上向外布散,肺之肃降作用则向下输布,并将其转输至全身;经过脾的运化,将水谷精微转化为气血等重要生命物质,以营养五脏六腑四肢百骸,以及皮毛、筋、肉等各个组织器官。

需要特别强调的是:脾在运输水谷精微的同时,也是调节人体水液代谢的关键环节。脾把人体所需要的水液(津液),通过心肺而运送到全身各组织中去,起到滋养濡润的作用。又把各组织器官利用后的水液,输送到膀胱,排泄于外,从而维持体内水液代谢的平衡。因此,脾运化水湿的功能健旺,能使体内各组织得到水液的充分濡养,不致使水湿过多而潴留;如果脾的运化水液功能减退,可导致水液在体内停滞,而产生水、湿、痰、饮等病理产物,这就是脾虚生湿,脾为生痰之源和脾虚水肿的发生机理。

3.1.2　脾主统血

统是统摄、控制的意思。脾主统血,指脾具有统摄血液,使之在经脉中运行而不溢出脉外的功能。脾统血的作用是通过气摄血的作用来实现的。脾为气血的生化之源,气为血帅,血随气行。脾的运化功能健旺,则气血充盈,气能摄血;气旺的固摄作用也强,血液也不会溢出脉外而发生出血现象。反之,如果脾失健运,气的

transforms and transports foodstuff essence to the heart and the lungs, distributing it up and outside through the dispersion of lungs. Then, the lungs depurate and descend the essence to the whole body; the spleen transforms and transports foodstuff essence into qi-blood and some other important substance to nourish the five- zang and six-fu organs, four limbs, bones, skin, body hair, tendons and muscles etc.

What should be emphasized here is that as the spleen transforms and transports foodstuff essence, it also plays a key role in regulating fluid metabolism. The spleen, through the heart and lungs, transports fluid (secretion) to all tissues around the body and plays a part of nourishing and moistening. Then, it transports the left over fluid used by tissues and organs to the bladder to be excreted, so that the balance of inside fluid metabolism is maintained through the spleen's transportation function. Thus, if the spleen's function of transforming and transporting fluid and moisture is sufficient, all the tissues inside the body will be nourished immensely, and there will be no retention of excessive fluid and moisture. If the spleen's function decays, it will cause retention of excessive fluid inside the body, and some pathogenic substances, such as water, moisture and phlegm will occur. That is the genesis mechanism of "deficient spleen inducing dampness," "the spleen being the origin of phlegm" and "deficient spleen inducing edema."

3.1.2　Spleen dominating blood

The spleen dominating blood means that the spleen controls blood circulation inside vessels and prevents it from overflowing. The spleen's function of dominating blood is realized through qi dominating blood. The spleen is the source of qi-blood, with qi dominating blood and blood circulating with qi. If the function that spleen governing transformation and transportation is sound, qi-blood will be abundant and qi can control blood; the more vibrant qi will be, the better the astriction effects are, and blood will not

固摄作用减退,可使血溢出脉外而见各种出血,如便血、尿血、崩漏等。

overflow to hemorrhage. Contrarily, if the spleen's function is deficient, qi's astriction effects will decay and blood will spill out of vessels, and different kinds of hemorrhages, such as hemafecia, hematuria and metrorrhagia, will happen.

3.2 与体窍液时等的关系

3.2 Relations of Spleen with Body, Orifices, Fluid and Seasons

3.2.1 在体合肌肉,主四肢

3.2.1 Spleen linking to muscles in body to dominate four limbs

肌肉需要气血来营养,才能丰满健壮,活动有力。脾为气血生化之源,所以人体肌肉的健壮与否,与脾的运化功能密切相关。若脾的运化功能不足,人就会消瘦,肌肉软弱无力,甚至萎弱不用。

Qi-blood's nourishment is necessary for muscles' strength, thickness and energy. The spleen is the source of qi-blood, so robust muscles are closely associated with the spleen's function of transformation and transportation. If the spleen's function is deficient, people will get thin and muscles will be weak, even be nerveless.

肌肉的强壮体现在四肢的运动。脾将饮食物的水谷精微,运化输送到四肢肌肉,则四肢轻劲,灵活有力。如果脾虚气弱,则四肢疲乏无力,萎弱不用。

Strong muscles manifest in the movement of four limbs. If the spleen transforms and transports foodstuff essence to the four limbs, they will be agile and forceful. If the spleen's function is deficient and qi is weak, four limbs will be forceless and nerveless.

3.2.2 在官窍为口,其华在唇

3.2.2 Spleen linking to mouth in orifice to reflect its brilliance on lips

饮食与脾运化功能有密切关系。脾气健运,则食欲口味正常;如果脾失健运,则食欲不振,口淡乏味,可觉口甜、口腻。如果脾有伏热,可循经上于口,发生唇口糜烂等。

Diet is closely connected with the spleen's function of transformation and transportation. If the spleen's function gets deficient, there will appear poor appetite and tastelessness, and sweet, greasy taste in the mouth. If there is heat latent in the spleen, it can climb up along meridian to the mouth to cause oral ulceration.

口唇的色泽,能反映全身气血的状况。脾为气血生化之源,所以口唇色泽不但是全身气血状况的反映,也是脾主运化功能的体现。正常脾气健运,气血充足,营养良好,口唇红润有光泽;脾失健运,气血衰少,营养不良,则

The color and luster of lips can reflect the condition of qi-blood of the whole body. The spleen is the source of generation and transformation of qi-blood, so the color and luster of lips not only reflect the qi-blood condition of the whole body, but also the spleen's function. If the spleen's function is normal, qi-blood will be abundant, nutritious enough, with lips red, moist and lustrous. If the spleen's function is abnormal, qi-blood will be deficient, with

口唇淡白无华,萎黄不泽。

3.2.3 脾在液为涎

唾液中较清稀的称为涎,具有保护口腔黏膜、润泽口腔的作用,在进食时分泌较多,有助于食物的吞咽和消化。在正常情况下,涎液上行于口,但不溢于口外。脾胃不和,则往往导致涎液分泌剧增,而发生口涎自出等现象。

3.2.4 脾在志为思

思,即思考、思虑,是人的精神意识思维活动的一种状态。正常的思考问题,对机体的生理活动并无不良影响,但在思虑过度、所思不遂等情况下,就会影响机体的正常生理活动。思虑太过又易伤脾,所以脾的生理功能与情志活动的"思"有关。

3.2.5 脾主长夏

长夏是一年中温度最高、雨水最多的季节,动植物生长快速,与脾主运化,为气血生化之源相似。脾运湿又恶湿,每年夏季因湿气太旺,湿邪伤脾,脾失健运,称为"湿困脾土"。吹空调、电扇,贪凉、贪吃生冷引起的感冒也大都可以归为湿困脾土。若脾为湿困,运化失职,可引起胸脘痞满、食少体倦、大便溏薄、口甜多涎、舌苔滑腻等。故长夏之时,处方遣药,常常加入藿香、佩兰等芳香化浊醒脾之品。

3.3 脾与胃相表里

胃,又称胃脘,位于腹腔内,

nutrition poor, lips pale, sallow and lusterless.

3.2.3 Spleen linking to saliva in secretion

Saliva is clear and thin slobber. Saliva can protect oral mucosa and moisten mouth. Saliva will be secreted while eating, which is conducive to swallowing and digesting food. Normally, saliva goes up to mouth, but it will not overflow the mouth. Malfunction of stomach and spleen will result in substantial secretion of saliva which will flow out of the mouth.

3.2.4 Spleen linking to thinking in emotion

Thinking is a state of mental activity of the human spirit. Normal thinking exerts no bad effects on physiological activities of the body. However, over-thinking, concern and depression will affect the normal physiological activities of the body. Over-thinking can hurt the spleen, so the physiological functions of the spleen is linked to thinking in emotion.

3.2.5 Spleen linking to long summer-qi

The attributes of long summer, a season when the temperature and rainfall volume are the highest of the year, and animals and plants grow fast, are similar to that the spleen governs transformation and transportation, and the spleen is the source of qi-blood's generation and transformation. In summer, excessive pathogenic dampness injures the spleen, so the dysfunction of the spleen is called "dampness invading spleen". Most of the cold diseases induced by being exposed to air conditioner, electric fan and taking excessive raw and cold food belong to "dampness invading spleen". Therefore, in the long summer, herbs of eliminating dampness with aromatics such as patchouli and eupatorium are always used in prescriptions.

3.3 Spleen and Stomach Forming an Internal-external Relationship

The stomach is also called gastral cavity. It is located in the abdomen, connecting with the esophagus in the

上接食道,下通小肠。胃的上口为贲门,又叫"上脘";下口为幽门,又叫"下脘";胃的中部叫"中脘",三部分统一称为"胃脘"。脾胃常合称为后天之本。

胃的生理功能有两方面:胃主受纳、腐熟水谷。

3.3.1 胃主受纳水谷

胃主受纳水谷是指胃接收和容纳水谷的作用。饮食入口,经过食道容纳并暂存于胃脘,这一过程称为受纳,所以称"胃为水谷之海"。机体生理活动和气血津液的化生,都需要饮食物的营养,所以又称胃为水谷气血之海。胃受纳功能的强弱,取决于胃气的盛衰,反映于能食不能食,能食则受纳功能强,不能食则受纳功能弱。

3.3.2 胃主腐熟水谷

腐熟是饮食物经过胃的初步消化,形成食糜的过程。胃接受由口摄入的饮食物并使其在胃中短暂停留,进行初步消化,依靠胃的腐熟作用,将水谷变成食糜。饮食物经过初步消化,其精微物质由脾之运化而营养全身,没被消化的食糜则下行于小肠,不断更新,形成胃的消化过程。如果胃的腐熟功能低下,就出现胃脘疼痛、食滞胃脘等症状。

中医学非常重视胃气,认为人以胃气为本,胃气强则五脏都盛,胃气弱则五脏俱衰,有胃气则

upper place and the small intestine in the lower place. The upper part of the stomach is cardia, also known as "shangwan"; the lower part of the stomach is pylorus, also known as "xiawan"; the middle part of the stomach is called "zhongwan". All of the three parts are called "gastral cavity". Both of the spleen and stomach are called the acquired foundation.

The physiological function of the stomach lies in two parts: receiving foodstuff and decomposing it.

3.3.1 Stomach receiving foodstuff

Receiving foodstuff means the stomach has the function of accepting and containing foodstuff. The process that foodstuff is taken in through the mouth and contained in the stomach through the esophagus and temporarily stored in the gastral cavity is called receiving, so the stomach is called "the sea of foodstuff". The physiological activity, transforming and transporting of qi-blood, and secretion needs food nutrients, so the stomach is also called "the sea of foodstuff and qi-blood".

The function of the stomach relies on the stomach-qi, reflecting in the appetite. Strong appetite signifies strong receiving and containing function and vice versa.

3.3.2 Stomach decomposing foodstuff

Foodstuff is digested by the stomach and transformed into chyme. The stomach takes in foodstuff through mouth and keeps it temporarily, conducts preliminary digestion and decomposes it into chyme. The essence of foodstuff through the preliminary digestion is sent to the whole body by the spleen. The undigested chyme goes down to the small intestine and is renewed again and again, forming the stomach's digestion process. Malfunction of the stomach in decomposing foodstuff causes epigastric pain and indigestion.

TCM attaches great importance to the stomach-qi, and believes it is the basis of body. Strong stomach-qi makes five internal organs strong and vice versa; people can live

生，无胃气则死。

3.3.3 脾与胃相表里

脾与胃同居中焦，以膜相连，足太阴经属于脾，络于胃，足阳明经属于胃，络于脾，两者构成表里配合关系。脾胃同为气血生化之源、后天之本，在饮食物的受纳、消化及水谷精微的吸收、转输等生理过程中起主要作用。脾与胃的关系，体现为水谷纳运相得、气机升降相因、阴阳燥湿相济三个方面。

水谷纳运相得：胃主受纳、腐熟水谷，为脾主运化提供前提；脾主运化、消化食物，转输精微，也为胃的继续摄食提供条件及能量。两者密切合作，才能维持饮食物的消化及精微、津液的吸收转输。若脾失健运，可导致胃纳不振，而胃气失和，也可导致脾运失常，最终均可出现纳少脘痞、腹胀泄泻等脾胃纳运失调之症。

气机升降相因：脾胃居中，脾气主升而胃气主降，相反而相成。脾气升则肾气、肝气皆升，胃气降则心气、肺气皆降，故为脏腑气机上下升降的枢纽。在饮食物的消化吸收方面，脾气上升，将运化吸收的水谷精微和津液向上输布，自然有助于胃气之通降；胃气通降，将受纳之水谷、初步消化之食糜及食物残渣通降下行，也有助于脾气之升运。脾胃之气升降相因，既保证了饮食纳运功能

with the stomach-qi or die without it.

3.3.3 Spleen and stomach forming an internal-external relationship

The spleen and stomach cohabit in middle-jiao, connecting each other by membrane. The meridian of foot-taiyin belongs to the spleen and the stomach; the meridian of foot yangming belongs to the stomach and the spleen; the two of them form internal-external and cooperative relationship. They are the sources of qi-blood and acquired foundation of the body. The relationship of them manifests in the commutative dependence of containing and transporting foodstuff, the coordination of ascending and descending qi, mutual supplementing between yin, yang, dryness, and moisture.

The stomach, receiving and decomposing foodstuff, provides premise for the spleen's function of transforming and transporting; the spleen's transforming, transporting and digesting foodstuff also provides energy for the stomach to continue to receive food. The close cooperation of them can maintain digestion of food, absorption and transference of essence and secretion. The malfunction of the spleen causes the disorder of containing function of the stomach; the disharmony of stomach-qi causes the malfunction of the spleen, even blockage of the stomach duct, abdominal distension, diarrhea and other diseases.

The spleen-qi governs ascending and the stomach-qi governs descending; they are contrary and complementary to each other. Ascent of the spleen-qi makes the kidney-qi and liver-qi ascend; descent of the stomach-qi makes the heart-qi and lung-qi descend. So they form the hub for regulating the qi movement of viscera. In the part of food digestion and absorption, ascent of the spleen-qi distributes the foodstuff essence and secretion to the upper place, so it is conducive to the descent of the stomach-qi; descent of the stomach-qi distributes the foodstuff, chyme and dross to the lower place, so it is conducive to the ascent of the spleen-qi. Cooperation of the ascent and descent of the spleen and stomach qi not only guarantees the normal function of

中医理论

Basic Theory of Traditional Chinese Medicine

的正常进行，又维护着内脏位置的相对恒定。若脾虚气陷，可导致胃失和降而上逆，而胃失和降，亦影响脾气升运功能，均可产生脘腹坠胀、头晕目眩、泄泻不止、呕吐呃逆或内脏下垂等脾胃升降失常之候。

阴阳燥湿相济：脾与胃相对而言，脾为阴脏，以阳气温煦推动用事，脾阳健则能运化升清，故性喜燥而恶湿；胃为阳腑，以阴气凉润通降用事，胃阴足则能受纳腐熟，故性喜润而恶燥。脾易湿，得胃阳以制之，使脾不至于湿；胃易燥，得脾阴以制之，使胃不至于燥。脾胃阴阳燥湿相济，是保证两者纳运、升降协调的必要条件。若脾湿太过，或胃燥伤阴，均可产生脾运胃纳的失常。如湿困脾运，可导致胃纳不振；胃阴不足，亦可影响脾运功能。脾湿则其气不升，胃燥则其气不降，可见中满痞胀、排便异常等症。

4 肝

肝者，将军之官，谋虑出焉。

肝的主要生理功能是肝藏血、肝主疏泄。肝在体合筋，其华在爪，在窍为目，在志为怒，在液为泪，与自然界春气相通应。胆

containing and transporting foodstuff, but also maintains the relatively stable position of the internal organs. Weak spleen-qi causes the stomach-qi to go the opposite way. The malfunction of the stomach-qi can also affect the function of the spleen-qi, and there will appear abdominal distension, dizziness, diarrhea, vomiting, hiccup, or visceral ptosis, and other symptoms triggered by malfunction of the spleen and stomach.

The spleen and stomach are both opposite and complementary. The spleen belongs to yin viscera, and warmth of yang-qi promotes it to work. Sufficient spleen yang can play a role in transformation and transportation and sending up the clear, so the spleen enjoys dryness and defies moisture; the stomach belongs to yang viscera, and coolness and moisture of the yin-qi promotes it to work. Sufficient stomach yin can play a role in receiving and decomposing, so it enjoys moisture and defies dryness. The spleen is easy to get wet, and the stomach-yang can get rid of its wetness; the stomach is easy to get dry, and the spleen-yin can get rid of its dryness. Cooperation of spleen-yin, stomach-yang and dryness, moisture is necessary to guarantee the normal function of the spleen and stomach. If the spleen is too wet, or the stomach is dry and hurts yin, their function will be abnormal. Wetness disturbs the spleen's transportation, resulting in the stomach's malfunction in containing; insufficient stomach-yin can also affect the spleen. Spleen wetness hinders spleen-qi's ascent while stomach dryness hinders stomach-qi's descent, resulting in fullness or distension in the stomach and abnormal defecation etc.

4 Liver

The liver, a general organ, decides people's intellectual level.

The main physiological function of the liver is that it stores blood and regulates the flow of qi. The liver is linked to tendons in body, manifesting its splendor in nails; it opens at eyes; it is linked to tears in fluid; it is linked

附于肝,肝与胆相表里。

肝藏血是女子经行的基本保证,气机调畅是女子行经能否通畅有度的重要条件,受肝气的疏泄功能的影响。治疗妇科病症,常以治肝为第一要法。由于肝的功能对女子的生殖机能尤为重要,故有"女子以肝为先天"之说。

4.1　生理功能

4.1.1　肝藏血

肝藏血是指肝具有贮藏血液、调节血量和防止出血的功能。当人体处于安静或情绪稳定状态时,机体外周需要量相对减少,部分血液就回流到肝脏贮藏起来;当人体进行剧烈活动或情绪激动时,肝内的血液被动员出来,运送到全身,供给各组织器官的需要。人动则血运于诸经,人静则血归于肝脏。肝的藏血功能失常,不仅会引起机体许多部分因血液濡养不足而导致病变,也有可能导致出血,同时肝藏血是女子经血的重要来源。

4.1.2　肝主疏泄

疏泄就是舒通、畅达的意思。人体各器官的生理活动,全靠气的升降出入活动正常进行。肝主疏泄是指肝脏能调畅气机,对全身气机的平衡起着调节作用。肝的疏泄功能不够会出现胸胁、两乳、小腹等部位胀痛的证候,肝气郁结、闷闷不乐、气机不

to anger in emotion; the liver and spring-qi are interlinked. The gallbladder is attached to the liver, and the liver and the gallbladder forms an internal-external relationship.

That the liver stores blood basically guarantees menstruation. Smooth qi is important for regular and smooth menstruation which is influenced by the liver's regulating flow of qi. The first step to treat gynecological diseases is to cure the liver disease. As the function of the liver is particularly important for women's reproductive function, so there is the saying "liver is essential for female " .

4.1　Physiological Function

4.1.1　Liver storing blood

The liver storing blood means the liver has the functions of storing blood, regulating blood volume and avoiding hemorrhage. When the body is in resting and calm state, blood volume will comparatively decrease around periphery and part of blood will flow back into the liver and be stored; when the body is in active and emotional state, blood in the liver will be mobilized and transported into the whole body to satisfy the needs of all the tissues and organs. Being active makes blood flow around meridians; on the contrary, being still makes blood flow back into the liver. Another connotation of "liver storing blood" lies in avoiding hemorrhage. Malfunction of the liver will lead to pathogenic changes due to deficient blood, even hemorrhage. At the same time, blood stored in the liver is an important source of menstruation.

4.1.2　Liver regulating flow of qi

The liver regulating flow of qi means the liver can dredge and smoothen qi. The physical activities of all the organs rely on normal activities of qi such as ascending, descending, exiting and entering. The liver can balance the whole body's qi dynamic. The liver's malfunction in regulating flow of qi causes the stagnated liver-qi and unsmooth qi, manifesting as depression, swelling pain on

畅。肝气升发太过会出现头目胀痛,面红耳赤,易怒等肝气上逆的证候。如果气升太过,血随气涌,甚至出现呕血、昏厥、不知人事等证候。

肝的疏泄功能主要体现在以下几方面:

调畅情志:肝气疏泄正常,气机调畅,气血平和,才能心情舒畅、开朗。如肝失疏泄,肝气郁结,人就会闷闷不乐,多愁善感;如肝气过亢,就会头昏脑涨、烦躁易怒、失眠多梦。外界的精神刺激,尤其是大怒最容易使肝失疏泄,因此有"暴怒伤肝"之说。

调节脾胃之气的升降和胆汁的分泌排泄:肝的疏泄功能正常,全身气机疏通畅达,有助于脾升胃降,促进对食物的消化、吸收。若肝的疏泄功能异常,影响脾的运化功能,在上则为眩晕,在下则为大便泻泄,称为肝气犯脾;影响胃的通降功能,在上则为呕吐,嗳气,在中则为脘腹胀痛,在下则为便秘等,称作肝气犯胃。

对血液和水液代谢的影响:血液的运行和水液的输布代谢有赖于肝气疏通、气机调畅。若肝失疏泄,气机郁滞,血运不畅,会停滞成为瘀血或肿块,在女子会出现月经不调,痛经等。肝气上逆,迫血上涌,又会出现咳血,吐血或脑出血等。气机失调会导致水液代谢失常,从而产生痰饮、水肿等病症。

促进男子排精、女子行经:

sternal ribs, breast and lower abdomen. Over-ascending of liver-qi will induce swelling pain on head and eyes, red complexion and ears, irritability. Blood welling with over-ascending of liver-qi will cause blood spitting, syncope, and coma.

The liver's function in regulating flow of qi is embodied in the following aspects.

As long as the liver is normal in regulating flow of qi, qi dynamic is smooth and qi-blood is even, the mood will be at ease. Abnormality of flow and stagnation of liver-qi will make people feel unhappy and sentimental; hyperactive rise of qi will cause dizziness, irritability, insomnia and dreamful sleep. The outside mental stimulation, especially rage is liable to cause failure of the liver to maintain free movement of qi, so there is the saying "outrage injures the liver".

Adjusting ascending and descending of spleen- and stomach-qi, secreting and excreting of bile: Normal liver functions in regulating flow of qi and smooth qi dynamic is conducive to spleen's ascending and stomach descending, promoting food digestion and absorption. Abnormal liver function affects the spleen's transformation and transportation, manifesting as dizziness and diarrhea, which is called liver-qi attacking spleen; it can also affect stomach's descent manifesting as vomit and eructation, distending pain inside stomach and abdomen and constipation.

Blood circulation and fluid transportation and metabolism rely on free flow of liver-qi and smooth qi dynamic. The failure of the liver in governing free flow of qi, stagnation of qi dynamic and blood will result in blood stasis or lump manifesting as irregular menstruation and menorrhalgia. Rise of liver-qi forces blood to well manifesting as hemoptysis, hematemesis and cerebral hemorrhage. Malfunction of qi dynamic will influence fluid metabolism manifesting as phlegm and edema.

Promoting ejaculation and menstruation: Ejaculation

中医理论

Basic Theory of Traditional Chinese Medicine

男子的排精、女子的排卵和月经来潮与肝的疏泄功能密切相关。男子精液的贮藏和施泄,是肝肾二脏闭藏和疏泄相互协调的结果。肝的疏泄功能正常,则精液排泄通畅有度;肝失疏泄,则排精不畅。女子月经及排卵同样受肝主疏泄的影响。肝的疏泄功能正常发挥,则月经周期正常,行经通畅;若肝失疏泄,月经周期就会紊乱,行经不畅,甚至痛经。

4.2 与体窍液时的关系

4.2.1 肝在体合筋,其华在爪

筋就是筋膜,有连接和约束骨节、肌肉、主持运动等功能。肝血充足,筋得以充分濡养。如果年老体衰,肝血不足,筋膜失养,会出现肢体痉挛、动作失灵、肢体麻木、屈伸不利等症状。由于肝藏血,能够濡养筋脉,使之耐受疲劳,是运动机能的根本,所以有"罢极之本"之称。

男子的阴茎亦属宗筋的范畴,与肝的疏泄密切相关。肝的疏泄功能好,性功能就正常,反之,则衰退。

爪,包括指甲和趾甲,实际上就是筋的延续,通过观察爪甲可以了解肝血的情况。肝血充盈,筋骨强健,爪甲坚韧;肝血不足,可见爪甲薄而软,易脆裂或变形。

in men and menstruation, ovulation in women are closely connected with the liver's function in governing free flow of qi. Sperm's storing and dredging rely on the coordinative work of storing and dredging for both the liver and kidneys. If the liver functions normally in governing free flow of qi, ejaculation will be smooth and proper while in contrast, ejaculation will be unsmooth. Menstruation and ovulation are also under the influence of the liver's function. If the liver functions normally in governing free flow of qi, menstruation cycle will be regular and smooth; if not, menstruation cycle will be irregular, unsmooth, even menorrhalgia will occur.

4.2 Relations of liver with Body, Orifice Fluid and Seasons

4.2.1 Liver linking to tendons in body manifesting its splendor in nails

Tendons, the fascias, connecting and constraining joints and muscles, command body movement. When liver-blood is sufficient, tendons will be immensely nourished. When people are getting old and infirm, liver-blood becomes deficient and tendons lose nourishment, spasm, inflexible movement, numbness of limbs and impeded flexion and extension will appear. The liver, storing blood, can nourish tendons and vessels to resist fatigue, which is the fundament of motor function, therefore it is known as "the root of physical stamina".

Men's phallus belongs to fascia associating closely with liver's function of governing free flow of qi. When the liver performs well, phallus will be vibrant or decay otherwise.

Nails include fingernails and toenails. In fact, nails are extensions of tendons, so the condition of liver-blood will be learned through surveying nails. Sufficient liver-blood makes tendons and bones strong, nails tough and tensile. Deficient liver-blood makes nails thin, soft, easy to crack and deform.

4.2.2 肝开窍于目

目，俗称眼睛，具有视觉功能。肝的精血充足，肝气调达，眼睛才能正常发挥视物辨色的功能。如果肝阴、肝血不足则见两眼干涩、视物不清、夜盲等；肝经风热，可见迎风流泪，目赤肿疼等；肝风内动，可见双目斜视上翻；肝气郁结，日久火动痰生可致二目昏蒙，目生翳障，视物不清。

4.2.3 肝在液为泪

肝开窍于目，泪从目出。肝血不足则见两眼干涩；肝经湿热，目眵增多，迎风流泪。

4.2.4 肝在志为怒

大怒或郁怒不解，既可以引起肝气郁结，气机不畅，造成血液津液运行输布障碍，导致痰饮瘀血阻滞；又会引起肝气上逆，发为出血或中风等病。需要注意的是：肝的精血不足，不能涵养肝气，人易发怒；肝阴不足，肝阳偏亢，稍有刺激，也易生气。

4.2.5 肝与春气相通应

肝主疏泄，喜调达而恶抑郁，与春天万物复苏、生机勃勃、一派欣欣向荣的景象相似。春季天气转暖，风气偏盛，人体肝气随之而旺，平素肝气偏旺、肝阳偏亢的人在春季容易出现眩晕、烦躁易怒、中风、情志不畅、焦虑，或两胁肋部疼痛等症状。

4.2.2 Liver associating with the eyes in orifice

Eyes possess visual function. If the liver-essence and blood are sufficient and the liver-qi is smooth, eyes can play the normal role of vision and color discrimination. Insufficient liver-yin and liver-blood results in dry eyes, blurred vision and night blindness; the flaring of liver-fire manifests itself in epiphora induced by wind and red eyes with distended pain; inside stirring of liver-wind manifests itself in strabismus and sursumversion; long-time stagnated liver-qi results in fire and phlegm, which causes blurred vision, eyes with nebula.

4.2.3 Liver linking to tears in fluid

The liver opens at eyes from which tears run. Insufficient liver-blood makes eyes dry; liver meridian invaded by damp heat will result in too much secretion and tears running irritated by wind.

4.2.4 Liver linking to anger in emotion

Outrage and depression can not only bring about unsmooth liver-qi and qi dynamic obstructing transformation and transportation of blood and body fluid, which causes phlegm and blood stasis or blocking, but can also irritate flaring of liver-qi manifesting as hemorrhage or stroke. Deficient essence and blood in the liver can't nourish liver-qi and makes people liable to blow out; deficient liver-yin and hyperactive liver-yang also makes people feel offended with slight irritation.

4.2.5 Liver and spring-qi interlinking

The liver regulates flow of qi. The liver, favoring optimistic openness and detesting depression, is similar to the prosperous scene in spring when everything revives with vigor and vitality. In spring, with weather getting warm and windy, liver-qi becomes vibrant. The person who usually has hyperactive rise of liver-qi and liver-yang is easy to get dizziness, restlessness, anger, stroke, depression, anxiety or pains on sternal ribs.

中医理论

Basic Theory of Traditional Chinese Medicine

4.3　肝与胆相表里

胆者,中正之官,决断出焉。

胆附着于肝,既是六腑之一,又是奇恒之腑。

胆的生理功能有:贮存和排泄胆汁、胆主决断。

4.3.1　贮存和排泄胆汁

胆汁生成于肝,味苦,呈黄绿色,贮存于胆,在消化食物过程中向小肠排泄,以帮助脾胃运化,尤其是脂类物质。胆汁的贮存和排泄有赖于肝的疏泄功能。肝的疏泄功能正常,有助于胆汁的正常贮存和排泄,促进饮食物的消化和吸收。如果肝失疏泄,肝气郁结,胆汁的排泄就不利,会出现胸胁胀满疼痛,食欲不振,厌食油腻,腹胀,便溏等症;胆汁上逆,可见口苦、呕吐黄绿苦水;胆汁外溢于肌肤,可出现黄疸。

4.3.2　主决断

胆在精神意识思维活动中,具有判断事物,做出决定的作用。胆主决断对于防御和消除某些精神刺激的不良影响,以维持和控制气血的正常运行,确保脏器之间的协调关系有着重要作用。

精神心理活动与胆之决断功能有关,胆能助肝的疏泄以调畅情志。肝胆相济,则情志和调稳定。胆气豪壮的人,剧烈的精神刺激对其所造成的影响不大,而且恢复很快。胆气虚弱的人,

4.3　Liver and the Gallbladder Forming an Internal–external Relationship

The gallbladder is like an upright official who is decisive.

Attached to the liver, the gallbladder is one of the six fu-organs, and the extraordinary organ.

The physiological function of the gallbladder is to store, excrete the bile and govern decision-making.

4.3.1　Storing and excreting bile

The bile is produced in the liver. It tastes bitter and appears yellow green. It is stored in the gallbladder. In the process of digesting food, the bile is excreted to the small intestine to help the spleen and stomach to transform and transport, especially lipid substances. The storage and excretion of bile depends on the liver's function of governing free flow of qi. When the liver functions normally, the bile will be stored and excreted normally to promote food digestion and absorption. When the liver functions abnormally and the liver-qi is blocked, the bile will be excreted unsmoothly, and there will appear distending pain in the hypochondrium, poor appetite, anorexia for the greasy, abdominal distension, diarrhea and other symptoms; if the bile goes adversely upward, there will appear bitter taste in mouth, vomiting bitter liquid in yellow and green; if the bile exudes out on the skin, there will be icteric.

4.3.2　Governing decision-making

In the mental activities, the gallbladder has the function to judge things and make decisions. The gallbladder, governing decision-making, is important to defend and eliminate bad effects of certain mental stimuli to maintain and control the normal operation of qi and blood to ensure the coordination between organs.

The mental activity relates to the governing function of the gallbladder, helping the liver govern free flow of qi to regulate emotion. Coordination between the liver and gallbladder makes smooth and stable emotion. The person with great gallbladder-qi can barely be affected by severe mental stimulation and recover soon once affected. When

中医理论

Basic Theory of Traditional Chinese Medicine

在受到精神刺激的不良影响时，容易形成疾病，表现为胆怯易惊、善恐、失眠、多梦等精神情志病变。

4.3.3 肝与胆相表里

肝胆同居右胁下，胆附于肝叶之间，足厥阴经属肝络胆，足少阳经属胆络肝，两者构成表里相合关系。肝与胆的关系，主要表现在同司疏泄、共主勇怯等方面。

同司疏泄：肝主疏泄，分泌胆汁；胆附于肝，藏泄胆汁。两者协调合作，使胆汁疏利到肠道，以帮助脾胃消化食物。肝气疏泄正常，促进胆汁的分泌和排泄，而胆汁排泄无阻，又有利于肝气疏泄功能的正常发挥。若肝气郁滞，可影响胆汁疏利，或胆腑湿热，也影响肝气疏泄，最终均可导致肝胆气滞、肝胆湿热或郁而化火、肝胆火旺之症。

共主勇怯：胆主决断与人的勇怯有关，而决断又来自肝之谋虑，肝胆相互配合，人的情志活动正常，遇事能做出决断。实际上，肝胆共主勇怯是以两者同司疏泄为生理学基础的。若肝胆气滞，或胆郁痰扰，均可导致情志抑郁或惊恐胆怯等病症。

the one with weak gallbladder-qi is affected by severe mental stimulation, he or she is easy to be sick, suffering from timidity, timorousness, insomnia, dreaminess and other mental diseases.

4.3.3 Liver and gallbladder forming an internal-external relationship

The liver and the gallbladder are located under the right hypochondrium, and the gallbladder attaches to the part between liver lobes. Meridian of foot-jueyin belongs to the liver and is affiliated with the gallbladder; meridian of foot-shaoyang belongs to the gallbladder and is affiliated with the liver; the liver and the gallbladder form an internal-external relationship; they together govern the free flow of qi and emotions as bravery and timidity.

The liver governs the free flow of qi and excretes the bile. The gallbladder is affiliated with the liver and stores, discharges the bile. Coordination and cooperation between the two sends the bile to the intestine to help the stomach digest food. Normal function of the liver can promote the bile's excretion and discharge. Smooth discharge of the bile is conducive to the liver's governing of free flow of qi. The stagnation of liver-qi can affect the bile's discharge, or the wet and hot gallbladder also can affect the function of the liver, which leads to the liver and gallbladder diseases, such as, qi stagnation, dampness and heat, or depression transformed into heat or flaring-fire.

The liver and gallbladder govern the emotions of bravery and timidity. That the gallbladder governs decision-making relates to the human's bravery and timidity, and decision making comes from the liver's tactics. Cooperation between the two maintains normal mental activities and decision making when things happen. In fact, the liver and gallbladder governing the free flow of qi is the physiological basis for governing the emotions of bravery and timidity. Qi stagnation of the liver and gallbladder or the depression of the bladder and sputum interference can lead to emotional depression or panic, timidity and other symptoms.

中医理论

Basic Theory of Traditional Chinese Medicine

5 肾

肾者，作强之官，伎巧出焉。

肾的主要生理功能是：主藏精，主水，主纳气。

由于肾藏先天之精，主生殖，为人体生命之本原，故称肾为"先天之本"。肾精化肾气，肾气分阴阳，肾阴与肾阳能资助、促进、协调全身脏腑之阴阳，故肾又称为"五脏阴阳之本"。

肾藏精，主蛰，又称为封藏之本。

肾在体合骨，生髓，通脑，其华在发，在窍为耳及二阴，在志为恐，在液为唾，与自然界冬气相通应。肾与膀胱相为表里。

5.1 生理功能

5.1.1 肾藏精

藏，就是闭藏。精，是指体内的精微物质，它是构成人体和维持人体生命活动的基本物质之一。肾藏精，是指肾有贮存、封藏精气的生理功能。肾把精气藏起来，促使精气不断充盈，还防止精气从体内无故流失，为精气在体内充分发挥作用创造必要的条件。肾中藏的精气，主要有两方面来源：一是来源于父母的生殖之精，就是我们通常说的"先天之精"；另外是来源于人出生后，机体从饮食物中摄取的营养成分和脏腑代谢所化生的精微物质，就是我们所说的"后天之精"。

5 Kidney

The kidney is like an official with strong ability and perfect skill.

The main physiological functions of the kidney are to store essence, govern water and receive qi.

Being the origin of human life, the kidney stores innate essence and governs reproduction, so it is called "the root of innateness". Kidney essence is transformed into kidney-qi which is divided into yin and yang. Kidney-yin and yang can assist, promote and coordinate yin and yang of viscera and body, so the kidney is also called "the root of viscera and yin and yang".

The kidney stores essence and governs hibernation, so it is called the root of sealing and storing.

Being linked to bones in body, the kidney generates marrow and reflects its brilliance in hair; it is linked to orifices in ears and genitalia and anus; it is linked to fear in emotion; it is linked to spittle in secretion. The kidney and winter-qi are interlinked. The kidney and the bladder form an external-internal relationship.

5.1 Physiological Functions

5.1.1 Kidney storing essence

Storing means sealing and keeping in storage. Essence refers to the subtle substances in the body. It is one of the basic components of the human body and essential in maintaining life activities. The kidney storing essence refers to the kidney's physiological function of storing and sealing essence-qi. The Kidney hiding the essence promotes essence being filled constantly, and also prevents the essence from flowing out of the body freely, creating the necessary condition for essence-qi to fully play its role in the body. The essence stored in the kidney has two main sources: the one from the parental reproductive essence is called the "congenital essence"; the other one, the nutrient acquired from diet after birth and subtle substance metabolized by viscera, is called "acquired essence".

中医理论

Basic Theory of Traditional Chinese Medicine

先天之精和后天之精虽然来源不同,但都同归于肾,两者是相互依存、相互为用、不可分割的。先天之精要靠后天之精的不断培育和充养,才能充分发挥生理作用;后天之精的化生,又要靠先天之精的资助,才能不断摄入和化生。二者在肾中的密切结合,组成了肾中的精气,从而维持人体的生命活动和生殖能力,因此称"肾为先天之本"。

机体的生、长、壮、老,与肾中精气的盛衰密切相关。人的齿、骨、发的生长状态是观察肾中精气的外候,是判断机体生长发育状况和衰老程度的客观标志。当精气不足时,小儿会出现生长发育迟缓;青年人的生殖器官发育不良,性成熟慢;中年人则性机能减退,或出现早衰;老年人会衰老得特别快。以上这些病理变化,临床上叫"肾精亏虚"。

肾的这种调节作用,就是通过肾中精气所含的肾阳和肾阴这两种物质的相互制约、相互依存、相互为用来实现的。肾阴肾阳平衡,全身的阴阳就平衡;如果肾阴肾阳发生偏盛偏衰,就会导致全身阴阳失调而引起疾病。

肾阴,又叫"元阴"、"真阴",主要有滋养、濡润和制约阳热等功能。肾阴到达全身脏腑、经络、形体、官窍,就变为脏腑、经络、形体和官窍之阴。肾阴对人的生命很重要。如果肾阴不足,则津液分泌减少,而见干燥、心烦意乱、潮热、五心烦热、口干咽燥、脉细

Although the congenital essence and acquired essence are different in sources, they both pertain to the kidney, and they are interdependent, mutually used and inseparable. Only when the congenital essence was cultivated and raised by acquired essence can it give full play to its physiological function; on the other hand, the metaplasia and intake of acquired essence relies on the supporting of the congenital essence. The close association between them composes the kidney essence so as to maintain the life activities and reproductive capacity. Hence, the kidney is called "the root of innateness".

The body's birth, growth, maturity and aging are closely related with the rise and fall of kidney essence. Kidney essence can be observed through the outside growing state of tooth, bone and hair which are the objective marks to judge the status of body growth and development and aging degree. Deficiency in essence will cause growth retardation to childen, reproductive organ dysplasia and slow maturity for young people; hypogonadism or premature aging for the middle-aged, and quick aging for the elderly. These pathological changes are clinically called "kidney essence deficiency".

The kidney's regulating function is fulfilled by the mutual restriction, interdependence and interavailability of kidney-yang and -yin contained in the kidney essence. The balance of kidney-yin and -yang determines the balance of the whole body's yin and yang; the imbalance of kidney-yin and -yang will lead to imbalance of yin and yang of the whole body and even diseases.

Kidney-yin, also called "vital yin" and "true yin", mainly nourishes, moistens and restricts heat of yang. Kidney-yin will become yin of viscera, meridians, body and orifices after reaching these places. Kidney-yin is very important for people's life. If the kidney-yin is deficient, body fluid will decrease leading to symptoms like dryness, upset mind, tidal fever, vexing heat in the chest, palms and

中医理论

Basic Theory of Traditional Chinese Medicine

数、舌干红少苔,此外还可见腰酸、腿软、阳事易举和遗精、早泄等表现。

肾阳,又叫"元阳"、"真阳"、"命门之火",主要有温煦、兴奋和化气的功能。肾阳到达全身的脏腑、经络、形体、官窍,就变为脏腑、经络、形体和官窍之阳。如果肾阳不足,则全身新陈代谢降低,产热能量减少,各脏腑、经络、形体和官窍的生理功能活动都减弱,临床上就会看到人的面色苍白、怕冷、肢冷、脉无力而迟缓,或者浮肿、精神萎靡、反应迟钝等。此外还可见腰酸、腿软、阴部清冷、生殖功能减退等症状。

5.1.2 肾主水

人体内水液(津液)的输布和排泄,依赖于脾的运化、肺的通调、膀胱的开合及肝脏的疏泄等作用,清的运行于人体各脏腑器官,浊的就转化为汗和尿排出体外。这些过程是靠肾阳与肾气来完成的,称为肾的气化作用。具体来说,一方面肾阳和肾气能使水液蒸腾上升,维持体内水液的正常需求;另一方面,肾阳肾气对水液具有推动作用,能使水液之浊者下降,生成尿液,并使之下注膀胱而排出体外。如果肾的阳气虚弱,气化作用失常,固摄不力,就可能发生小便量特多,以及遗尿、小便失禁等症;推动无力,还可能发生尿少、水肿等症。

soles, dry mouth and throat, thin pulse, dry and red tongue with little coating, backache, soft leg, spermatorrhea, premature ejaculation and so on.

Kidney-yang is also called "vital yang", "true yang" and "fire of life". It has the function of warming, exciting and producing qi. Kidney-yang becomes yang of viscera, meridians, body and orifices after arriving at these places. Deficiency of kidney-yang leads to the decrease of the body's metabolism, heat energy, and activities of physiological function of viscera, meridians, body and orifices. Clinically, the patients will show pale complexion, aversion to cold, cold limbs, weak and slow pulse, or edema, low spirit, slow action and so on. In addition, there will appear symptoms such as, backache, debility of the legs, soft leg, genital's coolness, reproductive dysfunction and so on.

5.1.2 Kidney governing water

The distribution and excretion of body fluid inside human body depend on the functions of spleen's transportation, the lung's regulation and the liver's dispersing. The clear substance works in human organs and the turbid is transformed into sweat and urine excreted out of the body. The above process is completed by the operation of kidney-yang and qi, which is called the kidney's gasification effect. Specifically, on the one hand, kidney-yang and qi can promote the liquid transpiration, maintaining the normal requirements of body fluid inside the body; on the other hand, kidney-yang and qi can promote the turbid fluid to descend, forming urine in the bladder to be excreted out of the body. If the kidney-yang is deficient, gasification effect is abnormal and the kidney's controlling function is inadequate, there may appear symptoms like excess urine volume, enuresis, and urinary incontinence. If the promoting effect of kidney-yang is weak, there may also appear symptoms like oliguria and edema disease etc.

5.1.3 肾主纳气

纳，就是接受和藏入的意思。肾主纳气，是指肾具有接受和藏入肺所吸入的清气的功能。这种功能，依赖于肾气的固摄作用。肾接受和纳入清气保证了肺的正常呼吸。如果肾气虚弱，纳气功能减退，就会出现呼吸表浅的气短，以及动辄气喘等症状，这就叫做"肾不纳气"。

5.2 与体窍液时的关系

5.2.1 肾主骨生髓，其华在发

肾精具有促进骨骼生长发育和化生骨髓、脑髓和脊髓的作用。肾藏精，精生髓。肾中精气充盈，骨髓、脑髓、脊髓就得到充养。髓海得养，脑的发育就正常；反之，肾中精气不足，则髓海失养，可出现骨骼脆弱无力，甚至发育不全，如小儿发育迟缓，骨软无力，不耐久立，或者容易发生骨折，或者经常出现腰膝酸软，步履不稳，无力等症。临床上老年痴呆病可以从肾脏上治疗。

齿与骨同出一源，牙齿也由肾中精气所充养。肾中精气充沛则牙齿坚固而不易脱落；肾中精气不足，则牙齿容易松动，甚至早期脱落。临床上有相当多的牙痛都是由肾虚引起的，不一定非用抗生素不可。

5.1.3 Kidney governing reception of qi

That the kidney governs the reception of qi means the kidney possesses the function of receiving and storing the fresh air inhaled by the lung. This function depends on the controlling and strengthening of kidney's qi. The kidney's function of receiving and storing the fresh air ensures the normal breath of the lung. If the kidney qi is deficient and the function of governing the reception of qi decreases, there will appear short and shallow breath and frequent gasp, which is called "the kidney can't govern the reception of qi".

5.2 Relations of Kidney with Body, Orifices, Fluid and Seasons

5.2.1 Kidney linking to bones in body; generating marrow and reflecting its brilliance in hair

This means the kidney essence possesses the function of promoting the growth and development of bones and generating bone, brain and spinal cord marrow. The kidney stores essence which generates marrow. If the essence in the kidney is sufficient, bone, brain and spinal cord marrow will be fully nourished. If the marrow sea is well raised, the development of brain will be normal. Conversely, insufficient essence-qi in the kidney will cause marrow sea undernourished, leading to fragile and weak bones, even hypoplasia, such as growth retardation for children, soft and weak bones, inability to stand for long, or being vulnerable to bone fractures, or frequent soreness and weakness of waist and knees, walking instability, weakness and other diseases. Clinically, Alzheimer's disease can be treated from the kidney.

Teeth and bones originate from the same source, and teeth are also nourished by essence-qi. If the essence-qi in the kidney is sufficient, teeth will be strong and not prone to fall off; if the essence-qi in the kidney is insufficient, teeth is easy to loosen, even fall off during young. Clinically, quite a lot of toothache is caused by kidney deficiency and is not necessarily treated with antibiotics.

中医理论 Basic Theory of Traditional Chinese Medicine

肾藏精,精又能化血,血又养发。肾精足则血旺,血旺则毛发黑而润泽,这就是其华在发。肾中精气虚衰,毛发就会发白、枯槁甚至脱落。实际生活中常看到的少白头和早脱发,除先天遗传外,大多是由于肾中精气虚衰所致。

5.2.2 肾开窍于耳和二阴

耳是听觉器官,肾开窍于耳,是指耳的听觉功能依赖于肾中精气的充养。肾中精气充足,髓海得养,听觉就好。如果肾中精气不足,髓海空虚,耳失所养,会出现耳鸣,听力减退,甚至耳聋等症。老年人由于肾中精气虚衰,所以多见听力下降。同样健康老人往往是耳聪目明。

二阴,指前阴(外生殖器)和后阴(肛门)。前阴有排尿和生殖的功能,后阴有排泄粪便的作用。尿液的贮存和排泄虽由膀胱所主,但需要肾的气化才能完成,而人的生殖机能同样由肾所主,如果肾的精气不足,就可能会出现遗精、遗尿、早泄、尿清长、尿频、尿少等症。大便的排泄同样与肾的气化作用有关。如果肾阳虚,脾失温煦,水湿运化就不正常,大便就溏泄;肾阴不足,大便就会秘结。

5.2.3 肾在液为唾

唾为口津,唾液中较稠厚的称作唾,能润泽口腔,辅助食物消

The kidney stores essence, the essence generates blood and blood nourishes hair. Abundant kidney-essence will bring about abundant blood and black, moist and lustrous hair, which means that the kidney reflects its brilliance in hair. If the kidney essence-qi is deficient, the hair will appear white, withered, and the hair may even fall off at youth. Young persons with grey hair and bald head are very common in daily life. In addition to heredity, it is mostly caused by deficiency of kidney essence-qi.

5.2.2 Kidney linking to orifices in ears and front and rear genitalias

The ear is the organ of hearing. That kidney linking to orifices in ears means hearing relies on kidney essence-qi. Sufficient kidney essence-qi and well-nourished marrow sea will bring about good hearing. If the kidney essence-qi is deficient, marrow sea is empty and ears are not well-nourished, there will appear tinnitus, hearing loss, and even deafness. The elderly who lack in kidney essence will suffer from hearing loss. The healthy elderly often have good hearing and eyesight.

Two yins, refer to the front yin (external genitals) and the rear yin (anus). The front yin has the function of urinating and reproducing, and the back yin has the function of excreting. Although the storage and excretion of urine is governed by bladder, it is fulfilled through the kidney gasification. People's reproducing function is also governed by the kidney. Deficient kidney essence-qi will cause nocturnal emission, enuresis, premature ejaculation, clear and long urine, frequent micturition, oliguria disease. Stool excretion is also associated with the kidney's gasification. Deficient kidney-yang and dysfunction of the spleen in warming will cause abnormal water transportation and diarrhea; deficient kidney-yin will cause constipation.

5.2.3 Kidney linking to spittle in secretion

Spittle, the thick secretion in mouth, can moisten mouth and promote food digestion. It is transformed from

化。中医学认为,唾为口津,为肾精所化,肾的经脉向上挟于舌本,肾阳气化阴液上腾,输于口腔。多唾或久唾易耗损肾精;肾阴不足则口干咽燥;肾阳不足见唾少口干而不欲饮等。所以古代一些导引家主张咽而不吐,以养肾精,方法是舌抵上腭,口腔就会有满口唾液,然后徐徐咽下。

5.2.4　肾在志为恐

恐,是人们对事物惧怕的一种情志活动,为不良刺激。恐惧太过可使上焦的气机闭塞不畅,气迫于下焦,使肾失封藏,可导致二便失禁、遗精、骨痿、瘫软等病症,所以说肾在志为恐。肾精亏虚,髓海失充者,易出现恐惧的情志病变,临床上多从肾论治。

5.2.5　肾与冬气相通应

冬季寒水当令,气候比较寒冷,万物归藏,与肾脏封藏有节,维持人体阴阳平衡,促进人体生长发育和脏腑气化的功能相通,故冬季以肾病、关节疾病较多为其特点。

5.3　肾与膀胱相表里

膀胱者,州都之官,津液藏焉,气化则能出矣。

膀胱的主要生理功能是贮存尿液、排泄小便。

the kidney-essence. Kidney meridian goes up to the basis of the tongue and yin secretion gasified from kidney-yang is transported to the mouth. Too much and prolonged spittle will be apt to consume the kidney-essence; deficient kidney-yin will cause dry mouth and throat; deficient kidney-yang will cause less spittle, dry mouth and not wanting to drink. So, some ancient health experts advocate swallowing spittle instead of spitting it out in order to nourish kidney-essence. The method is to put the tongue against the palate, then swallow the saliva slowly when the mouth is full of it.

5.2.4　Kidney linking to fear in emotion

Fear as an emotional activity is bad stimulation. Too much fear will make qi in the upper-jiao blocked, forcing qi to stay in the lower-jiao, which can make the kidney lose the function of sealing and storing, leading to incontinence, spermatorrhea, bone atrophy, paralysis and other diseases. So, the kidney is linked to fear in emotion. People with deficient kidney essence-qi and insufficient marrow sea are apt to getting emotional disease, such as fear. Clinically, many of them are treated from the kidney.

5.2.5　Kidney and winter-qi being interlinked

In winter, as it is cold, all the things return and hide. The phenomenon in winter is interlinked with the functions of sealing and storing of the kidney and with the functions of maintaining the balance of yin and yang, promoting the body's growth and development and viscera's gasification. Therefore, winter is featured with many kidney and joint diseases.

5.3　Kidney and the Bladder Forming an External–internal Relationship

The bladder is like an official of a state where the fluid and secretion stores, and qi transformation comes from.

The main physiological functions of the bladder are the storage and excretion of urine.

中医理论　Basic Theory of Traditional Chinese Medicine

5.3.1 贮存尿液

在人体津液代谢过程中,水液通过肺、脾、肾三脏的作用,布散全身,发挥濡润机体的作用。其被人体利用之后,下归于肾。经肾的蒸腾气化作用,升清降浊,清者回流体内,浊者下输于膀胱,变成尿液。尿为津液所化。小便与津液常常相互影响,如果津液缺乏,则小便短少;反之,小便过多也会丧失津液。

5.3.2 排泄小便

尿液贮存于膀胱,达到一定容量时,通过肾的气化作用,使膀胱开合适度,则尿液可及时从溺窍排出体外。

肾合膀胱,开窍于二阴,肾气足则化,肾气不足则不化。人气不化,则水归大肠而为泄泻。出气不化,则闭塞下焦而为癃肿。膀胱的贮尿和排尿功能,全赖于肾的固摄和气化功能。所谓膀胱气化,实际上属于肾的气化作用。若肾气的固摄和气化功能失常,则膀胱的气化失司,开合失权,可出现小便不利或癃闭,以及尿频、尿急、遗尿、小便不禁等。临床治疗小便异常,常从肾治之。

5.3.3 肾与膀胱相表里

肾为水脏,膀胱为水腑,足少阴经属肾络膀胱,足太阳经属膀胱络肾,两者构成表里相合关

5.3.1 Storing urine

In the process of body fluid metabolism, fluid is distributed to the whole body through the function of the lung, spleen and kidney, which plays a role in nourishing the body. After the fluid is used by the body, it is sent down to the kidney. Through the kidney's function of transpiration and gasification, ascending the clear and descending the turbid, the clear flows back to the body and the turbid flows down to the bladder and transforms into urine. Urine is transformed from fluid. Urine and fluid always interact with each other. Lack of body fluid will lead to oliguresis; on the other hand, too much urine will cause body fluid lose.

5.3.2 Excreting urine

When urine stored in the bladder reaches to a certain capacity, through the kidney's gasification, the bladder opens and closes properly, making the urine excreted from the drowning orifice in time.

The kidney, associating with bladder, opens into front and rear genitalias. When the kidney-qi is sufficient, gasification will occur, or vice versa. If there is no gasification, fluid will stay at the large intestine, leading to diarrhea, or it will block the lower-jiao, leading to focal swelling. The bladder's function of storing and excreting urine depends on the kidney's function of controlling, strengthening and gasification. In fact, the so-called gasification of the bladder belongs to the gasification of the kidney. If the kidney functions abnormally, the bladder will not govern gasification and will open and close disorderly, leading to dysuria or retention of urine, and frequent urination, urgency, enuresis and aconuresis. Clinical treatment of abnormal urine often starts from treating the kidney.

5.3.3 Kidney and bladder forming an external-internal relationship

The kidney is a water-zang; the bladder is a water-fu. The meridian of foot shao-yin affiliated with the bladder belongs to the kidney; the meridian of foot tai-yang affiliated with the kidney belongs to the bladder. The external-internal

系。肾与膀胱的关系,主要表现在共主小便方面。

肾为主水之脏,开窍于二阴;膀胱贮尿排尿,是为水腑。膀胱的贮尿排尿功能,取决于肾气的盛衰。肾气充足,蒸腾气化及固摄功能正常发挥,则尿液能够正常生成,贮于膀胱并有度地排泄。膀胱贮尿排尿有度,也有利于肾气的主水功能。因此,肾与膀胱相互协作,共同完成小便的生成、贮存与排泄。病理上,两者亦常相互影响。若肾气虚弱,气化无力,或固摄无权,可影响膀胱的贮尿排尿,而见尿少、癃闭或尿失禁。膀胱湿热,或膀胱失约,也可影响到肾气的气化和固摄,以致出现小便色质或排出的异常。

附: 命门

命门,人体生命的关键、根本,其部位至今尚无定论。中医学认为命门蕴藏先天之气,集中体现肾的功能,故对五脏六腑的功能发挥着决定性作用。一般认为命门主要藏"真火",因而称之为"命门火"或"命火"。火属阳,从这个意义上说,用命门二字就是突出肾阳的作用。肾阳是人体各脏腑阳气的根本,是人体生命活动的关键。

relationship they form mainly reflects in governing the urine.

The kidney as the water-zang opens into front and rear genitalias; the bladder as the water-fu stores and discharges urine. The bladder's function of storing and discharging urine relies on the ups and downs of kidney-qi. If the kidney-qi is sufficient and the kidney functions normally in gasifying, controlling and strengthening, urine will be produced normally and stored in the bladder and excreted orderly. If the bladder stores and excretes urine orderly, it is favorable for the kidney in governing fluid. Therefore, the kidney and bladder cooperates with each other to promote urine to be produced, stored and excreted. Pathologically, they influence each other. Insufficient kidney-qi, powerless gasification, weak controlling and strengthening can affect the bladder's function of storing and discharging urine, resulting in less urine, anuria and aconuresis. Damp and hot bladder or the bladder being out of control can also affect the kidney's function of gasification, controlling and strengthening, leading to abnormality of urine color and excretion.

Appendix: Vital Gate (GV4; DU4)

The Vital Gate (mingmen) is the fundament of human's life. Its position is still in dispute. According to the theory of TCM, the gate of vitality reserves natural gas and centrally embodies the kidney's function, so it plays a decisive role in the function of viscera. Generally, the gate of vitality mainly reserves "genuine fire", so it is called "the fire of the Vital Gate". The fire belongs to yang. In this sense, the term "the Vital Gate" highlights the function of kidney-yang which is the root of yang of the internal organs and key of life activities.

中医理论

Basic Theory of Traditional Chinese Medicine

第三章 气血津液
Chapter 3　Qi, Blood and Body Fluid

精、气、血、津液是构成人体和维持人体生命活动的基本物质。精，泛指人体内一切有用的精微物质；气，是人体内活力很强、运行不息、无形可见的极细微物质，是人体的重要组成部分及机体生命活动的动力；血，是红色的液态物质；津液，是人体内的正常水液的总称。精、气、血、津液，既是脏腑生理活动的产物，又是脏腑经络及组织器官生理活动的物质基础。

精、气、血、津液的生成和代谢，有赖于脏腑及组织器官的生理活动；而脏腑组织器官的生理活动，又必须依靠气的推动、温煦等作用，精、血、津液的滋养和濡润。因此，精、气、血、津液与脏腑经络及组织器官的生理和病理有着密切关系。因其是人体生命活动的物质基础，其运动变化规律也是人体生命活动的规律。

气与精、血、津液分阴阳，则气为阳。阳气主动，具有推动、温煦等作用，宜运行不息而不宜郁滞；精、血、津液为阴，阴主静，具

The essence, qi, blood and body fluid are the basic substances constituting human body and maintaining life activities. In a broad sense, the essence refers to all the useful refined nutritious substance; qi is a kind of active, invisible, tiny substance that is in constant movement, which is an important constituent of human body and motive power for life activities; blood is the red liquid substance; body fluid is the general term for the normal liquid inside human body. The essence, qi, blood and body fluid are not only the products of physiological activities of zangfu, but also the material basis for the physiological activities of zangfu, meridians and tissues.

The formation and metabolism of the essence, qi, blood and body fluid depends on the physiological activities of zangfu and tissues; and the physiological activities of zangfu and tissues must rely on the promoting and warming effect of qi and the nourishing and moistening effect of the essence, blood and body fluid. Therefore, the essence, qi, blood and body fluid are closely related to the physiology and pathology of zangfu, meridians and tissues. Since they are the material bases of human life activities, their law of movement and change is also the law of human life activities.

The essence, qi, blood and body fluid are divided into yin and yang. Qi belongs to yang. Yang-qi is active, and has the effect of promoting and warming; it should run ceaselessly without stagnating. The essence, blood and body fluid belong to yin which are calm, with the effect of

中医理论

Basic Theory of Traditional Chinese Medicine

有滋养、濡润作用,宜宁谧、秘藏而不宜妄泄。

气与精、血液、津液相对而言,则气无形,而精、血、津液有形,气与精、血、津液的相互化生与转化,体现了在生命活动中,形化为气,气化为形,形气相互转化的气化过程。精血同源、津血同源,精、津液化而为血,血涵蕴精与津液,故中医学对人体生命活动的基本物质,又常以气血概称。

气和血是构成人体和维持人体生命活动的两大基本物质,精、气、血、津液学说,以气血为要。气与血,异名同类,两相维附,气非血不和,血非气不运。但气血之中,尤以气为最,气为主,血为辅。

1 精

1.1 精的基本概念

中医学认为精气是最细微而能变化的气,是最细微的物质存在,是世界的本原,是生命的来源。

在精、气、血、津液学说中,精或称精气是一种有形的、多是液态的精微物质。其基本含义有广义和狭义之分。广义的精,泛指构成人体和维持生命活动的精微物质,包括精、血、津、液在内。狭义的精,指肾藏之精,即生殖之精,是促进人体生长、发育和生殖功能的基本物质。

nourishing and warming; it should be tranquil and hided secretly, and are not supposed to discharge carelessly.

Compared with the essence, blood and body fluid, qi is invisible and the latter are visible; their interaction and transformation reflect the process of the mutual transformation between qi and the visible in life activities: the visible can be transformed into qi, and qi can be transformed into the visible. The essence and blood share the same origin and body fluid and blood also share the same origin. The essence and body fluid can be transformed into blood; blood contains the essence and body fluid. Therefore, in TCM, the basic substance of life activities gets the general name qi-blood.

Qi and blood are the two basic substances which constitute human body and maintain life activities; the theory of the essence, qi, blood and body fluid mainly depicts qi and blood. Although they have different names, they are of the same kind and interlocked; qi cannot keep smooth without blood and blood cannot flow without qi. But qi assisted by blood possesses a predominant position.

1 The Essence

1.1 Basic Concept of Essence

In TCM, the essence-qi is the tiniest and most changeable qi, and the tiniest existing substance, which is the origin of the world and life.

In the theory of the essence, qi, blood and body fluid, essence or essence-qi is the visible refined nutritious substance mostly in liquid form. It has two meanings. In a broad sense, the essence refers to the visible refined nutritious substance which constitutes human body and maintains life activities, including essence, blood, and body fluid. In a narrow sense, it refers to the essence stored in the kidney—the reproductive essence that is the basic substance promoting growth, development and reproductive function of the human body.

1.2 精的生成

人之精根源于先天而充养于后天。从精的来源而言,则有先天与后天之分。

1.2.1 先天之精

人之始生,父母生殖之精结合,形成胚胎之时,便转化为胚胎自身之精,此即禀受于父母以构成脏腑组织的原始生命物质。胚胎形成之后,在女子胞中,直至胎儿发育成熟,全赖气血育养。胞中气血为母体摄取的水谷之精而化生。因此,先天之精,包括原始生命物质,以及从母体所获得的各种营养物质,主要秘藏于肾。

1.2.2 后天之精

胎儿足月离怀,出生之后,依赖水谷精微的充养,脾胃强健,脾胃运化水谷之精微,输布到五脏六腑而成为五脏六腑之精,以维持脏的生理活动,其盈余者藏于肾中。

1.3 精的功能

精是构成人体和维持人体生命活动的精微物质,其生理功能如下。

1.3.1 生殖

具有生殖能力的精称之为天癸。精气充盈而天癸产生,则具有生殖能力。男子二八天癸至,精气溢泻;女子二七而天癸至,月事应时而下。男女媾精,阴阳和调,胎孕方成,故能有子而繁衍

1.2 Production of Essence

The essence of human body is endowed by parents and nourished after birth. It can be classified into the innate and acquired essences viewing from the origin of production.

1.2.1 Innate essence

At the beginning of life, the reproductive essences from the parents combine and then transform into innate essence of the embryo that is the original life substance inherited from parents constituting zangfu and tissues. After the formation of an embryo in a uterus, it completely depends on the nourishing of qi-blood until the fetus matures. Qi-blood in the uterus is transformed from the essential substance in foodstuff assimilated by the mother. Therefore, the innate essence, including original life substance and nutritious substance acquired from the mother, is mainly stored in the kidney.

1.2.2 Acquired essence

After a fetus matures and is delivered, it depends on the nourishment of essence from foodstuff to strengthen the spleen and stomach which transport and transform the essence from foodstuff into the essence of zangfu to maintain its physiological activities and store the excess in the kidney.

1.3 Functions of Essence

The essence is the refined nutritious substance constituting the human body and maintaining life activities. Its physiological functions are as the following.

1.3.1 Reproduction

The essence bearing the reproductive ability is called tiangui. If the essence is sufficient, there will be tiangui and productive ability. When a male is sixteen years old, there will appear tiangui and spermatic ejaculation; when a female is fourteen years old, there will appear tiangui and menstruation. The reproductive essence of a couple

后代；等到年老体衰，精气衰微，天癸竭而地道不通，则丧失了生殖繁衍能力。由此可见，精是繁衍后代的物质基础，肾精充足，则生殖能力强；肾精不足，就会影响生殖能力。故补肾填精是临床上治疗不育、不孕等生殖机能低下的重要方法。

1.3.2　濡养

精能滋润濡养人体各脏腑形体官窍。

脏腑之精和肾精充盛，全身脏腑组织官窍得到精的充养，各种生理机能得以正常发挥。

若先天禀赋不足，肾精有损，则见生长发育迟缓或未老先衰；或后天之精化生有碍，如肺精不足，则见呼吸障碍、皮肤失润无泽；肝精不足，肝血不充，筋脉失养，则见肢体麻木、拘挛或抽搐等等。

如肾精亏虚，不能生髓，则骨骼失养，牙齿脱落松动；髓海不足，则头昏神疲，智力减退。

1.3.3　化血

精可以转化为血，是血液生成的来源之一。

肾精充盈，则肝有所养，血有所充。故精足则血旺，精亏则血虚。精作为精微的生命物质，既可单独存在于脏腑组织中，也可不断地融合于血液中。如心精融入心血中，肝精融入肝血中。

combine, and so yin harmonize with yang and produce a fetus; when people get old and weak, tiangui will dry up and they lose their reproductive ability. The essence, therefore, is the material basis for the reproduction; if the kidney essence is sufficient, the reproductive ability will be strong; if the kidney essence is insufficient, the reproductive ability will be affected. Therefore, nourishing the kidney essence is an important method for the treatment of infertility and other incapability of reproduction.

1.3.2　Nourishment

The essence can moisten and nourish viscera, body and orifices.

If the essence of viscera and kidney is sufficient, all the viscera, tissues and orifices will get necessary nourishment to perform their normal physiological functions.

Congenital deficiency and damage of kidney-essence will cause growth retardation or premature aging, or disturbed production of the acquired essence. For example, insufficient lung essence will lead to breathing disorder and lusterless skin; insufficient liver essence and blood, and tendons dystrophy will lead to numbness of limbs, spasm or convulsions and so on.

If the kidney essence is deficient and cannot produce marrow, bones will not get enough nourishment and teeth will get loose and fall off; insufficient marrow will cause dizziness, lassitude and mental deterioration.

1.3.3　Transforming into blood

The essence, one of the sources for blood production, can be transformed into blood.

If the kidney essence is sufficient, the liver will get enough nourishment. Therefore, sufficient essence will lead to enough blood and shortage of essence will cause blood deficiency. The essence, as the refined nutritious substance, can not only be stored in the viscera tissues alone, but also can gradually mix with blood. For example, the heart-essence mixes with the heart-blood and the liver-essence with the liver-blood.

中医理论　Basic Theory of Traditional Chinese Medicine

中医理论

Basic Theory of Traditional Chinese Medicine

1.3.4 化气

精可以化生为气。

先天之精可以化生先天之气(元气),水谷之精可以化生谷气,再加上肺吸入的自然界清气,综合而成一身之气。先、后天之精充盛,则其化生的一身之气必然充足;各脏腑之精充足,则化生的脏腑之气自然充沛。机体生命活动旺盛,身体健康,生殖功能正常,抗御外邪,祛病延年。

若脏腑之精亏虚,肾精衰少,则化气不足,机体正气虚衰,抗病和生殖能力下降。

1.3.5 化神

精能化神,精是神化生的物质基础。神是人体生命活动的外在总体表现,它的产生离不开精这一基本物质。只有积精,才能全神,这是生命存在的根本保证。

 气

2.1 气的基本概念

气在中国文化中是一个非常重要的概念,在中国传统哲学中. 气通常是指一种极细微的物质,是构成世界万物的本原。《黄帝内经》继承和发展了先秦气一元论学说,并将其应用到医学中来,逐渐形成了中医学的气学理论。

气是人体内活力很强运行不息的极精微物质,是构成人体和维持人体生命活动的基本物质之一。

1.3.4 Producing qi

The essence can generate qi.

The innate essence can generate the innate qi (primordial qi). The essence transformed from the foodstuff can generate the acquired qi which combines with the fresh air inhaled by the lung to form qi of the whole body. If the innate and acquired essence is sufficient, the generated qi of the whole body will be plentiful; enough viscera essence will produce sufficient viscera qi. Exuberant life activities make the human body healthy and reproductive function normal to resist the exogenous evil, eliminate disease and prolong life.

Deficient viscera essence and kidney essence cannot generate enough qi, leading to vital qi deficiency and decline of disease resistance and reproductive capacity.

1.3.5 Producing spirit

The essence is the material basis of spirit generation. The spirit, as the outside general reflection of the life activities, cannot exist without the essence. Only when the essence is sufficient can the spirit be sound, which is the basic assurance for life existence.

2 Qi

2.1 Basic Concept of Qi

In Chinese culture, qi is a very important concept. In traditional Chinese philosophy, qi usually refers to a very tiny substance constituting the basis of all things in the world. *Huangdi's Internal Classic* inherited and developed the qi monism theory of pre-Qin dynasty and applied it into medicine, which gradually formed the qi theory in Chinese medicine.

Qi is a kind of tiny substance inside the human body that is in constant movement, which is one of the basic materials constituting human body and maintaining life activities.

中医学中气的概念,可能源于古人对人体生命现象的观察,在古代哲学气学说的渗透和影响下形成的,如呼吸时气的出入、活动时随汗而出的蒸蒸热气,以及气功锻炼中体悟到的气在体内的运动等。

中医学的气是指在体内不断升降出入运动的精微物质,既是构成人体的基本物质,又对生命活动起着推动和调控作用。

2.2 人体之气的生成

人体之气来源于先天之精所化生的先天之气(即元气)、水谷之精所化生的水谷之气和自然界的清气,后两者又合称为后天之气(即宗气),三者结合而成一身之气。

先天之精是肾精的主体成分,先天之精所化生的先天之气(即元气),是人体之气的根本。

脾主运化,胃主受纳,共同完成对饮食水谷的消化吸收。水谷之精及其化生的血与津液,皆可化气,统称为水谷之气,布散全身脏腑经脉,成为人体之气的主要来源,所以称脾胃为生气之源。

肺主气,司呼吸。一方面,肺通过吸清呼浊的呼吸功能,将自然界的清气源源不断地吸入人体内,同时不断地呼出浊气,保证了体内之气的生成及代谢。另一方面,肺将吸入的清气与脾上输水谷精微所化生的水谷之气二者结合起来,生成宗气。

The concept of qi in TCM may originate from the ancients observing the phenomenon of human life and is formed under the influence of qi theory in ancient philosophy, such as inhaling and exhaling of qi, the hot qi from sweating and qi flowing inside the body which is learnt in qigong exercises.

Qi in TCM refers to the refined nutritious substance that is in constant movement, which is the basic substance constituting human body, and also promotes and regulates life activities.

2.2 Production of Qi

Qi in the human body originates from the innate qi (primordial qi) generated from the innate essence, the foodstuff qi from the foodstuff essence and the fresh air from the nature which are known as the acquired qi (pectoral qi). Combination of the three makes qi of the whole body.

The innate essence is the main component of the kidney essence, and the innate qi (primordial qi) generated from the innate essence is the basis of the qi of human body.

The spleen governs transformation and transportation; the stomach governs reception and containing; they complete the digestion and absorption of foodstuff. The foodstuff essence and blood and body fluid it generates can all produce qi, which is called the foodstuff qi collectively; it distributes around the viscera and meridians and is the main source of qi of human body, so the spleen and stomach are known as the source of qi.

The lung governs qi and controls respiration. On the one hand, the lung inhales the fresh air in the nature and exhales the turbid air out of the body to ensure generation and metabolism of qi inside the body. On the other hand, the fresh air and the foodstuff qi from the foodstuff essence ascended by the spleen are combined by the lung to produce the pectoral qi.

中医理论

Basic Theory of Traditional Chinese Medicine

中医理论

Basic Theory of Traditional Chinese Medicine

总之,肾与先天之气的生成关系密切,脾胃和肺与后天之气的生成关系密切。

2.3 气的运动

气是不断运动着的活力很强的极细微物质,它流行于全身,内至五脏六腑,外达皮毛肌腠,无处不到,推动和激发人体的各种生理活动。

气的运动称作"气机"。气的运动形式,通常可以归纳为升、降、出、入四种基本形式。升,是指气自下而上的运动;降,是指气自上而下的运动;出,是指气由内向外的运动;入,是指气自外向内的运动。升与降、出与入是对立统一的矛盾运动,广泛存在于机体内部。如呼吸,呼出浊气是出,吸入清气是入。从某个脏腑的局部生理特点来看,气机的升降出入各有所侧重,心肺位置在上,在上者宜降;肝肾位置在下,在下者宜升;六腑传化物而不藏,以通为用,以降为顺。其气的运动总体是降,降中寓升。

人体整个生命活动都离不开气的升降出入运动。人与自然环境之间的联系和适应,也离不开气的升降出入运动,如摄入食物和水液,排出粪便及尿液、汗液等等都是气运动的体现。只有人体之气的正常运动,各脏腑才能发挥正常生理功能。因此,气机升降出入的协调平衡是保证生命

In a word, the kidney is closely related with the generation of the innate qi; the spleen, stomach and lung are closely related with the generation of the acquired qi.

2.3 Movement of Qi

Qi is the very active and tiny substance which is in constant movement and flows around the whole body, including the inside five-zang and six-fu organs and the outside skin, hair and muscles to promote and activate physiological activities.

The movement of qi (also called "qi dynamic") can be summarized into four basic forms: ascending, descending, exiting and entering. Ascending means qi moves from the lower to the upper; descending means qi moves from the upper to the lower; exiting means qi moves from the interior to the exterior; entering means qi moves from the exterior to the interior. They are contradicted movements in the unity of opposites, which widely exist inside the human body. For instance, exhaling the turbid belongs to exiting and inhaling the fresh belongs to entering. As for the physiological characteristics of some internal organs, qi dynamic has different focus so far as its movement is concerned. For example, the heart and lung are in the upper position, so their qi tends to descend. The liver and kidney are in the lower position, so their qi tends to ascend. The six fu-organs transport and transform substances but do not hide them, so they should be kept smooth and descending. And the movement of their qi is always descending and occasionally ascending.

Life activities depend on the movement of qi. The contact and adaptation between people and natural environment also cannot be separated from the movement of qi. Intake of food and fluid, discharging feces and urine, sweating and so on are the embodiments of the movement of qi. Only when the movement of qi is normal, can the organs play a normal physiological function. Therefore, the coordination and balance among ascending, descending, existing and entering is important to ensure the normal life

活动正常进行的一个重要环节。

气一方面需要通畅无阻的运动；同时气的升降出入运动之间必须平衡协调，这种状态称之为"气机调畅"。反之，当气的运动出现异常变化，升降出入之间失去协调平衡时，概称为"气机失调"。

气机失调有以下几种表现：气的运动受阻而不畅通时，称为"气机不畅"；受阻较甚，局部阻滞不通时，称为"气滞"；气的上升太过或下降不及时，称为"气逆"；气的上升不及或下降太过时，称为"气陷"；气的外出太过而不能内守时，称为"气脱"；气不能外出而郁结闭塞于内时，称为"气闭"等。

2.4　人体之气的功能

气对于人体具有十分重要的作用，它既是构成人体的基本物质，又是推动和调控脏腑功能活动的动力。

2.4.1　推动作用

气的推动作用，指气具有激发和推动作用。

人体的生长发育和生殖功能以及脏腑经络，依赖气的推动以维持其正常的机能。生长发育与生殖和肾气的推动密切相关；水谷精微的化生依赖脾胃之气的推动；血液在经脉中循行，其动力来源于气。气行则血行，气滞则血滞，气升则血升，气降则血降；津液的输布和排泄同样依赖

activities.

On the one hand, qi needs unobstructed movement; on the other hand, the movement of qi must be kept balanced and coordinated. This state is known as "smooth qi dynamic". On the contrary, when the movement of qi is abnormal, the balance is lost, qi dynamic will be in disorder.

Disorder of qi dynamic has the following performance: blocked and unsmooth flow of qi is called "inhibited qi dynamic"; seriously blocked qi dynamic and local qi obstruction is called "qi stagnation"; hyper-ascending of qi or hypo-descending of qi is called "qi regurgitation"; hypo-ascending and hyper-descending of qi is called "qi sinking"; outside escape of qi due to its failure in holding itself inside is called "qi exhaustion"; failure of qi to exit and accumulation of qi in the interior is called "qi blockage".

2.4　Functions of Qi

Qi has a very important role in human body. It is not only the basic material constituting the body, but also the power promoting and regulating the functional activities of internal organs.

2.4.1　Promoting effect

The promoting effect of qi refers to its activating and regulating function.

Human body's function of growth, development and reproduction as well as internal organs and meridians depend on the promotion of qi to maintain its normal function. Growth, development and reproduction are closely related to the promotion of the kidney qi; transformation and generation of the foodstuff essence depends on the promoting function of the spleen and stomach qi; blood circulation in the vessels relies on the motive power from qi. Qi flowing makes blood circulate; qi stagnation leads to blood's stagnation; qi ascending makes blood ascend; qi descending leads to blood's descent. The distribution and excretion of body fluid also rely on the promotion of qi. Qi

中医理论

Basic Theory of Traditional Chinese Medicine

于气的推动,气行则水行,气滞则水滞。

2.4.2　温煦作用

气的温煦作用是指气有温暖作用。气是体内产生热量的物质基础,其温煦作用是通过激发和推动各脏腑组织的生理功能,促进机体的新陈代谢来实现的。气分阴阳,气的温煦作用是通过阳气的作用而表现出来的。

发挥温煦作用的气是人身之阳气。人体的体温、各脏腑、经络的生理活动,需要在气的温煦作用下进行;血和津液等液态物质,都需要在气的温煦作用下,才能正常循行,所以临床有血"得温则行、得寒则凝"之说。

气虚为阳虚之渐,阳虚为气虚之极。如果气虚而温煦作用减弱,则有畏寒肢冷、脏腑功能衰退、血液和津液的运行迟缓等寒性病理变化。

2.4.3　防御作用

气既能护卫肌表,防御外邪入侵,也能驱除侵入人体内的病邪。当邪气入侵人体时,机体正气就会聚集,发挥抗御邪气、驱邪外出的作用。因此,气的防御功能正常,则邪气不能轻易伤人;或虽有邪气侵入,也不易发病;即使发病,也易于治疗。

气的防御功能决定着疾病的发生、发展和转归。

2.4.4　固摄作用

固摄作用,是指气对于体内精、血、津液等液态物质的固护、统

flowing makes body fluid flow; qi stagnation leads to body fluid's stagnation.

2.4.2　Warming and moistening function

Qi is the material basis for heat production of the body. Its warming function is achieved through activating and promoting the physiological function of viscera and tissues to drive the body's metabolism. The warming effect of qi is displayed through the effect of yang-qi.

Qi playing the role of warming is yang-qi. The physiological activities of the human body's temperature, viscera and meridians can work under the warming effects of qi; blood, body fluid and other liquid materials function normally under the warming effects of qi. Therefore there is saying in clinic "blood circulates when it gets warmed by qi while coagulates when it gets cold by qi".

That yang gets deficient leads to qi deficiency and yang's deficiency leads to extremely deficient qi. If qi is deficient to an extent to weaken the warming effects, there will be aversion to cold, cold limbs, decline of viscera function, slow running of blood and body fluid and other cold pathological changes.

2.4.3　Defending function

Qi can not only protect the muscles from the invasion of exogenous evil, but also can get rid of the evil that invades into the body. When the evil invades the body, the vital qi will gather and work together to resist and expel the evil. Therefore, if the defending function of qi is normal, the evil cannot easily hurt the human body; or although the evil invades the body, illness can not attack easily; or even if the disease occurs, it is easy to cure.

The defensive function of qi determines the occurrence, development and outcome of diseases.

2.4.4　Controlling function

Controlling function means that qi can control liquid materials like the essence, blood, body fluid to preventing

摄和控制作用,从而防止这些物质无故流失,保证它们在体内发挥正常的生理功能。具体表现为:

固摄精液,防止其无故流失,气不固精,可以引起遗精、滑精、早泄等病症。

统摄血液,约束其在血管内正常运行,防止其逸出脉外。如气虚不能统摄血液,可以引起各种出血。

固摄汗液、尿液、唾液、胃液、肠液等,调控其分泌量或排泄量,防止其异常丢失。如果气不摄津,可以引起自汗、多尿、小便失禁、流涎、呕吐清水、泄泻滑脱等病症。

2.5　人体之气的分类

气是构成人体各脏腑组织并运行于全身的极细精微物质。它是由先天之精所化生之气、水谷之精所化生之气及吸入的自然界清气三者相融合而生成。

人身之气推动和调控着各脏腑经络形体官窍的生理活动,推动和调控着血、津液、精的运行、输布和代谢,维系着人体的生命进程。气分布于人体内部的不同部位,则有着各自的运动形式和功能特点,因而也就有了不同的名称。

2.5.1　元气

元气,是人体最根本、最重要的气,是人体生命活动的原动力,是指先天之气。

them from losing unduly so as to ensure their normal physiological functions inside the human body. The concrete performance is as the following.

Controlling sperm means qi can prevent sperm from losing unduly. If qi cannot control sperm, there will appear spermatorrhoea and premature ejaculation and other diseases.

Controlling blood means qi can make blood circulate normally inside the vessels to prevent it from overflowing out of vessels. If qi is weak and cannot control blood, there will appear various bleedings.

Qi controls sweat, urine, saliva, gastric juice and intestinal juice to regulate the secretion or excretion to prevent the abnormal loss. If qi cannot control body fluid, there will appear spontaneous sweating, polyuria, incontinence, salivation, clear water vomiting, diarrhea, slippage and other symptoms.

2.5　Classification of Qi

Qi is a kind of very tiny and refined nutritious substance which constitutes viscera and tissues and flows around the whole body. Qi is the combination of the innate qi produced from the innate essence, the foodstuff qi from the foodstuff essence and the fresh air from the nature.

Qi promotes and regulates the physiological activities of the zang and fu-organs, meridians, body and orifices; it promotes and regulates the operation, distribution and metabolism of blood, body fluid and essence and maintains the process of human life. Different kinds of qi distribute in different parts of the human body and have different forms of movement and functional characteristics, so they get different names.

2.5.1　Primordial qi

The primordial qi is the most fundamental and important qi which is the motive power of life activities. It is also called as the innate qi.

中医理论

Basic Theory of Traditional Chinese Medicine

1）生成与分布

元气主要由肾中所藏的先天之精所化生，通过三焦而布散全身，内而五脏六腑，外而肌肤腠理，无处不到，发挥其生理功能，成为人体最根本、最重要的气。人出生之后，则又依赖脾胃化生的水谷之精的滋养补充，方能保证充足的元气。因此，元气充盛与否，不仅与先天之精有关，也与脾胃功能、饮食营养等有关。若因先天之精不足而导致元气虚弱者，也可以通过后天的培育补充而使元气得到充实。

2）生理功能

元气的生理功能主要有两个方面：推动和调节人体的生长发育和生殖机能；推动和调控各脏腑、经络、形体、官窍的生理活动，与肾气的功能类同。

2.5.2　宗气

宗气是由谷气与自然界清气相结合而积聚于胸中的气，属后天之气的范畴。宗气的生成直接关系到一身之气的盛衰。宗气在胸中积聚之处，称为"气海"，又名膻中。

1）生成与分布

宗气的生成有两个来源：脾胃运化的水谷之精所化生的水谷之气；肺从自然界吸入的清气。二者相结合生成宗气。

因此，脾胃的运化水谷精微功能和肺主气、司呼吸的功能正

1) Production and distribution

The primordial qi is mainly generated from the innate qi stored in the kidney. Through the triple-energizer, it spreads all over the body including internal organs and external skin and gives full play to its physiological function, therefore it becomes the most fundamental and important part of the body. After birth, the nourishment and supplement of the foodstuff essence generated from the spleen and stomach ensure the primordial qi to be adequate. Therefore, the adequate primordial qi not only depends on the innate essence but relates with the function of the spleen and stomach, diet, nutrition and so on. If a person is deficient in innate essence and his innate qi is therefore deficient, his or her primordial qi can be enriched through the cultivation and complement after birth.

2) Physiological function

The physiological function of the primordial qi mainly has two aspects: to promote and regulate the growth, development and reproductive function of human body; to promote and regulate the physiological activities of viscera, meridians, body and the orifices. It is similar to the function of the kidney qi.

2.5.2　Pectoral qi

The pectoral qi accumulated in the chest is the combination of the foodstuff qi and fresh air from the nature, which belongs to the acquired qi. The generation of pectoral qi is directly related to the wax and wane of qi of the whole body. The position where the pectoral qi accumulates is called "the sea of qi", or danzhong.

1) Generation and distribution

The pectoral qi has two sources: the foodstuff qi generated from the foodstuff essence transported and transformed by the spleen and stomach and the fresh air inhaled by the lung from the nature. The combination of the two produces the pectoral qi.

Therefore, whether the spleen and stomach can function normally to transport and transform the foodstuff

常与否,对宗气的生成和盛衰有着直接的影响。

宗气聚于胸中,通过上出息道(呼吸道),贯注心脉及沿三焦下行的方式布散全身。宗气一方面上出于肺,循喉咙而走息道,推动呼吸;一方面贯注心脉,推动血行;三焦为诸气运行的通道,宗气还可沿三焦向下运行于脐下丹田,以资先天元气。

2)生理功能

宗气的生理功能主要有行呼吸、行血气和资先天三个方面。

宗气上走息道,推动肺的呼吸。凡是语言、发声、呼吸的强弱皆与宗气盛衰密切相关。宗气充盛则语言清晰、声音洪亮、呼吸徐缓而均匀。反之,则言语不清、声音低微、呼吸短促或微弱等。

宗气贯注于心脉,可以促进心脏推动血液运行。因此,可以依据心脏的搏动来测知宗气的强弱盛衰。宗气充盛则脉搏徐缓,节律一致而有力。反之,则脉来躁急,节律不规则,或微弱无力。若其搏动消失,则说明宗气亡绝。

另外,宗气作为后天生成之气,自上而下,蓄积于脐下丹田,对先天元气有重要的资助作用。

2.5.3 营气

营气是行于脉中而具有营养作用的气。营气在脉中,与血关系密切,可分不可离,是血液的重要组成部分,故常常将"营血"

essence, and the lung, to govern qi and control respiratory qi directly influences the generation, rise and fall of the pectoral qi.

The pectoral qi gathering in the chest spreads all over the whole body through pouring into heart vessels along upper respiratory tract and descending along the triple-energizer. On the one hand, the pectoral qi ascends out of the lung and flows into the respiratory tract through the throat to promote breath; on the other hand, it pours into the blood vessels to promote blood circulation. Triple-energizer is the channel which qi passes through. The pectoral qi can also descend to dantian below the belly button to assist the innate primordial qi.

2) Physiological function

The physiological function of the pectoral qi mainly lies in three aspects: managing breath and blood-qi and assisting the innate.

The pectoral qi ascends through respiratory tract to promote breath. Any speech, voice and breathing are closely related to the rise and fall of the pectoral qi. If the pectoral qi is adequate, the speech will be articulate, the voice will be loud and the breath will be slow and even. Otherwise, the speech will be unclear, the voice will be low and weak and the breath, short and weak.

The pectoral qi pours into the heart vessels to promote the heart to drive blood circulation. The state of the pectoral qi is sensed according to the heart beat. If the pectoral qi is adequate, the pulse will be slow, even and strong. Otherwise, the pulse will be rash, uneven or weak. If the pulse disappears, it is certain the pectoral qi vanishes.

In addition, as the acquired qi, the pectoral qi flows from the upper to the lower and gathers in dantian, which has an important role to assist the innate primordial qi.

2.5.3 Nutritive qi

The nutritive qi flowing in the vessel as an important component of blood is closely related to blood, so it is also called "nutritive blood". Compared in nature, function and

并称。营气与卫气从性质、功能和分布进行比较，则营属阴，卫属阳，所以又常常称为"营阴"。

1）生成与分布

营气来源于脾胃运化的水谷精微。水谷精微中的精华部分化生为营气，进入脉中循行全身。

2）生理功能

营气的生理功能有化生血液和营养全身两个方面。

营气行于脉中，是血液的重要组成部分，并随血脉流注于全身，营养五脏六腑、四肢百骸。

2.5.4 卫气

卫气是行于脉外而具有保卫作用的气。因其有卫护人体、抵御外邪入侵的作用，故称之为卫气。

卫气与营气相对而言属于阳，又称为"卫阳"。

1）生成与分布

卫气来源于脾胃运化的水谷精微。水谷精微中彪悍滑利部分化生为卫气，其运行于脉外，不受脉道的约束，外而皮肤肌腠，内而五脏六腑，布散全身。

2）生理功能

卫气有防御外邪、温养全身和调控肌腠的生理功能。

卫气昼行于阳，布散于肌表皮肤，起着保卫肌体，防御外邪入侵的作用。卫气盛则外邪不易

distribution with defensive qi, the former belongs to yin and the latter to yang, so it is often called "nutritive yin".

1) Generation and distribution

The nutritive qi originates from the foodstuff essence transported and transformed by the spleen and stomach. The best part of the foodstuff essence transforms into the nutritive qi, and comes into the vessels and circulates around the body.

2) Physiological function

The nutritive qi has two physiological functions: generating blood and nourishing the whole body.

The nutritive qi flowing in the vessels is an important part of blood. It circulates around the whole body along the blood vessels and nourishes the internal organs, limbs and bones.

2.5.4　Defensive qi

The defensive qi flowing outside the vessels has the function of protecting the body and resisting the invasion of exopathogens.

Opposite to the nutritive qi, the defensive qi belongs to yang, so it is also called "defensive yang".

1) Generation and distribution

The defensive qi originates from the foodstuff essence transported and transformed by the spleen and stomach. The sturdy and lubricating part of the foodstuff essence transforms into the defensive qi. It flows outside the vessel, so it is not bound by the pulse. It distributes around the whole body including skin and muscles and internal organs.

2) Physiological function

The defensive qi has the physiological functions of defending exopathogens, warming and nourishing the body and regulating muscles.

The defensive qi flows in the yang in daytime and spreads over muscle and skin to resist exopathogens from invading. The body won't be subject to exopathogens if the defensive qi is adequate where as exopathogens can easily

侵袭,卫气虚则易于感受外邪而发病。

卫气的温煦作用,体现在内而脏腑,外而肌肉皮毛,卫气无处不到,从而保证了脏腑肌表的生理活动得以正常进行。卫气充足,机体得以温养,则可维持人体体温的相对恒定;卫气虚亏则温煦之力减弱,多四肢不温,畏寒怕冷。

卫气能够调节控制腠理的开合,促使汗液有节制地排泄。通过对汗液排泄的控制,维持肌体相对恒定温度,从而保证了机体内外环境之间的协调平衡。卫气虚弱,调控肌腠功能失职,会出现无汗、多汗或自汗等病理现象。

卫气的三个功能之间是相互联系和协调一致的。若腠理疏松,汗液自出,则畏寒怕风怕冷,易于遭邪气侵犯;而腠理致密,则邪气难以入侵。

营气与卫气,既有联系,又有区别。两者都来源于水谷精微,均由脾胃所化生,但营卫二气在性质、分布、功能上均有一定区别:营气性质精纯,富有营养,卫气漂疾滑利,易于流行;营气行于脉中,卫气行于脉外;营气有化生血液和营养全身的功能,卫气有防卫、温养和调控腠理的功能。概而言之,即营属阴,卫属阳。营卫调和才能维持

attack the body and sickness occur if the defensive qi is deficient .

The warming function of the defensive qi reflects inside in viscera and outside on muscles, skin and body hair. The defensive qi is ubiquitous to ensure that the viscera and muscles function normally. If the defensive qi is sufficient, the body can keep warm and nourished to maintain relatively constant temperature of the body; if the defensive qi is deficient, the warming function will weaken resulting in lack of warmth in the limbs and cold intolerance.

The defensive qi can regulate and control the opening and closing of the striae to promote moderate excretion of sweat, which maintains the body temperature constant to ensure the balance and coordination between the internal and external environment of the body. Deficiency of defensive qi will lead to dysfunction of regulating the striae, and there will appear adiaphoresis, hidrosis or spontaneous perspiration and other pathological phenomena.

The three functions of the defensive qi are interrelated and coordinated. If the striae are loose leading to spontaneous perspiration, there will appear cold and wind intolerance and the pathogens will invade the body easily; if the striae are dense, it will be difficult for the pathogens to invade the body.

The nutritive qi and defensive qi are both related with each other, and different from each other. Both of them originate from the foodstuff essence transported and transformed by the spleen and stomach. However, they are different in nature, distribution and function: the former is refined, pure and rich in nutrition and the latter is active and powerful and easy to flow; the nutritive qi flows inside the vessels and the defensive qi flows outside the vessels; the former has the function to generate blood and nourish the whole body and the latter has the function to defend, warm and regulate the striae. In a word, the former belongs to yin and the latter, to yang. The coordination between the nutritive qi and defensive qi can maintain normal

中医理论

Basic Theory of Traditional Chinese Medicine

正常的体温和汗液分泌,若二者失和,则可能出现抗病能力低下,容易出现恶寒发热、无汗或汗多等感冒症状。

3 血

3.1 血的基本概念

血,即血液,是循行于脉中而富有营养的红色液态物质,是构成人体和维持人体生命活动的基本物质之一。

脉是血液运行的管道,又称为"血府"。

3.2 血的生成

水谷精微和肾精是血液化生的基础。它们在脾胃、心、肺、肝、肾等脏腑的共同作用下,得以化生为血液。其中,脾胃的生理功能尤为重要。

脾胃所化生的水谷精微物质营气和津液,是血液的主要组成部分。因此,中医认为脾胃是气血生化之源。若中焦脾胃虚弱,不能运化水谷精微,或化源不足,往往导致血虚。临床上治疗血虚,首先要调理脾胃。

水谷精微所化生的营气和津液,要上输于心肺,与肺吸入的清气相结合,贯注心脉,在心气的作用下变化而成为红色血液。

肾藏精,精生髓,精髓是化生血液的基本物质之一。肾中精气充足,则血液化生有源,若肾精

Basic Theory of Traditional Chinese Medicine

中医理论

temperature and excretion of sweat; the incompatibility between them may lead to lower disease resistance and be easy to get aversion to cold, fever, adiaphoresis and hidrosis and other cold symptoms.

3 Blood

3.1 Basic Concept of Blood

Blood is a red liquid substance which is rich in nutrition and one of the basic substances constituting human body and maintaining life activities.

The vessel is the channel that blood flows through, which is also known as "the house of blood".

3.2 Generation of Blood

The foodstuff and kidney essence are the basis of blood generation. They generate blood under the joint action of the spleen, stomach, lung, liver, kidney and other viscera. Among them, the physiological function of the spleen and stomach is particularly important.

The nutritive qi and body fluids, which are the refined nutritious substance transported and transformed by the spleen and stomach, are the important parts of blood. Therefore, in TCM, it is believed that the spleen and stomach are the sources of blood generation. If the spleen and stomach in the middle place are weak, which cannot transport and transform the foodstuff essence or are in lack of generation, there will occur blood deficiency. In clinic, to treat blood deficiency needs to regulate the spleen and stomach first.

The nutritive qi and the body fluids ascend to the heart and lung, and then combine with the fresh air inhaled by the lung and pour into the heart vessel, and at last turn into blood under the function of the heart-qi.

The essence stored in the kidney produces the marrow which is one of the basic substances to generate blood. When the kidney essence is sufficient, blood generation will be guaranteed; if the kidney essence is deficient or the

第三章 气血津液

不足,或肾不藏精,则可能导致血液亏虚。因此,临床会采用补肾益精方法治疗血虚病症。

肝主疏泄而藏血。肝脏是一个贮血器官。因精血同源,肝血充足,故肾亦有所藏,精有所资,精充则血足,同时肝脏也是一个造血器官。

3.3 血的循行

脉为血之府,脉管是一个相对密闭的管道系统。血液在脉管中运行不息,流布于全身,环周不休,以营养人体的周身内外上下。血液循行的方式为"阴阳相贯,如环无端","营周不休"。血液的正常运行受着多种因素的影响,同时也是多个脏腑功能共同作用的结果。

3.3.1 影响血液运行的因素

血行脉中,脉为"血府"。脉道的完好无损与通畅无阻是保证血液正常运行的重要因素。

血液的质与量,包括清浊及黏稠状态,都可影响血液自身的运行。

血属阴而主静,血的运行需要推行的动力,这种动力主要依赖于气的推动作用和温煦作用。

血行脉中,而不致逸出脉外,主要依赖于气的固摄作用。

气的推动与固摄作用之间、温煦与凉润作用之间的协调平衡是保证血液正常运行的主要因素。

阳盛则推动血行力量太过,

kidney does not store the essence, there will appear blood deficiency. Therefore, in clinic blood deficiency syndrome will be treated by the method of nourishing the kidney to enrich the essence.

The liver regulates qi flowing and stores blood. Especially, it is an organ that stores blood. The essence and blood are of the same source, so if the liver-blood is sufficient and the storage function works normally, the essence will be adequate. The liver is also a hematopoietic organ.

3.3 Circulation of Blood

The vessels as the house of blood are a relatively airtight pipeline system. Blood circulates endlessly in the vessels spreading over the whole body like "a ring without an end". The normal blood circulation is influenced by many factors and at the same time it is also the result of several organs cooperating with each other.

3.3.1 Factors affecting blood circulation

Blood circulates in the vessels which are called "the house of blood". The intact and smooth vessels play an important role in ensuring the normal blood circulation.

The quality and quantity of blood, such as the state of being clear and turbid, and viscous, can affect blood circulation.

Blood belongs to yin and is quiet. Blood circulation needs motive power which mainly relies on the promoting and warming function of qi.

That blood circulating in the vessels but not overflowing the vessels mainly depends on the controlling function of qi.

The coordination and balance between promoting and controlling function, and warming and cooling function of qi guarantees normal blood circulation.

If yang is excessive, it will promote blood to circulate

中医理论

Basic Theory of Traditional Chinese Medicine

77

血液妄行，或灼伤脉道，易使血逸脉外而出血。阴邪侵袭，或寒从中生则脉道涩滞不利，血行缓慢，甚至出现瘀血。

3.3.2　相关脏腑功能

血液的正常运行，与心、肺、肝、脾等脏腑的功能密切相关。

心主血脉，心气推动血液在脉中运行全身。心脏、脉管和血液构成了一个完整的循环系统。心气的充足在血液循行中起着主导作用。

肺朝百脉，司呼吸而主一身之气，调节着全身的气机，辅助心脏，推动和调节血液的运行。通过宣发与肃降，吐故纳新，完成了人体内外的气体交换，通过血液循行，把自然界清气输送到全身各处，把体内代谢后的浊气排出体外。

肝主疏泄，调畅气机，可以促进和调节血液循行；肝贮藏血液、调节血量和防止出血。

脾主统血。五脏六腑之血全赖脾气统摄，脾统血，与脾为气血生化之源关系密切。脾气健旺，气血旺盛，则能控摄血液在脉中运行，防止血逸脉外。

由上可见，心气的推动、肺气的宣发肃降、肝气的疏泄是推动和促进血液运行的重要因素。脾气的统摄及肝气的藏血是固摄控制血液运行的重要因素，而心、肝、脾、肺等脏器生理功能的相互协调与密切配合，共同保证了血

abnormally or burn the vessels and blood is easy to flow out of the vessels. If yin evil invades or the coldness generates, the vessels will be uneven and blood will circulate slowly, eventually there will even appear blood stasis.

3.3.2　Related function of viscera

The normal circulation of blood is closely related to the function of the heart, lung, liver, spleen and other zang- and fu- organs.

The heart governs blood and vessels; the heart qi promotes blood to circulate in the vessels and around the whole body. The heart, vessels and blood constitute an intact circulation system. Sufficient heart-qi plays a leading role in blood circulation.

The lung connects with vessels, controls respiration, governs qi and regulates the qi dynamic of the whole body, assists the heart and promotes and regulates blood circulation. By dispersing and descending, exhaling the turbid and inhaling the clear, gas exchange inside and outside the body is fulfilled; through blood circulation, fresh air from the nature is distributed around the whole body and the metabolized turbid gas is excreted out of the body.

The liver regulates qi flowing to promote and regulate blood circulation; the liver stores blood, regulates blood volume and prevents bleeding.

The spleen governs blood. The viscera blood depends on the spleen to govern, which is closely related to the spleen as the source of qi and blood. If the spleen qi is adequate, qi and blood will be sufficient to control the blood circulation in the vessels and prevent it from flowing out of the vessels.

Therefore, the promoting function of the heart-qi, the dispersing and descending function of the lung-qi and the distributing function of the liver-qi are the important factors to promote blood circulation. The governing function of the spleen-qi and the storing function of the liver-qi are the important factors to control blood circulation. Therefore, mutual coordination and close cooperation of the physiological functions of the heart, liver, spleen, lung

液的正常运行。其中任一脏器的生理功能失调,都可以引起血行失常的病变。

气的推动与固摄作用之间、温煦与凉润作用之间的协调平衡是保证血液正常运行的主要因素。

3.4 血的功能

血主要具有营养和化神两个方面的功能。

3.4.1 营养

血液由水谷精微所化生,含有人体所需的丰富的营养物质。血循行于脉内,沿脉管循行于全身,为全身各脏腑组织的功能活动提供营养。血在脉中循行,内至五脏六腑,外达皮肉筋骨,不断地对全身各脏腑组织器官起着濡养和滋润作用,以维持各脏腑组织器官发挥生理功能,保证人体生命活动的正常进行。

血的濡养作用表现在面色、肌肉、皮肤、毛发、感觉和运动等方面。血量充盈,濡养功能正常,则面色红润,肌肉壮实,皮肤和毛发润泽,感觉灵敏,运动自如。若血虚血亏,濡养功能减弱,则面色萎黄,肌肉瘦削,肌肤干涩,毛发不荣,肢体麻木或运动无力失灵等。

3.4.2 化神

血是机体精神活动的主要物质基础。人体的精神活动必须得到血液的营养,才能产生充沛而舒畅的精神情志活动。

血液充盛,则精力充沛、神

and other organs guarantee the normal blood circulation. Any physiological maladjustment of any organ can cause disorder in blood circulation.

The coordination and balance between the promoting and controlling function, the warming and cooling function of qi are the main factors to ensure normal blood circulation.

3.4 Functions of Blood

Blood mainly functions to nourish and govern spirit.

3.4.1 Nourishing function

Blood generated from the essence of the foodstuff is rich in nutrients. Blood circulates in the vessels spreading over the whole body and provides nutrition for the functional activities of viscera and tissues. Circulating in the vessels and spreading to the inside viscera and the outside skin, muscles, tendons and bones, it constantly nourishes and moistens viscera so that all the viscera can function normally to ensure normal life activities of human body.

The nourishing function of blood is embodied in complexion, muscle, skin, hair, feeling and movement, etc. If blood is adequate and functions normally, there will appear ruddy complexion, strong muscles, moist skin and hair, acute senses and free movement. If blood is deficient and functions abnormally, there will appear yellow complexion, thin muscles, dry skin, withered hair, numb or impaired movement of limbs, etc.

3.4.2 Governing spirit

Blood is the main material basis of one's mental activity. One's mental activity must be nourished to achieve vigorous and happy spirit and emotion.

If blood is adequate,one will be full of vitality, alert in consciousness, acute in senses and thinking. If blood

志清晰、感觉灵敏、思维敏捷。血液亏虚则可能表现出不同程度的精神情志方面的病症，如精神倦怠、失眠、健忘、多梦，或烦躁、惊悸，甚至神志恍惚、谵妄、昏迷等。

4 津液

4.1 津液的基本概念

津液，是人体一切正常水液的总称，包括各脏腑官窍的正常体液和正常分泌物，习惯上也包括代谢产物中的尿、汗、泪等。津液以水分为主体，含有大量营养物质，是构成人体和维持生命活动的基本物质之一。

津和液虽同属水液，但二者之间在性状、分布和功能上有所不同，一般来说，质地清稀，流动性大，布散于体表皮肤、肌肉和孔窍，并能渗入血脉之内，起滋润作用的，称之为津；质地较浓稠，流动性较小，灌注于骨节、脏腑、脑、髓等，起濡养作用的，称之为液。由于津液二者同属水液，且可以互补转化，故津和液常同时并称，不作严格区分。

4.2 津液的代谢

津液的生成、输布和排泄，涉及多个脏腑的生理功能，是多个脏腑相互协调配合的结果。"饮入于胃，游溢精气，上输于脾，脾气散精，上归于肺，通调水道，下输膀胱，水精四布，五经并行"（《素问·经脉别论》），是对津液

is deficient, there will appear a series of mental disorders, such as mental fatigue, insomnia, amnesia, dreaminess, or irritability, palpitation, even absent-mindedness, delirium and unconsciousness, etc.

4 Body Fluid

4.1 Basic Concept of Body Fluid

Body fluid is a general term for all normal liquids in human body including normal body fluid and excretion of all viscera and orifices, and also customarily including metabolites such as urine, sweat and tears, etc. Body fluid, with water as the main component, contains lots of nutrients, and is one of the basic substances for human body and life activities.

Though both belong to body fluid, the thick and thin fluid are different in characteristics, distribution and function. Generally speaking, the thin fluid is lucid and thin with more fluidity, spreading onto the skin, muscles and orifices, and seeping into the vessels to play the moistening and nourishing function; the thick fluid is dense and thick with less fluidity, pouring into the joints, viscera, brain and marrow to play the nourishing function. Both of them belong to body fluid, and can mutually supply and convert, so they are collectively termed and not strictly differentiated.

4.2 Metabolism of Body Fluid

The formation, distribution and excretion of body fluid involve the physiological function of many organs, which is the result of coordination and cooperation of many viscera. The process of body fluid metabolism is briefed as: "It is drunk into the stomach, overflown into the essence-qi, ascended into the spleen and dispersed, ascended into the lung to regulate fluid passage, descended into the bladder, and so water-essence spreads and five meridians move together." (*Plain Questions: Special Discussion on*

代谢过程的简要概括。

4.2.1 津液的生成

津液来源于饮食水谷,通过脾、胃、小肠和大肠消化吸收饮食中的水分和营养而生成。

胃为水谷之海,主受纳腐熟,赖胃气而吸收水谷中部分精微;脾主运化,赖脾气之升清,将胃肠吸收的谷气与津液上输于心肺,而后输布全身。

小肠主液。小肠泌别清浊,吸收饮食物中大部分的营养物质和水分,上输于脾而布散全身,并将水液代谢产物经肾输入膀胱,把糟粕下输入大肠。

大肠主津。大肠接受小肠下注的饮食物残渣,将其中部分水分重新吸收,使残渣形成粪便而排出体外。

津液的生成主要与脾、胃、小肠、大肠等脏腑的生理活动有关。

总之,津液的生成取决于如下两方面的因素:其一是充足的水饮类食物,这是生成津液的物质基础;其二是脏腑功能正常,特别是脾胃、大小肠的功能正常。其中任何一方面因素的异常,均可导致津液生成不足,引起津液亏乏的病理变化。

Channels and Vessels).

4.2.1 Generation of body fluid

Body fluid is generated from foodstuff and formed through digestion and absorption of water and nutrients in the foodstuff by spleen, stomach and intestines.

The stomach, as the sea of foodstuff, receives and decomposes foodstuff, absorbs part of the essence in foodstuff depending on stomach-qi; the spleen governs transportation and transformation, carries the essence derived from foodstuff and body fluid up to the heart and lung, and then spreads them over the whole body depending on the spleen-qi's ascending and clearing function.

The small intestine governs the thick fluid. The small intestine separates the clear from the turbid, absorbs most of the nutrients and water from foodstuff, and ascends them to the spleen to be spreaded over the whole body, delivers the water metabolites to the bladder via the kidney, and transports the waste down to the large intestine.

The large intestine governs the thin fluid. The large intestine receives foodstuff debris delivered from the small intestine and reabsorbs most of the water from the debris, and then excretes feces formed by the debris out of the body.

The generation of body fluid is mainly related to the physiological activities of the spleen, stomach, small intestine and large intestine.

In short, the generation of body fluid depends on the following two aspects: on the one hand, there should be enough foodstuff as the material basis to generate body fluid; on the other hand, viscera, especially the spleen and stomach, function normally. Any abnormal factor will lead to insufficient generation of body fluid and result in pathological changes henceforth.

中医理论 Basic Theory of Traditional Chinese Medicine

4.2.2　津液的输布

津液的输布主要是依靠脾、肺、肾、肝和三焦等脏腑生理功能的协调配合来完成的。

脾主运化，一方面脾将津液上输于肺，通过肺的宣发肃降，将津液布散全身。另一方面，脾可以将津液直接向四周布散至全身各脏腑。《素问·至真要大论》说："诸湿肿满，皆属于脾。"

肺主行水，通调水道。肺一方面通过宣发，将脾转输来的津液向身体外周体表和上部布散，一方面通过肃降，将津液向身体下部和内部脏腑输布，并将脏腑代谢后产生的浊液向肾和膀胱输送，故称"肺为水之上源"。若肺气宣发肃降失常，津液运行障碍，水停气道可发为痰饮，甚则水泛为肿。

肾为水脏，一方面是指肾气对人体参与水液输布代谢的脏腑具有推动和调控作用。从胃肠道吸收水谷精微，到脾气运化水液，肺气宣降津液，肝气疏利津行，三焦决渎通利，乃至津液的排泄等等，都离不开肾阳温煦蒸腾的激发作用。另一方面，由脏腑代谢产生的浊液，经过肾气的蒸化作用，将其中的清者重新吸收，将其浊者化为尿液排出体外。这一升

4.2.2　Distribution of body fluid

Body fluid distribution mainly depends on the coordination of the physiological function of the spleen, lung, kidney, liver and triple-energizer, etc.

The spleen governs transportation and transformation. On the one hand, the spleen delivers body fluid up to the lung and through the lung's dispersing and descending, the body fluid is spread over the whole body. On the other hand, the spleen can deliver body fluid directly around to the viscera, as what is said in *Plain Questions: Discussion on the Most Important and Abstruse Theory*: "all the symptoms such as dampness and swelling are caused by the abnormal function of the spleen."

The lung governs water transportation and regulates the water passage. On the one hand, the lung through dispersing carries body fluid transferred from the spleen to the peripheral surface and then ascends it; on the other hand, through descending, body fluid is delivered to the lower part of the body and the inside viscera, and then the turbid fluid metabolized by the viscera is carried to the kidney and bladder, so the lung is called "the source of upper water". If the lung-qi functions abnormally, body fluid cannot flow smoothly and the water passage is blocked, which will lead to phlegm and even edema.

The kidney is called the water organ. On the one hand, kidney-qi can promote and regulate the viscera involved in distributing and metabolizing water. The kidney-yang is necessary for the following conductions such as, absorption of cereal essence from the gastrointestinal tract, the spleen-qi transforming and transporting body fluid, the lung-qi dispersing and descending body fluid, the liver-qi dredging the fluid passage, the triple-energizer smoothing blockage and body fluid excretion. On the other hand, the turbid fluid metabolized by viscera is steamed by the kidney-qi to reabsorb the clear and transform the turbid into urine and excrete it out of the body. The function of ascending the clear and descending the turbid is significant to maintain

清降浊作用对维持整个水液输布代谢的平衡协调有着重要意义。

肝主疏泄,调畅气机,气行则水行,保持水道畅通,促进津液输布的通畅。若肝失疏泄,往往影响津液的输布,产生痰饮、水肿以及痰气互结的梅核气、瘿瘤、臌胀等病症。

心主血脉。津液和血液赖心气之动力,方能正常运行,环周不休。

三焦为水液和诸气运行的通路。若三焦气化不利,也会导致水液停聚,发为多种病症。

综上所述,津液在体内的输布依赖于多个脏腑生理功能密切协调、相互配合,是人体生理活动的综合体现。

4.2.3 津液的排泄

津液的排泄主要通过排出尿液来完成。汗液、呼气和粪便也将带走部分水分,涉及的脏腑主要有肾、肺、脾等。

肾为水脏,肾气的蒸化作用,将脏腑代谢产生浊液分为清浊两个部分:清者重新吸收布散至全身,浊者则成为尿液,所以尿液的产生依赖于肾气的蒸化功能。

尿液贮存于膀胱,有赖于肾气的固摄作用;当贮存的尿液达到一定量时,则在肾气的推动激发作用下排出体外。

尿液的生成和排泄均依靠肾气的蒸化等作用,肾在维持人体津液代谢平衡中起着至为关键

the balance and coordination of fluid distribution and metabolism.

The liver governs dredging and regulating the qi dynamic. Smoothness of qi makes the liquid flow smoothly, so keeping the water passage open can promote body fluid distribution unblocked. If the liver cannot govern dredging, body fluid distribution will be affected, leading to phlegm, edema and even globus hystericus, gall, swelling and other diseases.

The heart governs blood. Body fluid and blood rely on the heart-qi dynamic to run normally and circulate in the vessels endlessly.

The triple-energizer is the passage of body fluid and qi. If the triple-energizer steams abnormally, there will appear fluid accumulation and a variety of diseases.

In summary, body fluid distribution depends on the close coordination and cooperation of the physiological function of several viscera, which is a comprehensive reflection of human physiological activities.

4.2.3 Excretion of body fluid

The excretion of body fluid is completed mainly through excreting urine. Sweat, exhalation and stool will also take away part of the liquid, which mainly involves kidney, lung, spleen and other organs.

The kidney is the water organ. The steaming function of the kidney-qi divides the metabolized fluid into the clear and turbid parts: the clear is reabsorbed and spread over the whole body; the turbid becomes urine, so urine generation depends on the steaming function of the kidney-qi.

The urine stored in the bladder depends on the controlling function of the kidney-qi; when the stored urine reaches to a certain amount, it is excreted out of the body by the promoting and activating function of the kidney-qi.

Urine generation and excretion depends on the steaming function of the kidney-qi. The kidney plays a key role in maintaining the metabolism balance of the

中医理论 Basic Theory of Traditional Chinese Medicine

的作用。临床上尿少、尿闭、水肿等津液排泄障碍的病变,常常与肾气的蒸化作用失常有关,

肺气宣发,将津液外输于体表皮毛,津液在气的蒸腾激发作用下,形成汗液由汗孔排出体外。肺在呼气时也会带走一些水液,这也是津液排泄体外的一个途径。

正常情况下粪便中所含水液的量很少。胃肠功能失常,则粪便稀薄,带走大量水分,甚至连胃液、肠液也随之丢失,引起体内津液的损耗,发生伤津或脱液的病变。

综观津液的生成、输布和排泄过程,是诸多脏腑相互协调、密切配合而完成的,其中尤以脾、肺、肾三脏的综合调节为首要。

4.3　津液的功能

4.3.1　滋润濡养

津液是含有营养物质的液体。津的质地较清稀,其滋润作用较明显,而液的质地较浓稠,其濡养作用较明显。其滋润和濡养二者作用之间相辅相成,难以分割。

布散于体表的津液能滋润皮毛肌肉,渗入体内的能濡养脏腑,输注于孔窍的能滋润鼻、目、口、耳等官窍,渗注骨、脊、脑的能充养骨髓、脊髓、脑髓,流入关节的能滋润骨节屈伸等。

body fluid. Clinically, diseases concerning fluid excretion disorder such as oliguria, anuria, edema, etc. are attributable to kidney-qi's dysfunction of steaming.

The lung-qi disperses to deliver body fluid to skin and body hair. Under the steaming and activating function of qi, body fluid transforms into sweat which is excreted out of the body through pores. Some liquid is taken away when the lung exhales, which is also a way the body fluid is excreted out of the body.

Under normal circumstances, the amount of liquid contained in feces is very small. Gastrointestinal dysfunction leads to thin stool which takes away a lot of liquid and even the gastric and intestinal juice, causing loss of body fluid to bring about lesions such as deficiency or drainage of fluid.

In the process of the generation, distribution and excretion of body fluid, many organs coordinate and cooperate closely with each other, and especially the comprehensive regulation of the spleen, lung and kidney is of primary importance.

4.3　Function of Body Fluid

4.3.1　Moistening and nourishing

Body fluid is the liquid containing nutritious substance. The fluid which is clear and thin has the more obvious moistening function; the fluid which is viscous and thick has the more obvious nourishing function. The nourishing and moistening functions are supplementary to each other, which is hard to separate.

Body fluid spreading on the surface of the body can moisten the skin, body hair, and muscles; the one seeping into the body can nourish the viscera; the one pouring into the orifices can moisten the nose, eyes, mouth, ears and other orifices; the one seeping into the bone, spine and marrow can nourish the bone marrow, spinal cord and brain; the one seeping into the joints can moisten the condyle to be flexible.

4.3.2 充养血脉

津液入脉,成为血液的重要组成部分。津液和营气共同渗注于脉中,化生为血液,以循环全身发挥滋润、濡养作用。

津液渗入脉中为血,出于脉外为津液。当肌体血液亏虚时,津液就渗入脉中补充血液。当机体的津液亏少时,血中之津液可以从脉中渗出脉外以补充津液。由于津液和血液都是水谷精微所化生,而且脉内外的津液互相渗透,故有"津血同源"之说。

此外,津液的代谢可以调节机体内外环境的阴阳相对平衡。气候炎热或体内发热时,津液化为汗液向外排泄以散热,而天气寒冷或体温低下时,津液因腠理闭塞而不外泄,如此则可维持人体体温相对恒定。

5 精、气、血、津液之间的关系

精、气、血、津液均是构成人体和维持人体生命活动的基本物质,均赖于脾胃化生的水谷精微不断补充,它们之间又相互渗透、相互促进、相互转化。在生理功能上,又存在着相互依存、相互制约和相互为用的密切关系。

5.1 气与血的关系

气与血是人体内的两大类基本物质,在人体生命活动中占有重要地位,气是血液生成和运

4.3.2 Filling and nourishing vessels

Body fluid coming into the vessels becomes an important part of blood. Both of body fluid and the nutritive-qi seeping into the vessels are transformed into blood which circulates in the body to play a role of moistening and nourishing.

Body fluid seeping into the vessels is blood and the one seeping out of the vessels is body fluid. When the body is short of blood, body fluid will seep into the vessels to supplement body fluid. Both of the body fluid and blood are transformed from foodstuff essence and body fluid inside and outside the vessels penetrate into each other, so there is the saying "body fluid and blood are of the same origin".

In addition, body fluid metabolism can adjust the relative balance of yin and yang in the internal and external environments of the body. When the climate is hot or the body generates heat, body fluid is transformed into sweat excreted out to dissipate heat. When the weather is cold and temperature is low, body fluid will not flow out because of the closed striae to maintain body temperature relatively stable.

5 Relationship between Essence, Qi, Blood and Body Fluid

Essence, qi, blood and body fluid are the basic substances constituting the human body and maintaining life activities, which are constantly supplemented by foodstuff essence generated from the spleen and stomach. They are mutually penetrated, promoted and transformed. As for the physiological function, they are closely related in terms of mutual interdependence, restraint and use.

5.1 Relationship between Qi and Blood

Qi and blood, as the two basic substances in human body, play an important role in life activities. Qi is the power of blood generation and circulation and blood is the

中医理论 Basic Theory of Traditional Chinese Medicine

行的动力,血是气的化生基础和载体,因而有"气为血之帅,血为气之母"的说法。

5.1.1　气为血之帅

气为血之帅,包含气能生血、气能行血、气能摄血三个方面。

气能生血,是指血液的化生离不开气的推动和激发作用。当然气能生血还包含了营气在血液生成中的作用。

临床上治疗血虚的病变,在使用补血药的同时常常以补气药配合,取得较好疗效,即是源于气能生血的理论。

气能行血,是指血液的运行有赖于心气的推动、肺气宣降及肝气的疏泄调畅等。气行则血行。气亏虚无力推动血行,气机郁滞不通使血不能行,都容易产生血瘀的病变。如果气的运行发生逆乱,升降出入失常,也会影响血液的正常运行,出现血液运行异常的病变,如血随气逆之吐血、咳血;血随气下崩漏、便血等。所以临床上在治疗血液运行失常时,根据气能行血的理论,常常配伍补气、行气、降气、升提的药物。

气能摄血,是指气能控制约束血液循行于脉中的作用。气能摄血主要体现在脾主统血的生理功能之中。脾气充足,统摄血液行于脉中而不致逸出脉外,从而保证了其濡养功能的发挥。如若脾气虚弱,失去统摄,往往导致各种慢性或下部出血,临床上称为

basis and carrier of qi generation, so there is the saying "qi is the commander of blood and blood is the mother of qi".

5.1.1　Qi as the commander of blood

Qi as the commander of blood means qi can generate, circulate and control blood.

Qi generating blood means blood generation depends on the promoting and activating function of qi and the nutritious qi plays a role in blood generation.

In the clinical treatment of blood deficiency disease, the prescriptions of supplementing blood are used together with the prescriptions of supplementing qi to achieve better curative effect, which is derived from the theory of qi generating blood.

Qi can circulate blood means blood circulation depends on the promotion of the heart-qi, the dispersing and descending of the lung-qi and dredging and smoothing of the liver-qi. Qi circulation promotes blood circulation. Qi deficiency cannot promote blood circulation and obstructed qi leads to blood blockage, which is liable to get lesions of blood stasis. If qi flows abnormally in ascending, descending, existing and entering, the normal blood circulation will be affected and there will appear lesions of abnormal blood circulation, such as hematemesis and hemoptysis due to blood inverse following qi inverse, and uterine bleeding and hematochezia due to blood descending following qi descending. So, in the treatment of blood circulation disorders, compatibility of medicines for supplementing, circulating, descending and ascending qi are used according to the theory of qi circulating blood.

Qi controlling blood means qi can control and constrain blood circulation in the vessels, which mainly embodies the physiological function of the spleen controlling blood. The sufficient spleen-qi controls blood to circulate in the vessels instead of flowing out of the vessels, which ensures its nourishing function. If the spleen is deficient and out of control, it will lead to chronic or lower-part bleeding, which is called "qi failing to control blood" or "spleen

"气不摄血"或"脾不统血"。临床中治疗这些出血病变时,常用健脾补气摄血的方法,甚至发生大出血时,用大剂补气药物以摄血,也是这一理论的应用。

气能生血、行血和摄血的三个方面体现了气对于血的统率作用,故概括地称之为"气为血之帅"。

5.1.2 血为气之母

血为气之母,包含血能养气和血能载气两个方面。

血能养气,是指在人体各个脏腑组织官窍中,血不断地为气的生成和功能活动提供支撑帮助。血足则气旺。人体脏腑、组织、形体、九窍等任何部位,一旦失去血的供养,即可出现气虚衰少甚至气的功能丧失。血虚的病人往往见有气虚的表现,其道理即在于此。

血能载气是指气存于血中,依附于血而不致散失,赖血之运载而运行全身。气需依附于血而得以存在体内,并以血为载体而运行全身。临床上血液亏虚往往兼有气虚的症状,而大失血的病人,往往出现气的涣散不收,漂浮无根的气脱病变,称为"气随血脱"。

血能养气与血能载气,体现了血对气的基础作用,故概括地称之为"血为气之母"。总之,血属阴,气属阳。气血阴阳之间协调平衡,生命活动得以正常进行。因此,调整气血之间的关系是治疗疾病的常用法则之一。

cannot govern blood"in clinic. In the clinical treatment of the bleeding lesions, methods of strengthening spleen, nourishing qi and controlling blood are used. Even massive hemorrhage can be controlled by large dose prescription of supplementing qi, which is also the application of this theory.

That qi generating, circulating and controlling blood reflects the governing function of qi, so there is the saying "qi is the commander of blood".

5.1.2 Blood as the mother of qi

Blood is the mother of qi means blood can nourish qi, and blood can carry qi.

Blood nourishing qi means that in the organs, tissues and orifices, blood constantly provides support and assistance for the generation and functional activity of qi. Sufficient blood leads to vigorous qi. Once any part of the body such as, organs, tissues, body and nine orifices, loses support from blood, there can appear qi deficiency and even functional loss. That's why the patient with blood deficiency always has qi deficiency.

Blood can carry qi means it is stored in and is attached to blood so that it will not disperse, and flows over the body depending on the carrying function of blood. Qi needs to be attached to blood for staying inside the body. Clinically, blood deficiency usually leads to the symptom of qi deficiency. The patient with massive blood loss often has disorganized qi inside his body and qi prostration called "exhaustion of qi resulting from hemorrhea".

That blood nourishing and carrying qi shows blood is the basis of qi, so there is the saying "blood is the mother of qi". In short, blood belongs to yin and qi, to yang. The Coordination and balance between qi and blood, yin and yang ensures normal life activities. Therefore, adjusting the relationship between qi and blood is one of the common rules for curing diseases.

5.2 气与津液的关系

气属阳,津液属阴。气与津液的关系类似于气与血的关系,津液的生成、输布和排泄,有赖于气的激发、推动、固摄等作用,而气的功能发挥及在体内的存在也离不开津液的滋润和运载。

5.2.1 气能生津

气是津液生成的动力,津液的生成依赖于气的激发和推动作用。从饮食水谷变成人体的津液,需要经过脾胃运化、小肠分清别浊、大肠主津等诸多脏腑之气的作用,尤其是脾胃、肾。临床上遇到津液不足的病变,可以采取补气生津的治法。

5.2.2 气能行津

气是津液在体内正常输布运行的动力,津液的输布、排泄等代谢活动离不开气的激发、推动作用。津液通过气的升降出入运动,推动津液输布到全身各处;代谢后所产生的废液可以转化为汗、尿或水汽排出体外,这一过程同样离不开气的激发和推动。

若气虚,推动作用减弱,气化无力进行,或气机郁滞不畅,气化受阻,可以引起津液的输布、排泄障碍,并形成痰、饮、水、湿等病理产物,病理上称为"气不行水",也可称为"气不化水"。

5.2 Relationship between Qi and Body Fluid

Qi belongs to yang and the body fluid, to yin. The relationship between qi and body fluid is similar to that of qi and blood. The generation, distribution and excretion of body fluid depend on the activating, promoting and controlling function of qi. However, qi relies on the moistening and carrying functions of body fluid to function normally and stay inside the body.

5.2.1 Qi generating body fluid

Qi is the power of body fluid generation which depends on the activating and promoting function of qi. The body fluid transformed from the foodstuff essence needs the coordinated effects of lots of viscera-qi, such as the small intestine separating the clear from the turbid and the large intestine governing body fluid, especially the spleen and stomach transforming and transporting the foodstuff essence. The lesions caused by deficient body fluid can be treated by supplementing qi to generate body fluid.

5.2.2 Qi impelling body fluid to flow

Qi impels body fluid to circulate inside the body. The distributing and discharging and other metabolizing activities of body fluid count on qi's activating and promoting effects. Body fluid flows over the whole body through qi's ascending, descending, existing and entering movements; the metabolized waste water transforms into sweat, urine or vapor excreted out of the body, the process of which cannot do without qi's activation and promotion.

If qi is deficient, the promoting effect will be reduced and gasification will be difficult to carry out; or if the qi dynamic is unsmooth or blocked, there will appear distributing and discharging barrier of body fluid causing the formation of phlegm, drink, water, moisture and other pathological products, which is known as "qi cannot circulate fluid" or "qi cannot gasify fluid".

5.2.3 气能摄津

气通过对分泌物和排泄物的有效控制，可以防止体内津液无故地大量流失，维持着体内津液量的相对恒定。

若气虚，固摄津液力量减弱，则会出现诸如自汗、盗汗、遗尿、二便失禁等病症。

5.2.4 津能生气

由饮食水谷化生的津液，在输布过程中受到各脏腑阳气的蒸腾温化，可以化生为气，以输布于全身各处以滋润、濡养各脏腑、组织、形体、官窍，使其发挥正常的生理活动。临床上津液亏耗不足，也会引起气的衰少。

5.2.5 津能载气

津液是气运行的载体之一，气的运行必须依附于津液，否则也会使气漂浮失散而无所归。因此当大汗、大吐、大泻等津液大量丢失时，必定导致气的损耗，甚至气亦随之大量外脱，称之为"气随津脱"。

5.3 精血津液之间的关系

精、血、津液都是液态物质，与气相对而言，其性质均归属于阴。精、血、津液三者都来源于水谷精微，而且它们之间存在着互相化生、互相补充的关系。病理上，三者之间也往往发生互相影响。这种关系集中体现在"精血同源"和"津血同源"的理论之中。

5.3.1 精血同源

精与血都由水谷精微化生和充养，化源相同；两者之间又

5.2.3 Qi controlling body fluid

Through the effective control of the secretion and excretion, qi can prevent body fluid from losing and maintain a relatively constant amount of body fluid.

If qi is deficient, the power of controlling body fluid will be weakened, leading to spontaneous sweating, night sweating, enuresis, urinary and fecal incontinence.

5.2.4 Body fluid generating qi

Body fluid transformed from foodstuff in the process of spreading is steamed, warmed and resolved by yang-qi in viscera and transformed into qi spreading over the whole body to moisten and nourish viscera, tissues, body and orifices to function normally. Clinically, insufficient body fluid will cause decline of qi.

5.2.5 Body fluid carrying qi

Body fluid is one of the carriers for the flowing of qi, which must depend on body fluid. Otherwise, it will float and scatter. Therefore, sweating, vomiting, diarrhea and other losses of body fluid will cause qi deficiency, even massive loss of qi known as "qi's loss following body fluid deficiency".

5.3 Relationship between Essence and Body Fluid

The Essence, blood, body fluid are liquid substances. In contrast to qi, their properties belong to yin. All of them are derived from foodstuff essence and mutually generated and supplemented and pathologically interacted. This relationship is embodied in "essence and blood being of the same origin" and "body fluid and blood being of the same origin" theory.

5.3.1 Essence and blood being of the same origin

The Essence and blood, transformed and nourished by the foodstuff essence, have the same source. They promote

中医理论　Basic Theory of Traditional Chinese Medicine

互相滋生,互相转化,并都具有濡养和化神等作用。精与血的这种化源相同而又相互滋生的关系称为精血同源。因肾藏精,肝藏血,也可称为"肝肾同源"。

血能生精,血旺则精充,血亏则精衰。临床上血虚者往往有肾精亏损之象。

精髓是化生血液的重要物质基础。精足则血足,所以肾精亏损可导致血虚。目前治疗白血病、再生障碍性贫血等血虚之症,用补肾填精之法,就是以精可化血为理论依据的。

5.3.2 津血同源

血和津液都由饮食水谷精微所化生,都具有滋润濡养作用,二者之间可以相互滋生,相互转化,故有"津血同源"之说。

津液与营气是血液化生的组成部分。血液行于脉中,脉中津液可以渗出脉外而化为津液,脉外津液可以进入血管之内化为血液,而津液可化为汗液排泄于外,故又称"血汗同源"。

当大汗、大吐、大泻,或严重烧烫伤时,脉外津液不足,血管内的津液渗出脉外,可以补充津液的亏耗,这时候不能再用放血或破血疗法,以防血液和津液的进一步耗伤,故《灵枢·营卫生会》说:"夺汗者无血。"

and transform into each other and have the function of nourishing and generating spirit. So, they are of the same origin. Because the kidney stores essence and the liver stores blood, so there is the saying "liver and kidney are of the same origin".

Blood can generate essence; sufficient blood makes essence abundant; deficient blood leads to the decline of essence. Clinically, one with blood deficiency is always deficient in kidney essence.

Essence is the important material basis of blood. Sufficient essence makes blood abundant, so deficiency of the kidney essence can lead to blood deficiency. At present the treatment of leukemia, aplastic anemia and other blood deficiency syndrome is to nourish the kidney and fill the essence according to the theoretical basis of essence generating blood.

5.3.2 Body fluid and blood being of the same origin

Blood and body fluid transformed from the foodstuff essence both have the function of moistening and nourishing. They can promote and transform into each other, so there is the saying "body fluid and blood are of the same origin".

Body fluid and nutritious qi is a part of blood generation. Blood circulating in the vessels can ooze out to transform into body fluid; at the same time, body fluid outside of the vessels can enter the vessels to transform into blood and it can also transform into sweat excreted out of the body, so there is the saying "blood and sweat are of the same origin".

When profuse sweating, vomiting, diarrhea, or severe burns happen, body fluid outside the vessels is deficient, and body fluid inside the vessels oozes out to supplement the loss of body fluid. At this time, the therapy of bloodletting and blood-breaking is no longer to be used in order to prevent further consumption and loss of blood and body fluid, so there is the saying in *The Spiritual Pivot: The Production and Convergence of Yingqi*, "polyhidrosis shunning hemorrhagia".

若血亏液耗,尤其是在失血时,脉中血少,不能化为津液,反而需要脉外津液进入脉中,此时,不能再使用发汗的治疗方法,以防津液与血液进一步耗竭的恶性后果,故《灵枢·营卫生会》说:"夺血者无汗。"《伤寒论》说"衄家不可发汗"和"亡血家不可发汗"。

If blood and body fluid are deficient, especially bleeding happens, blood inside the vessels is too deficient to transform into body fluid, and even the outside body fluid is needed to supplement. At this time, the therapy of sweating is no longer used to prevent vicious consequences caused by further depletion of body fluid and blood, so there is the saying in *Miraculous Pivot (Lingshu): The Production and Convergence of Yingqi*, "polyhidrosis shunning hemorrhagia". There are also the sayings in *Treatise on Cold Damage Diseases (Shanghan Lun)* "the person with frequent nose bleeding cannot be induced perspiration" and "the person prone to bleed cannot be induced perspiration".

中医理论

Basic Theory of Traditional Chinese Medicine

第四章 十四经络

Chapter 4 Fourteen Meridians

经脉者,所以决死生,处百病,调虚实,不可不通。

Normal function of the meridians determines the person's life and plays a key role in treating illnesses and adjusting deficiency and excess, so they must be kept smooth.

中医理论

Basic Theory of Traditional Chinese Medicine

1 经络的概念

经络,是运行气血、联络脏腑形体官窍、沟通内外上下、感应和传导信息的一种特殊的通路系统。

经络是经脉和络脉的总称。经,又称经脉,有路径之意。经脉大多循行于人体的深部,且有一定的循行部位。经脉贯通上下,沟通内外,是经络系统中纵行的主干。络,又称络脉,有网络之意,是经脉别出的分支,较经脉细小。

经络相贯,遍布全身,形成一个纵横交错的联络网,通过有规律的循行和复杂的联络交会,组成了经络系统,把人体五脏六腑、肢体官窍及皮肉筋骨等组织紧密地联结成统一的有机整体,从而保证了人体生命活动的正常进行。

1 Concept of Meridians

The meridians as a special pathway system can circulate qi-blood, connect viscera, body and orifices, link the inside with outside, the upper with the lower, and sense and conduct information.

The meridians as a general term include the channels and collaterals. The channels mean passages. They circulate in the deep location of human body along with certain running courses. The channels which link the upper with the lower, the inside with the outside are the main column in the meridian system. The collaterals, as the branches of channels, are like networks, thinner and smaller than channels.

The meridians throughout the body form a crisscrossed network. Through their regular cycling and complex contact, viscera, limbs, orifices, skin, flesh, tendons and bones are closely linked as an organic whole to ensure the normal life activities.

2 经络系统

经络系统是由经脉、络脉及其连属部分构成的。经脉是它的主体,在经脉中,尤其十二经脉和

2 Meridian System

The meridian system is constituted by channels, collaterals and its affiliated portions, among which the channels are the principal part. And among the channels,

任、督二脉最为重要,通常合称为"十四经脉"。人体穴位也主要集中在这十四经脉。

2.1 经脉系统

经脉系统主要有十二经脉、十二经别、十二经筋、十二皮部和奇经八脉等。

2.1.1 十二经脉

包括手三阴经、足三阴经、手三阳经、足三阳经。它们归属于五脏(外加心包络)六腑,脏腑经脉相互络属,在人体中交接分布很有规律,是针灸、腧穴等经络运用中的主体部分,习惯称之为十二正经。

2.1.2 十二经别

经别是十二经脉别出的正经,它们分别起于四肢,循行于体内,联系脏腑,上出颈项浅部。阳经的经别从本经别出而循行体内,上达头面后,仍回到本经;阴经的经别从本经别出而循行体内,上达头面后,与相为表里的阳经相合。为此,十二经别不仅可以加强十二经脉中相为表里的两经之间的联系,而且因其联系了某些正经未循行到的器官与形体部位,从而补充了正经之不足。

2.1.3 十二经筋

经筋是十二经脉之气"结、聚、散、络"于筋肉、关节的体系,是十二经脉的附属部分,是十二

the twelve meridians, ren and du meridians are the most important ones, and they are collectively called the "fourteen meridians" in which acupoints mostly gather.

2.1 Channel System

The channel system mainly contains the twelve meridians, the twelve meridian divergences, the twelve meridian musculatures, the twelve skin areas and the eight extra meridians.

2.1.1 Twelve meridians

Twelve meridians include three yin meridians of hand, three yin meridians of foot, three yang meridians of hand, three yang meridians of foot. They belong to five-zang (plus heart envelope) and six-fu organs. The viscera meridians are affiliated with each other whose joint and distribution are very regular. As the main part in the meridian application such as acupuncture and acupoints, they are customarily called the twelve meridians.

2.1.2 Twelve meridian divergences

Twelve meridian divergences are the meridians separating out from the twelve meridians. Originating respectively from the four limbs, they run through the body, associate with viscera and reach up to the superficial part of the neck. The yang meridian divergence separates out from the meridians-proper, runs through the body, reaches up to the head and face and then returns to the meridians-proper. Therefore, the twelve meridian divergences can not only reinforce the external-internal relationship between the two meridians in the twelve meridian divergences, but also supplement the defects of the meridians-proper, because they connect the organs and the parts of body around which the twelve meridians do not circulate.

2.1.3 Twelve meridian musculatures

The meridian musculatures are the system of tendons and joints where qi of the twelve meridians "concentrate, accumulate, distribute and connect". They are the affiliated

中医理论

Basic Theory of Traditional Chinese Medicine

经脉循行部位上分布于筋肉系统的总称,它有连缀百骸、维络周身、主司关节运动的作用。

2.1.4 十二皮部

十二皮部是十二经脉在体表一定部位上的反应区。全身的皮肤是十二经脉的功能活动反映于体表的部位,所以把全身皮肤分为十二个部分,分属于十二经,称为"十二皮部"。

2.1.5 奇经八脉

奇经八脉即督脉、冲脉、任脉、带脉、阴跷脉、阳跷脉、阴维脉、阳维脉八条经脉。由于八脉与脏腑无直接络属关系,八脉之间无表里配合关系,且八脉的分布不像十二经脉分布遍及全身,人体的上肢无八脉的分布,故为奇经,合称奇经八脉。奇经八脉有统率、联络和调节全身气血盛衰的作用。在临床医疗保健、针灸推拿中,人们比较熟悉和常用的是任、督二脉。

2.2 络脉系统

络脉有别络、浮络、孙络之分。

2.2.1 别络

从经脉分出的支脉,大多分布于体表,有本经别走邻经之意。

十二经脉和任督两脉各别出一络,加上脾之大络,共十五条,称为"十五别络",若加上胃之大络又称"十六别络"。途径是由阴经别络走向阳经,阳经别络走

part of the twelve meridians and the general term of the circulation parts of the twelve meridians distributed in the tendon system; they play the role of connecting with bones, developing a network of the whole body and governing joint movement.

2.1.4 Twelve skin areas

Twelve skin areas are the reaction zone of twelve meridians in certain parts of the body. Skin is the part on body surface reflecting the functional activity of the twelve meridians, so skin is divided into twelve areas according to twelve meridians which are called "twelve skin areas".

2.1.5 Eight extra meridians

Du, chong, ren, dai, yinqiao, yangqiao, yinwei and yangwei meridians are collectively called eight extra meridians. They are not directly affiliated with viscera and there are no external-internal and cooperative relationships among them. Unlike twelve meridians around the body, they do not distribute on the upper limbs, so they are called the extra meridians. They play the role of governing, connecting and regulating the ups and downs of qi-blood of the whole body. Ren and Du meridians are widely known and used in the clinical health care, acupuncture and massage.

2.2 Collateral System

The collaterals are divided into the divergent, the superficial and the minute collaterals.

2.2.1 The divergent collaterals

They branch out from the channels and distribute around the surface of the body. They have the meaning that the meridian-proper diverges to nearby channels.

Each of the twelve meridians and Ren and Du meridian sprouts one extra collateral. In addition to the large collateral of the spleen meridian, there are altogether fifteen collaterals collectively called "the fifteen divergent collaterals". Together with the large collaterals of the

向阴经,所以,十五别络的功能是加强表里阴阳两经的联系与调节作用,统率其他络脉,加强了人体前、后、侧面的统一联系。

stomach, they are called "the sixteen divergent collaterals". They diverge from the yin channels to the yang channels or from the yang channels to the yin channels, so the function of the fifteen divergent collaterals is to strengthen the relation between external-internal yin and yang channels and their regulating effects, to command the other collaterals and to reinforce the unity and link of the anterior, posterior and lateral parts of human body.

2.2.2 浮络

浮络是络脉由深至浅、多浮行于浅表部位而常浮现的络脉。

2.2.3 孙络

孙络是络脉由大到小、络脉中最细小的分支。

2.2.2 The superficial collaterals

They are the collaterals starting from the deep to shallow and appearing superficially on the surface.

2.2.3 The minute collaterals

They are the smallest branch in collaterals which start from the big to the small.

3 十二经脉

3.1 十二经脉的名称

3.1.1 命名原则

十二经脉根据各经所联系的脏腑的阴阳属性以及在肢体循行部位的不同,具体分为手三阴经、手三阳经、足三阴经、足三阳经四组。

脏为阴,腑为阳:内脏为阴,六腑为阳。每一阴经分别隶属于一脏,每一阳经分别隶属于一腑,各经都以脏腑命名。

内为阴,外为阳:阴经分布于肢体内侧面,阳经分布于肢体外侧面。一阴一阳衍化为三阴三阳,称为太阴、厥阴、少阴、阳明、少阳、太阳。

上为手,下为足:分布于上肢的经脉,在经脉名称之前冠以"手"字;分布于下肢的经脉,在

3 Twelve Meridians

3.1 Nomenclature of Twelve Meridians

3.1.1 Nomenclature principle

According to the yin-yang attributes of the organs associated with the twelve meridians, they are divided into three yin and yang meridians of hand, three yin and yang meridians of foot respectively.

Zang organs are yin and fu organs are yang: every yin meridian is affiliated to every zang organ and every yang meridian is affiliated to every fu organ.

The inside is yin and the outside is yang: the yin meridians distribute on the inside lateral part of the limbs and the yang meridians distribute on the outside lateral part of the limbs. Yin is divided into taiyin, jueyin and shaoyin and yang is divided into yangming, shaoyang and taiyang.

The upper is hand and the lower is foot: the meridians of the upper limbs are entitled the word "hand" before the name of meridians; the meridians of the lower limbs are

中医理论

Basic Theory of Traditional Chinese Medicine

经脉名称之前冠以"足"字。

3.1.2　具体名称

循行分布于上肢内侧的称为手三阴经：手太阴肺经、手厥阴心包经、手少阴心经。

循行分布于上肢外侧的称为手三阳经：手阳明大肠经、手少阳三焦经、手太阳小肠经。

循行分布于下肢内侧的称为足三阴经：足太阴脾经、足厥阴肝经、足少阴肾经。

循行分布于下肢外侧的称为足三阳经：足阳明胃经、足少阳胆经、足太阳膀胱经。

3.2　十二经脉的走向和交接规律

3.2.1　十二经脉的走向规律

手之三阳，从手走头；手之三阴，从脏走手；足之三阳，从头走足；足之三阴，从足走腹。

3.2.2　十二经脉的交接规律

经络交接与走向之间密切联系：手三阴经，从胸走手，交手三阳经；手三阳经，从手走头，交足三阳经；足三阳经，从头走足，交足三阴经；足三阴经，从足走腹（胸），交手三阴经，构成一个"阴阳相贯，如环无端"的循行径路。

entitled the word "foot" before the name of meridians.

3.1.2　Specific names

The meridians of the inside lateral part of the upper limbs are called three yin meridians of hand: the lung meridian of hand taiyin, the pericardium meridian of hand jueyin and the heart meridian of hand shaoyin.

The meridians of the outside lateral part of the upper limbs are called three yang meridians of hand: the large intestine meridian of hand yangming, the triple-energizer meridian of hand shaoyang and the small intestine meridian of hand taiyang.

The meridians of the inside lateral part of the lower limbs are called three yin meridians of foot: the spleen meridian of foot taiyin, the liver meridian of foot jueyin and the kidney meridian of foot shaoyin.

The meridians of the outside lateral part of the lower limbs are called three yang meridians of foot: the stomach meridian of foot yangming, the gallbladder meridian of foot shaoyang and the bladder meridian of foot taiyang.

3.2　Regularity in Course and Connection of Twelve Meridians

3.2.1　Regularity in course

Three yang meridians of hand start from hands to head; three yin meridians of hand start from the chest to hands; three yang meridians of foot start from head to feet; three yin meridians of foot start from feet to belly.

3.2.2　Twelve meridians run and connect as the following

Twelve meridians run and connect as the following: the three yin meridians of hand start from the chest to hands and connect three yang meridians of hand; three yang meridians of hand start from hands to the head and connect three yang meridians of foot; three yang meridians of foot start from the head to the feet and connect three yin meridians of foot; three yin meridians of foot start from the feet to the belly (chest) and connect three yin meridians of hand. They form a circulatory route in which "yin and yang meridians communicate with each other".

互为表里的三阴经与三阳经在四肢部衔接。如手太阴肺经在食指端与手阳明大肠经相交接；手少阴心经在小指与手太阳小肠经相交接；手厥阴心包经由无名指端与手少阳三焦经相交接；足阳明胃经从大趾与足太阴脾经相交接；足太阳膀胱经从足小趾与足少阴肾经相交接；足少阳胆经从大趾与足厥阴肝经相交接。

同名的阳经在头面相交接。如手足阳明经都通于鼻翼旁，手足太阳经皆通于目内眦，手足少阳经皆通于目外眦。

手、足三阴经在胸腹相交接。如足太阴经与手少阴经交接于心中，足少阴经与手厥阴经交接于胸中，足厥阴经与手太阴经交接于肺中等。

3.3 十二经脉的分布规律

3.3.1 头面部

手三阳经与足三阳经在头面部交接，所以说："头为诸阳之会"。十二经脉在头面部的分布规律是：阳明在前，少阳在侧，太阳在后。

3.3.2 躯干部

足三阴与足阳明经分布在胸、腹部（前），从里到外依次是：足少阴肾经、足阳明胃经、足太阴脾经、足厥阴肝经；背部有足太

The external three yin meridians and the internal three yang meridians connect in the four limbs. For example, the lung meridian of hand taiyin connects the large intestine meridian of hand yangming at the end of the index finger; the heart meridian of hand shaoyin connects the small intestine of hand taiyang at the little finger; the pericardium meridian of hand jueyin connects the triple-energizer meridian of shaoyang of hand at the end of the ring finger; the stomach meridian of foot yangming connects the spleen meridian of foot taiyin at the big toe; the bladder meridian of foot taiyang connects the kidney meridian of foot shaoyin at the little toe; the gallbladder meridian of foot shaoyang connects the liver meridian of foot jueyin at the big toe.

The yang meridians sharing same names connect at the head and face. For example, the yangming meridians of hand and foot connect at the sides of nose; the taiyang meridians of hand and foot connect at the inner canthus (BLI); the shaoyang meridians of hand and foot connect at the outer canthus (GBI).

The three-yin meridians of hand and foot connect at the chest and belly. For example, the taiyin meridian of foot and the shaoyin meridian of hand connect at the heart; the shaoyin meridian of foot and the jueying meridian of hand connect at the chest; the jueyin meridian of foot and the taiyin meridian of hand connect at the lung.

3.3 Regularity in distribution of twelve meridians

3.3.1 Head and face

The three-yang meridians of hand and foot connect at the head and face, so there is the saying "the head is the gathering place of all yangs". Regularity in distribution of twelve meridians on the head and face is as the following: the yangming meridian is at the front, the shaoyang meridian is at the side and the taiyang meridian is at the back.

3.3.2 Torso

The three-yin meridian of foot and the three-yang meridian of foot distribute on the chest and belly as the following from the inside to the outside: the kidney meridian of foot shaoyin, the stomach meridian of foot yangming, the

中医理论 Basic Theory of Traditional Chinese Medicine

阳膀胱经(后)，足少阳胆经(侧)。

spleen meridian of foot taiyin, the liver meridian of foot jueyin; the bladder meridian of foot taiyang is at the back and the gallbladder meridian of foot shaoyang is at the side.

3.3.3 四肢部

阴经分布在四肢的内侧面，由前往后依次是太阴、厥阴和少阴经；阳经分布在外侧面，由前往后依次是阳明、少阳和太阳经。上(手经)、下肢(足经)同理。

3.3.3 Four limbs

The yin meridians distribute in the inner side of the limbs as the following from the front to the back: the taiyin, jueyin and shaoyin meridian; the yang meridians distribute at the outer side of the four limbs as the following from the front to the back: the yangming, shaoyang and taiyang meridian. The upper limbs (hand meridians) and the lower limbs (foot meridians) are the same.

3.4 十二经脉的流注次序

流注，是人身气血流动不息，向各处灌注的意思。作为气血运行的主要通道。十二经脉从手太阴肺经开始，依次流至足厥阴肝经，再流至手太阴肺经，阴阳相贯，如环无端，循环灌注，分布于全身内外上下，构成了十二经脉的气血循环，又名十二经脉的流注。

3.4 Flow Order of Twelve Meridians

Qi-blood flows ceaselessly over the body. As the main channel of qi-blood circulation, twelve meridians flow from the lung meridian of hand taiyin to the liver meridian of foot jueyin and then to the lung meridian of hand taiyin. Yin and yang meridians communicate with each other around the whole body, forming a qi-blood circulatory route of twelve meridians, also known as the flow order of twelve meridians.

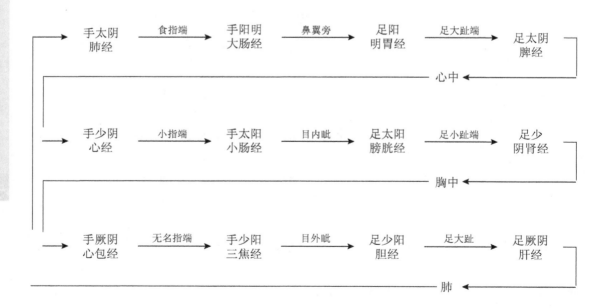

中医理论

Basic Theory of Traditional Chinese Medicine

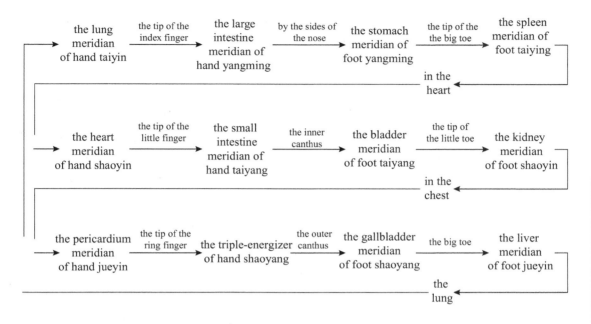

4 奇经八脉

奇经八脉,是督脉、任脉、冲脉、带脉、阴跷脉、阳跷脉、阴维脉、阳维脉的总称。奇经是与正经相对而言的,由于其分布不如十二经脉那样有规律,与五脏六腑没有直接的属络联系,相互之间也没有表里关系,不同于十二正经,故曰"奇经",又因其数有八,故曰"奇经八脉"。

奇经八脉的共同生理功能为:

进一步加强十二经脉之间的联系:如督脉总督一身之阳经;任脉总任一身之阴经;带脉约束纵行诸脉;二跷脉主宰一身左右的阴阳;二维脉维络一身表里的阴阳。

调节十二经脉的气血:十二经脉气有余时,则蓄藏于奇经八

4 Eight Extra Meridians

Extra meridians are of eight, namely du, ren, chong, dai, yinqiao, yangqiao, yinwei and yangwei meridians. The eight extra meridians are relative to the meridian-proper. However, their distribution is not as regular as the twelve meridians and they are not directly affiliated to viscera and there is no external-internal relationship among them, so they get the name "extra meridians". Since there are eight of them, they are also called "eight extra meridians".

Physiological functions of eight extra meridians are as the following.

They further reinforce the relation among the twelve meridians. For example, the du meridian governs the yang channels of the whole body; the ren meridian governs the yin channels of the whole body; the dai meridian constrains the longitudinal meridians; the two-qiao meridians govern the left and right yin and yang of the whole body; the two-wei meridians connect the external-internal yin and yang.

Regulate qi-blood of the twelve meridians: when qi of twelve meridians is excessive, it will be stored in eight extra

脉；十二经脉气血不足时，则由奇经"溢出"及时给予补充。

督、任、冲三脉皆起于胞中，同出于会阴，主要能调节人的生殖机能，带脉束腰如带，能约束纵行诸经，所以督、任、冲、带与妇女的经、带、胎、产关系密切，因此调理冲任是治疗妇科病的重要原则。

4.1　督脉

4.1.1　循行部位

督脉起于小腹内，下出会阴，向后至尾骶部的长强穴，沿脊柱上行，经项部至风府穴，进入脑内，属脑，沿头部正中线，上至巅顶的百会穴，经前额下行鼻柱至鼻尖的素髎穴，过人中，至上齿正中的龈交穴。

4.1.2　生理功能

调节阳经气血：督有总督、统率、督促的意思。督脉循行属于身体阳位的背部；手、足三阳经共六条阳经与督脉交会于大椎穴，督脉对诸阳经有调节作用，有"阳脉之海"之称。

反映脑、肾及脊髓的功能：督脉属脑，络肾。肾生髓，脑为髓海。督脉与脑、肾、脊髓的关系十分密切。

主生殖功能：督脉络肾，与肾气相通，肾主生殖，故督脉与生殖功能有关。

中医理论

Basic Theory of Traditional Chinese Medicine

meridians; when qi-blood of twelve meridians is deficient, it will "spill" out of eight extra meridians to give the timely supplement.

The du, ren and chong meridians all originate from the interior of the lower abdomen and emerge at the perineum mainly to regulate reproductive function. The dai meridian is around the waist like a belt to constrain the longitudinal meridians, so the du, ren, chong and dai meridians are closely related to the female's menstruation, leucorrhea, pregnancy and partum, thus nursing the ren meridian is important in treating gynecological diseases.

4.1　Du Meridian

4.1.1　Running route

The du meridian originates from the interior of the lower abdomen, emerges at the perineum and moves back to the changqiang (DU1) point at the sacrococcygeal region. Ascending along the spine, via the neck, it reaches at the fengfu (GV16) point. Then it enters the brain, and along the midline of the head it reaches the baihui point (DU20) on the top of the head. Via the forehead, it further moves down the stem of the nose to the suliao point (DU25) at the tip of the nose. At last, via philtrum, it arrives at the yinjiao point (DU28) in the middle of the upper teeth.

4.1.2　Physiological functions

"Du" has the meaning of governing, commanding and urging. The du meridian circulates on the back which belongs to the yang position of the body; six yang meridians of hand and foot meet the du meridian at the dazhui point. It regulates the yang meridians and is called the "sea of the yang meridians".

The du meridian, belonging to the brain, is affiliated with the kidneys. The kidneys produce the marrow and the brain is the "sea of marrow". The du meridian is closely related to the brain, the kidneys and the spinal cord.

The du meridian is affiliated with the kidneys and interlinks with kidney-qi. The kidney governs reproduction, so the du meridian is related to the reproductive function.

4.2 任脉

4.2.1 循行部位

任脉起于胞中，下出于会阴，经阴阜，沿腹部正中线上行，经咽喉部（天突穴），到达下唇内，左右分行，环绕口唇，交会于督脉之龈交穴，再分别通过鼻翼两旁，上至眼眶下（承泣穴），交于足阳明胃经。

4.2.2 生理功能

调节阴经气血：任有总任、妊娠之意。任脉循行于腹部正中线，腹为阴；另外，足三阴经在小腹与任脉相交，手三阴经借足三阴经与任脉相通，因此任脉对阴经气血有调节作用，有"阴脉之海"之称。

调节月经，妊养胎儿：任脉起于胞中，具有调节月经，促进女子生殖功能的作用。

5 经络理论的运用

5.1 阐释人体病理变化

在正常生理情况下，经络有运行气血、感应传导的作用。所以在发生病变时，经络就可能成为传递病邪和反映病变的途径。

一般认为，外邪从皮毛腠理而入，传变于五脏六腑，其传变途径就是经络。通过经络的传导，内脏的病变也可以反映于外，表现于某些特定的部位或官窍。如因为足厥阴肝经抵小腹、布胁肋，

4.2 Ren Meridian

4.2.1 Running route

The ren meridian originates from the interior of the lower abdomen, emerges at the perineum. Then, via the mons pubis, it ascends along the midline of the abdomen and via the throat (RN.22), arrives at the inside of the lower lip. It further curves around the lips, arriving at the yinjiao point of the du meridian. At last, through the nose sides, it ascends under the eyes (ST1), and arrives at the stomach meridian of foot yangming.

4.2.2 Physiological functions

"Ren" has the meaning of pregnancy. The ren meridian circulates at the midline of the abdomen which belongs to the yin; besides, the three-yin meridian of foot meets the ren meridian at the lower of the abdomen. The three-yin meridian of hand and the ren meridian are interlinked through the three-yin meridian of foot. Therefore, the ren meridian, regulating qi-blood of the yin meridians, is called "the sea of the yin meridians".

The ren meridian, originating from the interior of the lower abdomen, can regulate menstruation, nourish the fetus and promote reproductive function.

5 Application of Meridian Theory

5.1 Interpreting Pathological Changes

Under normal physiological conditions, the meridian has the function of running qi-blood, induction and conduction. Therefore, when a disease occurs, the meridians may be the way to transfer pathogens and reflect pathological changes.

Generally, pathogens via the meridians go from the skin, body hair and the texture of the subcutaneous flesh to the viscera. Through the meridian's conduction, the pathological changes of the viscera can be reflected on certain exterior areas and orifices. For example, since the liver meridian of foot jueyin enters the lower abdomen,

所以肝气郁结常见两胁、少腹胀痛；因为手少阴心经行于上肢内侧后缘，所以真心痛(心肌梗死)不仅表现为心前区疼痛，且常引及上肢内侧后缘。其他如胃火炽盛见牙龈肿痛，肝火上炎见目赤等与之同理。

经络还是脏腑之间疾病病变相互影响的途径。如肝病犯胃出现胃疼、呕吐，犯肺出现咳逆等，是由于足厥阴肝经挟胃、注肺中；肾虚水泛可凌心、射肺出现咳逆，不能平卧也是因为足少阴肾经入肺、络心。至于相为表里的两经，更因脏腑是相互络属，在病理上常相互影响，如心火可下移小肠，既有口舌生疮，又见小便不利；大肠实热，腑气不通，可使肺气不利而喘咳胸满等等。

这是中医诊断望、闻、问、切的理论依据："有诸内，必行诸外"。

5.2　指导疾病的诊断

由于经络有一定的循行部位和络属的脏腑，在临床上，就可以根据疾病所出现的症状，结合经络循行的部位及其联系的脏腑，作为诊断疾病的依据。例如：两胁疼痛，多为肝胆疾病；缺盆

spreads its branches over the costal and hypochondriac region, stagnation of liver qi may lead to pains of the hypochondria and lower abdomen; as the heart meridian of hand shaoyin runs at the back of the inner side of the upper limbs, genuine heartache (myocardial infarction) not only shows pains in the precordial region but also at the back of the inner side of the upper limbs. Excessive stomach fire shows gingival swelling and pain, while up-flaming of liver qi shows red eyes.

The meridians are also the routes through which the pathological changes of organs influence each other. For example, the liver disease can invade the stomach resulting in gastric pains, vomiting and can invade the lung leading to cough with dyspnea due to the liver meridian of foot jueyin running into the stomach and the lung; kidney deficiency can invade the heart and affect the lung leading to cough with dyspnea; the patient with heart disease can not lie on his or her back, because the kidney meridian of foot shaoyin enters the lung and spreads its branch over the heart. The external-internal meridians often interact with each other pathologically, because viscera are affiliated with each other. For example, the heart fire descends to the small intestine showing mouth sores and difficulty in micturition; excess heat in the large intestine and bowel gas barrier make lung-qi unsmooth, showing cough and fullness in the chest etc.

This is the theoretical basis for the diagnosis of TCM—observing, listening, questioning and feeling the pulse: "Changes inside the human body is bound to reflect on the external".

5.2　Guiding Diagnosing Diseases

The meridians have certain running routes and affiliated viscera. Clinically, the doctor can take the symptoms together with the running routes of the meridians and affiliated viscera as the basis for the diagnosis of the disease. For example, pains in the hypochondria often indicate diseases of the liver and gallbladder; pains in the supraclavicular fossa often indicate the lesion of the lung.

中痛，常是肺的病变。头痛常按疼痛部位来诊断，如痛在前额者，多属阳明经；痛在两侧者，多属少阳经；痛在后头部及项部者，多属太阳经；痛在巅顶者，多属厥阴经。《伤寒论》的六经辨证与经络的三阴经、三阳经同出一辙。

在临床实践中，观察在经络循行的通路上或某些穴位处，是否有明显的压痛或有结节状、条索状的反应物，或局部皮肤的形态变化，也常有助于疾病的诊断。如肺脏病人在其肺俞穴或中府穴会出现结节或压痛，肠痈病人的阑尾穴会有压痛，脾胃不好的病人可在脾俞穴见到异常变化等。

5.3　指导疾病的治疗

经络学说被广泛地用以指导临床各科的治疗，特别是对针灸、按摩和药物治疗，更具有重要指导意义。

针灸与按摩疗法，必须按经络学说，根据经络的循行分布路线和联系范围来选穴，这就是"循经取穴"。根据某一经或某一脏腑的病变，通过针灸或按摩病变的邻近部位或经络循行的远端穴位，调整经络气血的功能活动，从而达到治疗的目的。

药物治疗也离不开经络。在长期临床实践中，根据某些药物对某一脏腑经络有特殊作用，确定了"药物归经"理论，金元时期的医家更是提出了"引经报使"药，如治太阳经头痛，可用羌活，

Headache is diagnosed according to the location of the pain. For example, front headache usually relates to the yangming meridian; lateral headache usually relates to the shaoyang meridian; occipital headache and nape pain often relate to the taiyang meridian; vertical headache often relates to the jueyin meridian. Differentiation of syndromes according to the theory of six meridians in *Treatise on Cold Damage Diseases* is the same as the three- yin and yang meridians.

Clinically, observing whether there is apparent tenderness or nodular, reactant cords or morphological changes on the skin along the running routes and some points is conducive to diagnosis of the disease. For example, patients with the lung disease may have the nodule and tenderness in feiyu point and zhongfu point; patients with abdominal carbuncle may have tenderness in lanwei point (EX21); patients with weak spleen and stomach may have an unusual change in piyu point.

5.3　Guiding Treatment of Disease

The meridian theory is widely used to guide the clinical treatment of diseases in various departments, especially in acumoxibustion, massage and pharmacotherapy.

Acumoxibustion and massage therapy must rely on the meridian theory to select points according to the running routes and contact points of the meridians, which is called "selecting points according to the meridians". On the basis of lesions of one meridian and organ, the functional activities of the meridians and qi-blood are adjusted by acupuncture or massage of the adjacent parts of the lesion or distal points of the running routes to meet the treatment aim.

Pharmacotherapy also depends on the meridians. In the long-term clinical practice, the theory of "meridian-tropism of medicinal" is founded according to the special effects of some medicine on a certain organ or meridian. Doctors in Jin and Yuan dynasties put forward "channel conduction" drugs, which means that certain drugs can guide other drugs to reach the lesion site or a meridian. For

中医理论

Basic Theory of Traditional Chinese Medicine

治阳明经头痛用白芷,治少阳经头痛用柴胡等。

此外,针刺麻醉,以及耳针、电针、穴位埋线、穴位结扎等等治疗方法,都是在经络学说的指导下进行的,并使经络学说得到一定的发展。

经络系统遍布全身,气、血、津液通过经络,才能输布人体各部,发挥其濡养、温煦作用。脏腑之间,脏腑与各形体官窍之间,也是通过经络维持其密切联系,使其各自发挥正常的功能。所以经络的生理功能,主要表现在运行气血、沟通人体内外、联络人体上下,将人体各部组织器官联结成为一个有机的整体,通过经络的调节作用,保持人体正常生理活动的平衡协调。同时经络又是人体的信息传导系统,它能够接受和传导各种信息。

example, notopterygium root is used to cure headache of the taiyang meridian, angelica root is used to cure headache of the yangming meridian and bupleurum root can be used to cure headache of the shaoyang meridian.

Besides, acupuncture anesthesia and auricular needling, electroacupuncture, catgut implantation at acupoint, acupoint ligation and other treatments are carried out under the guidance of meridian theory and at the same time, they promote the development of meridian theory.

The meridian system covers the whole body through which qi, blood and body fluid can be transported to each part of the body and processes the function of nourishing and warming. The close contact among the organs, and the connection between the organs, the body and orifices are maintained by the meridians; their normal functions are also guaranteed by the meridians. So, the physiological functions of the meridians mainly reflect on running qi and blood, contacting the inside of the body with the outside, relating the upper part of the body with the lower, connecting all the tissues and organs together as an organic whole. Through the adjustment of the meridians, the balance and coordination of the normal physiological activities of the body can be maintained. At the same time, the meridians as the conductive system of the body can accept and conduct various information.

第五章　病因病机

Chapter 5　Etiology and Pathomechanism

凡能破坏人体生理动态平衡而导致人体发生疾病的原因，称之为病因。

致病因素多种多样，如气候异常、瘟疫流行、精神刺激、饮食劳倦、虫兽所伤等。为便于了解和把握，历代医家提出不同的分类方法。《黄帝内经》把风雨寒暑等外来病因归属于阳，把饮食喜怒等内生病因归属于阴。

宋·陈无择把病因与发病途径结合起来，把六淫外感归为外所因，七情内伤归为内所因，饮食劳倦、虫兽金刃等归为不内外因，明确提出了三因学说，对后世医家影响较大，现代中医病因依然以此分类。

在疾病的发生发展过程中，原因和结果是相互作用、相互影响的。某一阶段中的病理结果，有可能成为另一阶段中致病的原因。如痰饮、瘀血等，是脏腑气血功能失调所形成的病理产物，又会成为新的病因，导致其他病理变化，出现各种症状和体征。

All that causes disharmony in the dynamic balance of the human body's physiology and leads to diseases are called pathogenic factors.

There are many and varied pathogenic factors, such as abnormal climate changes, plagues, emotional stimulation, improper diet, overstrain and insect or animal bites. The ancient physicians proposed different classifications for people to better understand and grasp them. *Huangdi's Internal classic* attributes external causes such as wind, rain, cold and summer-heat to yang, and the internal factors such as improper diet, joy and anger to yin.

Chen Wuze of the Song dynasty combined the pathogenic factors with the way of disease occurrence and clearly put forth "the doctrine of three causes", i.e., exogenous pathogens (invasion by the six climatic factors), endogenous pathogens (internal injury caused by emotional factors) and non-exo-endogenous pathogens (injury due to improper diet, overstrain, insect or animal bites and traumatic wound), which influenced later physicians greatly. The modern TCM etiologies are still classified based on this theory.

In the development of diseases, cause and effect are always interacting with and thus influencing each other. An effect in a pathological stage may be a cause in another pathological stage. Examples are phlegm-stagnant-fluid and blood stasis, which are pathological outcomes of a disturbance of the functions of viscera, qi and blood, may become factors of new diseases leading to other pathological changes and various symptoms and physical signs.

中医病因学有以下两个特点：

整体观念：在天人相应统一整体观的指导下，中医学将人体与自然环境，人体内部各脏腑组织的功能联系起来，用整体的、联系的、发展的观点，探讨致病因素在疾病发生、发展、变化中的作用，辩证地探讨了气候变化、饮食劳倦和精神活动等在发病过程中的作用，奠定了中医病因学的理论基础。如肝属木，在四时应春，在六气为风，在五味为酸，在志为怒，在体合筋，开窍于目，与胆相表里。故气候异常变化的"风"，情志过激的"怒"，饮食失调的"酸"等均与肝脏病变密切相关。

辨证求因：中医临床是根据疾病反映出来的临床表现，通过分析疾病的症状和体征来推求病因，为治疗用药提供理论依据。这种方法称为"辨证求因"或"审症求因"。如自然界风性善行，风胜则动。临床但凡见到周身游走性疼痛或瘙痒，就可以确认其病因为"风"邪。不管实际致病因素多么复杂，只要人体出现了"风"这种反应状态，就可以用"风邪"来概括之。治疗时只要采用相应的"祛风"药物，就可使临床症状缓解或消失。

本章根据疾病的发病途径及形成过程，将病因分为外感病因（六淫、疫疠）、七情内伤、病理产物性病因（痰饮、瘀血），

TCM Etiology has two characteristics.

Conception of holism: Under the guidance of the correspondence between nature and humanity, TCM explores the roles of pathogenic factors in the process of disease occurrence, development and change, by connecting the natural environment with the human body, and the functions of organs and tissues inside the body. It explores the effects of climate change, improper diet, overstrain and mental activities and sets the theoretical foundation of TCM etiology. To name just one example: the liver pertains to wood in five elements and associates with spring in four seasons, with wind in six natural factors and acid in five flavors, with anger in emotion and tendons in constituent, with eyes in orifice, and forms an exterior-interior relationship with gallbladder. Therefore, abnormal changes of climate— "wind", emotional excesses of "anger," eating disorders of "acid" are all closely related to liver disease.

Inferring the cause by syndrome differentiation: TCM Clinic provides theoretical basis for clinical treatment and prescription by observing the clinical manifestations and analyzing the symptoms and physical signs of the disease to infer the cause. The process is called "inferring the cause by syndrome differentiation". For example, in the nature wind is characterized by constant movement, so when wind pathogen prevails, movement occurs. Clinically, whenever there is migratory pain or pruritus changeable in location all over the body, it can be identified as wind pathogen. However complicated the pathogenic factors might seem, as long as the symptom of "wind" occurs, it can be categorized as "wind pathogen". The clinical symptoms will be eased or disappear by using the appropriate "wind expelling" medicine.

This chapter puts pathogenic factors into four categories based on ways of disease outbreak and formation process: exogenous etiology (six climatic factors, pestilence), internal injury caused by emotional factors, pathological product

以及其他病因(饮食、劳倦、外伤等)四类。

etiology (phlegm-stagnant-fluid, blood stasis), and other pathogenic factors (improper diet, overstrain, trauma).

1 六淫

1.1 六淫的基本概念

1.1.1 六气

是指风、寒、暑、湿、燥、火六种正常的自然界气候。六气的变化是万物生长的条件。人类通过自身的调节机制产生了一定的适应能力,从而使人体的生理活动与六气的变化相适应。所以,正常的六气一般不易于使人生病。

1.1.2 六淫

六淫,是风、寒、暑、湿、燥、火六种外感病邪的统称。阴阳相移、寒暑更作、气候变化都有一定的规律和限度。如果气候变化异常,六气发生太过或不及,或非其时而有其气(如春天当温而反寒,冬季当凉而反热),以及气候变化过于急骤(如暴寒暴暖);或有人因其适应能力低下,气候变化超过了其适应的限度,就会导致疾病的发生。于是,对人体无害的六气就转化为能导致机体发生疾病的"六淫",又称"六邪"。

1.2 六淫致病的共同特点

1.2.1 季节性

由于六淫本为四时主气的太过或不及,故容易形成季节性

1 The Six Climatic Pathogens

1.1 The Concepts of Six Climatic Pathogens

1.1.1 Six climatic factors

They refer to six kinds of normal climate factors of wind, cold, summer-heat, dampness, dryness and fire. The change of six climatic factors is the basic prerequisite for the growth of everything. Human beings evolve certain ability through their own regulatory mechanism to adapt to the change. So, normally the six climatic factors do not cause diseases.

1.1.2 Six climate pathogens

They are a collective term used for six kinds of exogenous pathogens of wind, cold, summer-heat, dampness, dryness and fire. With the transferrence of yin and yang and change of winter and summer, the climate changes according to certain regulations and within certain limits. They will cause diseases only when the climate changes abnormally, the climatic factors are excessive or weak, or occur in the wrong season (e.g.: It's supposed to be warm in spring while it's too cold instead, and it's supposed to be cold in winter yet it's too hot instead.), or there is a sudden and sharp climate change (e.g.: The weather gets too cold or too hot suddenly.); or when some people are weak in adaption and the climate change is beyond their resistance. In this way, six climatic factors harmless to the human body are transformed into "six climatic pathogens" that can cause diseases, which are also called "six evils".

1.2 Common Pathogenic Characteristics of Six Climatic Pathogens

1.2.1 Seasonality

The six climatic pathogens are the excess or deficiency of the four main seasons, so they tend to cause seasonal

中医理论

Basic Theory of Traditional Chinese Medicine

的常见病、多发病。如春季多伤风,夏季多中暑,长夏易伤湿病,秋季多干燥,冬季多寒病等。但是,气候变化是复杂的,不同体质对外邪的感受性不同,所以同一季节可以有不同性质的外感病发生。

diseases such as catching cold in spring, heat stroke in summer, wet disease in summer, dry disease in autumn, cold disease in winter. However, since climate change is complex, and different people have different physical sensitivity of external evil, therefore different exogenous diseases occur in the same season.

1.2.2 地域性

地域性指不同地域如工作或居处环境不同,有不同的发病特点,如北方气候寒冷,多病痹痛;南方气候炎热多雨,多病湿热、温病;久处潮湿环境多有湿邪;干燥环境多燥邪;高温环境常有火热之邪等。

1.2.2 Regionalism

Different areas, including work or living conditions, have different morbidity characteristics. For example, it is cold in the north, so there occur more diseases like arthralgia; it is hot and rainy in the south, so there occur damp and hot and febrile diseases; staying in damp and wet condition for a long period can cause damp evil; there occurs more dry evil in dry conditions; there usually occur fire and hot evil in high temperature environment, etc.

1.2.3 外感性

六淫之邪多从肌表或口鼻而入,侵犯人体,故六淫致病,多有由表及里的传变过程。

1.2.3 External perception

The six climatic pathogens always invade human beings from the body surface or the nose and mouth. The diseases caused by climatic pathogens mainly develop from the outside to the inside.

1.2.4 相兼性

六淫邪气既可单独致病又可相兼为害,如风寒感冒、湿热泄泻、风寒湿痹等。

1.2.4 Combination

The six climatic pathogens can cause diseases separately and jointly, such as, common cold of wind-cold type, diarrhea due to damp-heat and arthralgia due to wind-cold dampness and so on.

1.2.5 转化性

六淫致病以后,在疾病发展过程中,其病理性质可向不同于病因性质的方向转化,如六淫皆可化火等。

1.2.5 Transformation

In the course of disease development after the disease occurrence caused by the six climatic pathogens, their pathological nature can transform into the direction different from the etiological properties. Such as, all of the six climatic pathogens can transform into fire.

1.3 六淫的性质及其致病特点

1.3 The Nature and Pathogenic Characteristics of the Six Climatic Pathogens

1.3.1 风

风具有轻扬开泄,善动不居

1.3.1 Wind

The wind is characterized by dispersing and constantly

的特性,为春季主气。

风邪具有一系列性质和致病特点。

轻扬开泄:风为阳邪,其性轻扬升散。所以风邪致病,容易伤人上部、肌表等阳位。因其性开泄,使肌腠疏松,汗孔开张,而出现汗出、恶风等症状。

善行数变:风善动不居,易行而无定处。"善行"是指风邪致病有病位游移、行无定处的特性,如风疹、荨麻疹之发无定处,此起彼伏;行痹(风痹)之四肢关节游走性疼痛等,均属风气盛的表现。"数变",是指风邪致病具有变化无常和发病急骤的特性,如风疹、荨麻疹之时隐时现,中风之猝然昏倒、不省人事等。总之,风邪致病,无论是外感还是内伤,一般都具有发病急、变化多、传变快等特征。

风性主动:风邪致病具有动摇不定的特征,如眩晕、震颤、四肢抽搐、角弓反张、直视上吊等症状,故称"风胜则动"。

风为百病之长:风虽为春季的主气,但终岁常在,四时皆有。风邪又是外感病因的先导,寒、湿、燥、热等邪,往往都依附于风而侵袭人体,如风寒、风热、风湿等,故称风为百病之长,六淫之首。

1.3.2 寒

寒具有寒冷、凝结特性,为

moving. It prevails in spring.

The nature and pathogenic characteristics of wind will be discussed in the following sections.

Dispersing: Wind is a yang pathogen and is characterized by dispersing. Therefore, wind pathogen tends to invade the upper part of the body, body surface and other yang portions. It loosens the striae of the skin and muscles and open the pores leading to sweating and aversion to wind.

Constant movement and rapid change: Wind is characterized by constant movement and instability. "Constant movement" means the diseases caused by wind pathogen possess the feature of emigration. For example, rubella and nettle rash migrate around one after another without a certain location. In a migratory arthralgia or wind arthralgia syndrome, the pain migrates in limbs and joints, which is a sign of wind pathogen prevalence. "Rapid change" denotes that diseases caused by wind pathogen are characterized by sudden attack and quick transformation, such as the rising and going of rubella and nettle rash, the sudden faint of stroke without consciousness and so on. In a word, diseases caused by wind pathogen, be it external or internal, feature rapid onset, various change and quick transformation.

Activity: Wind is characterized by activity and restlessness, such as dizziness, tremor, twitching limbs and opisthotonos and other wind syndromes, so there is the saying, "domination of wind pathogen may disturb the body".

Wind is the first and foremost factor of diseases. Wind as the dominant qi of spring, remains in four seasons. Cold, dampness, dryness and heat pathogens often follow wind pathogen which is a leading exopathic factor invading the body, such as wind-cold, wind-heat and wind-dampness. So wind is the first and foremost factor of diseases, and is the most common factor among the six climatic pathogens.

1.3.2 Cold

Cold, characterized by coldness and condensation, is

冬季主气。

寒邪具有以下性质和致病特点。

寒易伤阳：寒为阴气，"阴盛则寒"，"阴盛则阳病"。所以寒邪伤人，阳气受损，肌体失于温煦，故全身或局部可出现明显的寒象。如寒邪束表，则恶寒、无汗；若肺脾受寒，则咳嗽喘促、痰液清稀或水肿；寒伤脾肾，则畏寒肢冷、腰脊冷痛、尿清便溏、水肿腹水等；若心肾阳虚，寒邪直中少阴，则可见恶寒蜷卧、手足厥冷、下利清谷、精神萎靡、脉微细等。

寒性凝滞：凝滞，凝结阻滞。人体气血津液有赖阳气的温煦推动，才能运行输布全身。寒邪侵犯人体，使气血凝结阻滞，涩滞不通，不通则痛，故疼痛是寒邪致病的重要特征。因寒而痛，其痛得温则减，逢寒剧增。

寒性收引：是指寒邪具有收引拘急之特性。"寒则气收"。寒邪侵袭人体，可使气机收敛，腠理闭塞，经络筋脉收缩而挛急；若寒客肌表，则毛孔收缩，故恶寒而无汗；若寒客经络关节，则筋脉收缩拘急，以致拘挛作痛、屈伸不利。

1.3.3 暑

暑为夏季主气，有明显的季节性，主要发生在夏至以后，立秋以前。暑邪独见于夏令，纯属外

prevalent in winter.

Cold pathogen is apt to attack yang. Cold pertains to yin. "Excessive yin leads to cold" and "excessive yin leads to yang diseases". Cold pathogen invading the body leads to damage of yang-qi and failure in warming the body, so there appear evident cold syndromes around the whole body or at local parts. For example, cold pathogen invading the exterior can lead to aversion to cold and no sweating; cold pathogen invading the lung and spleen can lead to cough, dyspnea, thin sputum or edema; cold pathogen hurting the spleen and kidney can lead to aversion to cold and cold limbs, cold pain in the lumbar spine, clear urine, loose stool, edema and abdominal dropsy; yang deficiency of the heart and kidney and cold pathogen hitting shaoyin can lead to aversion to cold, cold hands and feet, watery diarrhea with indigested food in the stool, listlessness and faint and thin pulse.

Cold is characterized by condensation, stagnation, and obstruction. Qi, blood and body fluid rely on the warming and promoting function of yang-qi to distribute around the body. Cold pathogen invading the body makes blood condense and stagnate, leading to pains, which are the most important signs of cold pathogen causing diseases. Pains caused by cold alleviate with warmth and aggravate with cold.

Cold is characterized by contraction, traction and constriction. "Cold makes qi contract." Cold pathogen invading the body may depress qi dynamic, constrict the striae, tighten the meridians, tendons and vessels. If cold pathogen invades the body surface, pores will be contracted and there will appear aversion to cold and no sweating. If cold pathogen attacks meridians and joints, tendons and vessels will tighten, and there will appear spasm and pain and impaired movement.

1.3.3 Summer heat

Summer heat, with obvious season characteristics, hosts qi for summer time. It mainly occurs before autumn and after summer solstice. Summer-heat pathogen exclusively exists in summer time, purely refers to external

中医理论

Basic Theory of Traditional Chinese Medicine

邪,无内暑之说。

暑邪具有以下性质和致病特点。

暑性炎热。暑为夏月炎暑,具有酷热之性,属阳邪。暑邪伤人多表现出一系列阳热症状,如高热、心烦、面赤、烦躁、脉象洪大等,称为伤暑(或暑热)。

暑性升散。升,指暑邪易于上犯头目,内扰心神;散,指暑邪为害,易于伤津耗气;故暑邪侵犯人体,可致腠理开泄而大汗出,汗多伤津则可出现口渴喜饮,唇干舌燥,尿赤短少等。在大量出汗同时,往往气随津泄,而导致气虚,可见到气短乏力。

暑热之邪,不仅耗气伤津,还可扰动心神,引起心烦闷乱而不宁,甚则突然昏倒、不省人事等症。

暑多挟湿:暑季常多雨而潮湿,热蒸湿动,湿热弥漫。暑邪为患除发热、烦渴等暑热症状外,常兼见四肢困倦、胸闷呕恶、大便溏泄不爽等湿阻症状。

暑邪致病的基本特征为热盛、阴伤、耗气,又多挟湿。所以,临床上以壮热、阴亏、气虚、湿阻为特征。

1.3.4 湿

湿具有重浊、黏滞、趋下特性,为长夏主气。亦可因涉水淋

evil rather than internal heat.

Its nature and pathogenic characteristics can be manifested as follows.

Summer heat is characterized by burning heat. Summer heat is a yang pathogen since summer is scorching-hot. It hurts people mostly in a series of yang heat symptoms, manifesting as high fever, vexation, flushed face, dysthesia and rapid large surging pulse, which is called summer-heat injury.

Summer heat by nature ascends and dissipates. Ascending means that summer-heat pathogen is apt to invade the head and disturb the internal spirit; dissipating refers to its consumption of qi damages liquid as a harmful pathogen. Therefore, the invasion of the summer-heat pathogen may open the striae and lead to heavy sweating, which will impair the body fluid, manifesting as thirst for water, dry lips and tongue and scanty dark yellow urine. While there is heavy sweating, qi flew away along with the loss of body fluid, resulting in qi deficiency, short breath and fatigue.

Summer-heat pathogen causes not only the consumption of qi and damage of body fluid, but also the disturbance of the internal spirit, resulting in sudden faint and unconsciousness.

Summer heat often combines with dampness. It is often rainy and damp in summer with heat and steam filling the air. Except for summer heat symptoms such as fever, vexation and thirst, some damp obstruction syndromes including fatigued cumbersome limbs, oppression in the chest, vomiting and loose stools are all triggered by summer-heat pathogen.

Because the basic pathogenic characteristics are exuberant heat, damage to yin and consumption of qi, as well as dampness in the heat pathogen, the clinical syndromes are characterized by vigorous heat, yin depletion, qi deficiency and damp obstruction.

1.3.4 Dampness

Dampness, being prevalent in late summer, is characterized by heaviness and turbidity, stickiness and

中医理论

Basic Theory of Traditional Chinese Medicine

雨、居处伤湿,或以水为事。

　　湿邪具有以下性质和致病特点。

　　湿为阴邪,易阻气机,损伤阳气:湿性类水,水属于阴,故湿为阴邪。湿邪侵及人体,最易阻滞气机,从而使气机升降失常。湿阻胸膈则胸闷;湿困脾胃,则不思饮食、脘痞腹胀、便溏不爽。"湿胜则阳微",由湿邪郁遏使阳气不伸者,当用化气利湿通利小便的方法,使气机通畅,水道通调,则湿邪可从小便而去,湿去则阳气自通。

　　湿性重浊:所谓"重",即沉重、重着之意。湿邪致病,其临床症状有沉重的特性,如头重身困、四肢酸楚沉重等。所谓"浊",即秽浊垢腻之意。湿邪为患,易于出现排泄物和分泌物秽浊不清的现象,如面垢、眵多、下痢脓血、小便浑浊、带下过多以及湿疹、脓水秽浊等。

　　湿性黏滞:黏滞是指湿邪致病具有黏腻停滞的特性,主要表现在两个方面:一是症状的黏滞性,即湿病症状多黏滞而不爽,如大便黏腻不爽,小便涩滞不畅,以及分泌物黏浊和舌苔黏腻等。二是病程的缠绵性。因湿性黏滞,蕴蒸不化,胶着难解,故起病缓慢隐袭,病程较长,往往反复发作或缠绵难愈。如湿温、湿疹、湿痹(着

stasis and downward sinking. Dampness damage also involves wading through water and getting soaked in the rain, living in dampness or doing water-based work.

Its nature and pathogenic characteristics can be manifested as follows.

As the yin pathogen, dampness obstructs qi dynamic and damages yang qi. Dampness is called as a yin pathogen because its nature is like water, which belongs to yin. The invasion of damp-pathogen to our body can easily obstruct qi dynamic, triggering abnormal ascending and descending of qi dynamic. Damp retention in the chest can result in thoracic oppression; damp retention in the spleen and stomach can lead to no appetite, abdominal distention and loose stool. Exuberance in dampness leads to yang debilitation. The insufficiency of yang qi caused by damp-pathogen depression can be treated by promoting qi transformation and removing dampness to alleviate water retention to free the qi dynamic and waterway, so dampness can be removed along with urinating and yang qi will be smooth.

Dampness by nature is heavy and turbid. "Heaviness" refers to ponderosity. Clinically, the damp-pathogen is characterized by heaviness, such as heavy head, fatigued body and aching limbs. "Turbidity" refers to dirtiness and greasiness. Damp-pathogen is a factor to cause turbid excreta and secretion, for instance, grimy facial complexion, much eye discharge, dysentery with pus and blood, turbid urine, excessive vaginal discharge, eczema and foul pus.

Dampness is viscous by nature. Viscosity means that the damp-pathogen is characterized by stickiness and stagnancy. It can be manifested in two aspects. Firstly, symptoms with viscosity. The damp disease is always sticky and stagnant, such as ungratifying sticky defecation, inhibited stagnant urine, foul pus and slimy tongue fur. Secondly, the course of disease is lingering. Damp disease is slow in occurence and long in course because of the humid viscosity and sticky conglutination. They cannot be quickly cured due to their dampness, such as damp warmth, eczema and damp impediment (fixed impediment).

痹）等，因其湿而不易速愈。

湿性趋下：湿类于水，其质重浊，故湿邪有下趋之势。其病如带下、小便浑浊、泄泻、下痢等多见下部的症状。

1.3.5　燥

燥具有干燥、收敛清肃特性，为秋季主气。燥邪为病，有温燥、凉燥之分。夏末初秋燥与热相合多病温燥。深秋近冬燥与寒合多病凉燥。

燥邪的性质和致病特点：

燥易伤津：燥与湿对，其性干涩枯涸，故曰"燥胜则干"。燥邪为害，最易耗伤人体的津液，形成阴津亏损的病变，表现出各种干涩的症状和体征，诸如皮肤干涩皲裂、鼻干咽燥、口唇燥裂、毛发干枯不荣、小便短少、大便干燥等。

燥易伤肺：肺喜清肃濡润而恶燥。肺主气而司呼吸，直接与自然界大气相通，且外合皮毛，开窍于鼻，燥邪多从口鼻而入。燥为秋令主气，与肺相应，故燥邪最易伤肺，从而出现干咳少痰，或痰黏难咳，或痰中带血，以及喘息胸痛等。

1.3.6　火（热）

火具有炎热特性，旺于夏季。

火邪的性质和致病特点：

Dampness by nature descends. Dampness and water are alike. Because of its heavy and turbid nature, damp-pathogen tends to descend. Most symptoms occur in the lower body, for instance, vaginal discharge, turbid urine, diarrhea and dysentery.

1.3.5　Dryness

Dryness, characterized by constraining and purging, hosts qi for the autumn. Dry-pathogen is divided into warm and cool dryness. Dryness combining with heat mostly belongs to warm character in the end of the summer and at the outset of the autumn, while with cold, mostly cool character at the late autumn.

Its nature and pathogenic characteristics can be manifested as follows.

Dryness tends to damage body fluid. Dryness is the opposite of dampness, which by nature is dry and astringent. There is saying that "when dryness prevails, there is aridity". It is apt to impair body fluid as a harmful pathogen, forming insufficiency of yin liquid and manifesting as various dry symptoms, such as skin rhagades, dry nose and throat, cracked lips, hair xerasia, short voidings of scant urine and stool xerosis.

Dryness tends to damage the lung. The lung loves to be clear and hates to be dry. It governs qi and controls respiration, directly communicates with the atmosphere from the nature, associates with skin, body hair and with nose in orifice. Dry-pathogen usually invades through the mouth and nose. It can easily damage the lung because dryness hosts qi for the autumn and corresponds with the lung. Symptoms are followed as dry cough with scant phlegm, stick phlegm difficult to expectorate, phlegm containing blood or panting and chest pain.

1.3.6　Heat (fire)

Heat is the prominent climate factor in summer.

The following is the brief description of the nature and characteristics of heat in causing disease.

中医理论

Basic Theory of Traditional Chinese Medicine

火性炎上：炎，热也。故火邪致病，临床上表现出高热、恶热、脉洪数等热盛之证。上指火为阳邪，其性升腾向上，故火邪致病多表现于上部，如心火之舌尖红赤疼痛、口舌糜烂、生疮；肝火上炎之头痛如裂、目赤肿痛；胃火炽盛之齿龈肿痛、齿衄等。

伤津耗气：火热之邪，蒸腾于内，最易迫津外泄，消烁津液，使人体阴津耗伤。故火邪致病，其临床表现除热象显著外，往往伴有口渴喜饮、咽干舌燥、小便短赤、大便秘结等津伤液耗之症。阳热亢盛之壮火，最能损伤人体正气，此外，火迫津泄，津液虚少无以化气，亦可导致气虚，可见少气懒言、肢体乏力等气虚之症。

生风动血：火热之邪侵袭人体，耗伤津血，使筋脉失于濡养，而出现四肢抽搐、颈项强直、角弓反张、目睛上视等风证。火热之邪，灼伤脉络，并使血行加速，迫血妄行，易于引起各种出血，如吐血、衄血、便血、尿血，以及皮肤发斑，妇女月经过多、崩漏等。

易扰心神：心主血脉而藏神。火热之邪，迫血妄行，故最易扰乱神明，轻则心烦失眠，狂躁妄动，甚则神昏谵语，危及生命。

易致肿疡：火热之邪入于血分，聚于局部，腐肉败血，则发为痈肿疮疡。临床表现以疮疡局部红肿热痛为特征。

Heat tends to flame up. Heat pertains to yang. So the disease caused by the pathogenic heat is marked by high fever, aversion to heat, extreme heat and large and rapid pulse. Heat tends to flame up. So the pathogenic heat attacks the upper body with the syndrome of red and painful tongue with erosion and sores, pathogenic lung-heat with the syndrome of severe headache and swollen red eyes, stomach-heat with the syndrome of swollen teeth and bleeding from the gum.

Heat tends to consume qi and impair body fluid. Heat tends to consume yin-fluid. It will drive body fluid out of the body. So the disease caused by the pathogenic heat is often accompanied with thirst, dry throat and tongue, dark and scanty urine and retention of dry feces due to consumption and impairment of body fluid. The pathogenic heat as a hyperactive fire consumes the healthy qi. Besides, exuberance of heat also impairs the healthy qi causing the deficiency of vital qi with the syndromes of physical weakness and no desire to speak.

Heat tends to produce wind and disturb blood. When heat invades the body, it usually scorches the liver meridians, consumes body fluid and deprives the tendons of moisture and nourishment, leading to occurrence of convulsion of the four limbs, stiff neck, opisthotonos and upward view. But if the heat is excessive, it will drive blood to flow very fast or scorch the vessels, leading to various hemorrhages, such as hematemesis, epistaxis, hematochezia, hematuria, skin spots, menorrhea, and metrorrhagia.

Heat tends to disturb mind. Heart dominates blood and meridians, and also possesses mind. Pathogenic heat forces blood to move frenetically, so it's apt to disrupt the minds, resulting in symptoms ranging from irritability, insomnia, mania to coma and delirium, and so threatening life.

Heat tends to cause swelling and ulceration. When heat invades blood phase and accumulates in local area, it will putrefy blood and muscles, causing abscess, furuncle and ulceration, manifesting clinically as local redness, swelling, heat and pain.

2 疠气

2.1 疠气的基本概念

疠气是一类具有强烈传染性的病邪,又名戾气、疫疠之气、毒气、异气、杂气、乖戾之气等。疠气通过空气和接触传染。

2.2 疠气的性质及其致病特点

发病急骤,病情危笃:疫疠之气具有发病急骤、来势凶猛、病情险恶、变化多端、传变快的特点,且易伤津、扰神、动血、生风。疠气与火热之邪致病相似,但毒热较火热为甚,而且常挟有湿毒、毒雾、瘴气等秽浊之气,故其致病作用更为剧烈险恶,死亡率也高。

传染性强,易于流行:疫疠之气具有强烈的传染性和流行性,无论男女老幼,身体强壮与否,触之即可发病。这一点与六淫区别甚大。其发病可散在,也可以大面积流行。如大头瘟、蛤蟆瘟、疫痢、白喉、烂喉丹痧、天花、霍乱、鼠疫等,实际包括现代医学许多传染病和烈性传染病。

症状相似,一气一病:疠气种类不同,所致之病各异,但每一种疠气均有各自独特的临床特征和传变规律,一气一病,症状相似。

3 七情

七情是指喜、怒、忧、思、悲、恐、惊等七种情志活动,是人体对外界事物的情感反应。七情一般

2 Pestilence

2.1 The Basic Concept of Pestilence

Pestilence is a strong infectious pathogenic disease. It is also known as pathogenic factor, pestilence qi, poison qi, abnormal qi, mixed qi, surly qi and etc. Pestilence is infected through air and contact.

2.2 The Nature and Pathogenic Characteristics of Pestilence

Pestilence features acute onset and severe pathological condition. Pestilence qi is marked by an acute onset, severe pathological condition, changeable and quick transmission characteristics, and it is apt to consume body fluid, disturb mind, move blood and produce wind. It is quite similar to the pathogenic heat in the six pathogenic climate factors in nature, but toxic heat is more serious, often carrying damp toxicity, toxic smog, malaria and other turbid qi, so its pathogenic role is more violent and dangerous with high mortality.

Pestilence qi has strong infection and epidemicity. Everyone, regardless of age, sex, or physical condition can suffer from it once they contact it. This is very different from the six climatic pathogens. It can be scattered, and be epidemic in a large area including bulk disease, plague, frog ekiri, diphtheria, scarlet fever, smallpox, cholera, pestis and so on, including many infectious diseases and other severe infectious diseases in modern medicine.

Pestilence has similar symptoms while one pestilence qi corresponds to one disease. Different pestilence qi causes different diseases. Each kind of pestilence qi has its own unique clinical features and transmission.

3 The Seven Emotions

Seven emotions refer to joy, anger, worry, thinking, sorrow, fear and fright. They are emotional reaction of the body to the things outside. They generally do not cause

中医理论 Basic Theory of Traditional Chinese Medicine

不会使人致病。只有强烈、持久或突然的情志刺激，超过人体本身的正常生理活动范围，使人体气机紊乱，脏腑阴阳气血失调，才会导致疾病的发生。七情因其由内发病，故又称"内伤七情"。七情的致病特点如下：

3.1 直接伤及脏腑

人体的情志活动与脏腑有密切关系，所以情志刺激最易伤及脏腑。七情损伤脏腑，主要有三种情况，一是特异性损伤，即根据五脏和五志的联系，如喜伤心、怒伤肝、思伤脾、悲忧伤肺、恐伤肾。二是心藏神，肝主疏泄、调畅情志，脾藏意，情志所伤，数情交织，多伤及心肝脾。三是情志所伤，多伤及潜病之脏腑。

3.2 影响脏腑气机

七情致病主要是导致脏腑气机紊乱，阴阳失调。

怒则气上。气上，气机上逆之意。暴怒伤肝，使肝气疏泄太过而上逆为病。肝气上逆，可见头晕头痛、面赤耳鸣，甚至呕血或昏厥。肝气横逆，犯脾可见腹胀、飧泄。犯胃可出现呃逆、呕吐等。

喜则气缓。气缓，心气弛缓之意。暴喜伤心，使心气涣散，神不守舍，出现乏力、懈怠、注

diseases. Only sudden, intense or prolonged emotional stimulation beyond the regulatory range of physiological activities of the body can cause disturbances of qi dynamic, disorders of yin-yang and qi-blood of the viscera, thus giving rise to the onset of diseases. As they trigger diseases from inside the body, seven emotions are also called "endogenous seven affects". The pathogenic characteristics of the Seven Emotions are as follows.

3.1 Direct Injury to the Viscera

Since emotional activities are closely related to viscera, emotional stimulation can easily hurt them. Seven emotions hurt viscera mainly in three conditions. First, special injury identified by the relations between five Zang-viscera and five emotions, for instance, over-joy hurts the heart, rage hurts the liver, over-thinking hurts the spleen, grief hurts the lung and great fear hurts the kidney. Second, the heart houses the spirit. The liver is in charge of free flow of qi and in control of emotions. The spleen houses wishes. If emotions mingle with each other and are damaged by emotional pathogens, they may mostly hurt the liver and spleen. Third, injuries caused by emotional pathogens will mostly hurt the viscera which house the diseases.

3.2 Influencing Qi Dynamic of the Viscera

Diseases triggered by seven emotions are mainly disturbances of qi dynamic of viscera, and dysfunctions of yin and yang.

Rage causes qi to go upward. Going upward means that qi dynamic goes adversely upward. Rage hurts liver, causing diseases due to over-adverse flow of qi. Dizziness, headache, flushed complexion, tinnitus, even hematemesis and syncope may occur as symptoms with reversed upward flow of the liver-qi. Invasion of the hyperactive liver-qi to spleen can cause distended abdomen and night diarrhea, and invasion to stomach can cause hiccups and vomiting.

Over joy causes qi to relax. Relaxed qi means slow flow of qi in the heart. Too much joy will hurt the heart. It will make the heart qi sluggish, and the spirit will be unable

中医理论

意力不集中,乃至心悸、失神,甚至狂乱等。

悲则气消。悲哀太过,耗伤肺气,使气弱消减,意志消沉,可见气短胸闷、精神萎靡不振和懒惰等。

思则气结。思虑太过,气结于中,见胃纳呆滞、脘腹痞塞、腹胀便溏,甚至肌肉消瘦等。思虑太过,既可伤脾,也会伤心,使心血虚弱,神失所养,而致心悸、怔忡、失眠、健忘、多梦等,临床称为"心脾两伤"。

恐则气下。恐惧伤肾,可见心神不安、夜不能寐、二便失禁、精遗骨痿等症。

惊则气乱。大惊则心气紊乱,气血失调,出现心悸、失眠、心烦、气短,甚则精神错乱等症状。

此外,喜、怒、忧、思、恐等情志活动失调,能够引起脏腑气机紊乱,郁而化火,出现烦躁、易怒、失眠、面赤、口苦,以及吐血、衄血等属于火的表现,称之为"五志化火"。

3.3 影响病情变化

情志异常,可以引起疾病,而且对整个病情的发展、变化都可以产生影响。不良情绪或异常的情感波动能够加重病情,或使其恶化,但良好的情感活动有助于治疗和保持健康。

to rest, manifesting as weakness, sluggishness, absent-mindedness and even heart palpitation, psychataxia, or mental confusion.

Grief causes qi to be consumed. Great sorrow will consume lung-qi, resulting in weak lung-qi and depression, marked by shortness of breath and oppression in the chest, listlessness and laziness.

Over-thinking causes qi to depress. Over-thinking will make qi stagnate in the middle and result in loss of appetite, abdominal distention and loose stool, even muscle symptosis. Over-thinking hurts both spleen and heart, making insufficiency of heart blood and loss of nourishment for spirit, manifesting as palpitation, fearful throbbing, insomnia, amnesia and dreaminess. Clinically, it can be called "heart-spleen deficiency".

Great fear causes qi to sink. Fear will hurt kidney, manifesting as disquieted spirit, inability to sleep at night, incontinence of urine and feces, spermatorrhea and weakness of the bone.

Great fright causes qi to be disordered. Great fright can cause disorder of heart qi, dysfunction of qi and blood, manifesting as palpitation, insomnia, vexation, shortness of breath and even entanglement.

In addition, dysfunctions of emotional activities including joy, anger, worry, thinking and fear can cause disorder of qi dynamic of the viscera and fire formation of the depression, manifesting as agitation, irascibility, insomnia, flushed complexion, bitterness in the mouth, blood ejection, and hemorrhinia, which can be called "fire formation due to excess among the five minds".

3.3 Influencing State of Illness

Abnormal emotions can cause diseases and influence the changes and development of the patients' conditions. Unhealthy emotions or mood swings may aggravate the patients' condition or rapidly exacerbate it, while healthy emotional activities can be advantageous to treatment and help people to keep fit.

4 病理产物性病因

在疾病发生和发展过程中，痰饮、瘀血等是疾病过程中所形成的病理产物。它们滞留体内又可成为新的致病因素，引起各种新的病理变化，又称继发性致病因素，或病理性致病因素。

4.1 痰饮

痰饮是机体水液代谢障碍所形成的病理产物。黏稠为痰，清稀为饮。两者同源而异流，常并称为痰饮。

痰饮多由外感六淫，或饮食及七情所伤等产生，使肺失宣降，津液不布，水道不利；脾失健运，水湿不化；肾不蒸腾气化；三焦不利等脏腑气化功能失常，水液不能正常输布，聚而为痰为饮。

痰饮的致病特点如下：

阻碍气血运行：痰饮随气流行，机体内外无所不至。若痰饮流注经络，会出现肢体麻木、屈伸不利，甚至半身不遂等。若结聚于局部，则形成肿块（瘰疬、痰核、流注等）。痰饮停肺，可出现胸闷、咳嗽、喘促等。痰饮停于胃，则出现恶心呕吐等。

影响水液代谢：痰饮本为水液代谢失常的病理产物，但形成

4 Pathogens from Pathological Products

Phlegm, stagnant fluid and blood are the pathological outcomes in the course of disease. Their retention in the body may become pathogenic factors causing new disorders, which lead to pathological changes. That is also called secondary pathogenic factors or pathological pathogenic factors.

4.1 Phlegm and Stagnant Fluid

Phlegm and stagnant fluid are the pathological products of fluid metabolism disorder. Phlegm is thick and turbid, and stagnant fluid is thin and clear. The two are from the same origin but differ in routes, so they are called phlegm and stagnant fluid.

Phlegm and stagnant fluid are usually caused by an exogenous invasion of six climatic pathogens, or dietary ignorance and seven emotions. Under many conditions may body fluid condense into damp resulting in phlegm and stagnant fluids, such as: when the lung fails both in dispersing and descending, body fluid fails to distribute and the water channel is not smooth. When the spleen loses its normal transporting function, water-damp fails to transform; the kidney fails in transpiration and vaporization; triple-energizer doesn't function well and other dysfunction of gasification for other viscera.

The pathogenic characteristics of phlegm and stagnant fluid are as follows.

Blocking circulation of qi and blood: phlegm and stagnant fluid may go to every part of the body. If they flow into meridians, numbness of the limbs, inhibited bending and stretching and hemiplegia may occur; if they stagnate in parts of the body, lump will be formed (i.e. scrofula, subcutaneous nodules and streaming sore); if they stagnate in the lung, oppression in the chest, cough and hasty panting will occur. When they stay in the stomach, nausea and vomiting may occur.

Influencing the metabolism of water: phlegm and stagnant fluid originally are the pathological products of

之后,又可以反过来作用于机体,进一步影响肌体的水液输布,使水液代谢障碍更为严重。

易于蒙蔽清窍:痰浊上扰,蒙蔽清阳,会出现头昏目眩、精神不振、痰迷心窍。痰火扰心、心神被蒙,可引起胸闷心悸、神昏谵妄,或引起癫狂、痫等疾病。

致病广泛,变幻多端:痰饮致病,无处不到,其临床表现也十分复杂。痰饮停留在不同的部位可表现出不同的症状,变化多端,故有"百病皆由痰作祟"、"怪病多痰"之说。

4.2 瘀血

瘀血指因体内血液停滞或血行不畅、阻滞于脏腑经络的血液。瘀血是血液运行失常的病理产物,又是具有致病性的"恶血"、"死血"。

4.2.1 瘀血的形成

离经之血。出血之后,未能及时消散或排出体外而为瘀。如跌打损伤、负重过度等各种内外伤造成的出血;气不摄血或血热妄行等所致的血行脉外。

各种影响血液运行的因素,使血液循行不畅,凝聚停留而为瘀血。常见因素有:气虚、气滞、血寒、血热、情志内伤和生活失宜等。

4.2.2 瘀血的致病特点

瘀血形成之后,不仅失去正

water metabolism disorder. After their formation, they may adversely have an effect on the body, further influencing the water transportation of the body, which may result in more severe water metabolism disturbance.

Being prone to disturb spirit: if phlegm and stagnant fluid rise upward, it may confuse the clear yang, manifesting as dizziness, devitalized essence-spirit and phlegm confounding the orifices of the heart. If the phlegm-fire harasses the heart to make the heart-spirit confused, diseases may occur such as choking sensation in chest, palpitation, clouded spirit and deliria, or mania.

Causing various and changeable diseases: diseases caused by phlegm and stagnant fluid may go to every part of the body and its clinical manifestation is really complex. Various and changeable symptoms may arise in different parts they stay in, thus sayings go that "hundreds of diseases arise out of phlegm", and "most weird diseases are caused by phlegm".

4.2 Stagnant Blood

Stagnant blood refers to static blood held within the body and viscera or meridian. Stagnant blood is the pathological outcome of improper circulated blood. It is also "malign blood" and "dead blood" with pathogenic factors.

4.2.1 Formation of stagnant blood

Stagnant blood is extravasated blood. One type of stagnant blood is due to wild flow of blood caused by various traumatic injuries or being overloaded. Other causes for stagnant blood include blood flowing out of vessels caused by deficiency of qi or qi failing to control blood.

Various factors affect blood circulation resulting in stagnated blood. The common factors include qi deficiency, disturbance of circulation of qi, blood-cold, blood-heat, and internal injury caused by emotional factors and inappropriate life.

4.2.2 Pathogenic characteristics of stagnant blood

As stagnant blood forms, it will lose the nourishment

中医理论

Basic Theory of Traditional Chinese Medicine

常血液的濡养作用，而且反过来可以导致新的病变发生，概括起来可分为以下几点：

疼痛：一般多刺痛，固定不移，且多夜间为重的特点。

肿块：体表肿块见色青紫或青黄，体内为癥积，固定不移。

出血：血色紫暗或夹有瘀块。

紫绀：面部、口唇、爪甲青紫。

舌质紫暗或有瘀点、瘀斑，是瘀血最常见的也是最敏感的指征。

脉细涩沉弦或结代。

除掌握上述瘀血特征外，在临床上可从以下几点判断是否有瘀血存在：

有外伤、出血、月经胎产史者；

瘀血征象虽不太明显，但屡治无效，或无瘀血证之前久治不愈者，中医有"久病入络"之说。

此外，面色黧黑、肌肤甲错、善忘、狂躁等怪病也多按瘀证论治。

5 饮食失宜

饮食水谷是化生气血，以维持人体生长、发育，完成各种生理功能，保证生命生存和健康的基本条件，所谓"民以食为天"，但"病从口入"也是不争的事实。饮食失宜不仅损伤脾胃，引起消化机能障碍，还能积滞生热、助湿生痰等等，成为疾病发生的一个重要因素。

of normal blood and adversely may cause the emergence of new pathology, which can be summarized as follows.

Pain: generally stabbing pains in fixed positions, normally severer at night;

Lump: on the body surface, greenish purple or greenish yellow lumps inside which enclosed mass accumulates in certain positions;

Hemorrhage: dark purple blood with lumps inside;

Cyanotic: the face, lips and fingers appearing greenish purple;

Tongue: dark purple or tongue with petechia and ecchymosis, which is the most sensitive and common physical sign;

The pulse is thin, rough, deep, wiry and intermittent.

Except for the characteristics above, stagnant blood can be identified in the clinic as follows.

People had traumas, hemorrhages, menstruation or childbirth experience.

The signs of blood stasis are not very obvious, but frequent treatments show no effect or the patient suffered long from a disease before there appears the blood stasis. In TCM, there is the saying "chronic illness enters the meridian".

In addition, most strange diseases are included in stagnant blood diseases, such as soot-black facial complexion, encrusted skin, amnesia and manic agitation.

5 Improper Diet

Food and drink can be transformed into qi and blood to maintain body's growth and development, fulfilling all physical functions and ensuring life existence and health. Hence the saying goes that "Food is the first necessity of the people." But it's also true that improper diet may cause diseases. Improper diet becomes an important factor of diseases. It not only damages spleen and stomach, causing digestive dysfunction, but also leads to food retention and heat accumulation, dampness and phlegm.

中医理论

Basic Theory of Traditional Chinese Medicine

5.1 饮食不节

按固定时间、有规律地进食，可以保证脾胃消化吸收功能有节奏地进行活动，使水谷精微化生有序，有条不紊地输布全身。

过饥：摄食不足，如饥不得食或脾胃虚弱，食不得入，致使气血衰少，脏腑功能减退；正气虚弱，抵抗力降低又易使外邪入侵。

过饱：饮食过量，如暴饮暴食，或脾胃虚弱而强食，可导致饮食阻滞，出现脘腹胀满、嗳腐泛酸、厌食、吐泻等食伤脾胃之病，所谓"饮食自倍，肠胃乃伤"。小儿脾胃较弱及消化原因，食积尤为多见。

饥饱失常：自古就有一日三餐，所谓"早饭宜好，午饭宜饱，晚饭宜少"。若饮食无时，饥一顿、饱一顿，最易损伤胃肠，变生他病。

5.2 饮食偏嗜

特别嗜好某些食物，可导致阴阳失调，或某些营养缺乏而发生疾病。

种类偏嗜：人的膳食结构应该以谷类为主，肉类为辅，蔬菜为充，水果为助，才能获得充足的营养，以满足生命活动的需要。若专嗜某类或厌恶不食某类食物，会造成肌体营养不全从而导致一些疾病的发生，如脚气病、瘿瘤、佝偻症、夜盲等。

5.1 Immoderate Diet

Regular food intake on a fixed time can ensure rhythmic digesting activities of spleen and stomach, orderly transformation and methodical distribution of grain and water essence through the whole body.

Insufficient food intake, like hunger or not being able to eat because of weak spleen and stomach may lead to waned qi and blood, subsiding zang-fu viscera functions, less vital qi and weakened immune systems, as well as more accessible external evil invasion.

An excess of food intake like voracious eating and drinking, or eating forcefully in spite of weak spleen and stomach may result in diseases of spleen and stomach like stagnation of food, manifesting as abdominal distention, putrid belching, pantothenic acid, loss of appetite, vomiting and diarrhea. As an old saying goes "overeating may hurt spleen and stomach", weakness in spleen and stomach for most children can be attributed to food stagnation.

It has been a tradition to eat three meals a day since the ancient times. As an old saying goes, "Eat well for breakfast, satiated for lunch and less for supper". Eating irregularly, or being full for one meal and staying hungry for another may damage the spleen and stomach, triggering other diseases.

5.2 Dietary bias

Special preference for certain food can lead to the imbalance between yin and yang, and certain nutritional deficiencies resulting in occurrence of diseases.

People's dietary structure should have cereals as staple food, meat as side food, vegetables as supplementary and fruit as auxiliary food, in order to obtain adequate nutrition and meet the needs of life. Being addicted to some kinds or neglect certain foods will cause defective nutrition, leading to the occurrence of some diseases, such as beriberi, goiter and tumor, rickets and night blindness.

中医理论

Basic Theory of Traditional Chinese Medicine

寒热偏嗜：过食生冷寒凉，可损伤脾胃阳气，寒湿内生，发生腹痛泄泻等症。偏食辛温燥热，可使胃肠积热，出现口渴、便秘，或酿成痔疮。

五味偏嗜：五味与五脏，各有其亲和性，如酸入肝，苦入心，甘入脾，辛入肺，咸入肾。长期嗜好某味食物，就会使该脏腑机能偏盛偏衰，久之甚至可以损伤他脏而发生疾病。只有"谨和五味"才能健康长寿。

5.3　饮食不洁

进食不洁，会引起多种胃肠道疾病，出现腹痛、吐泻、痢疾等；或引起寄生虫病，如蛔虫、蛲虫、寸白虫等；若进食腐败变质有毒食物，可致食物中毒，常出现腹痛、吐泻，重者可出现昏迷或死亡。随着时代的发展，相对感染病、寄生虫病发病率大大降低，但食品安全也是当代中国人最关心的问题之一。

6　劳逸失度

正常的劳动和必要的休息，是保证人体健康的必要条件。

6.1　过劳

劳力过度：劳力过度主要指超过体力负担和不适当的活动。劳力过度可出现少气无力、四肢困倦、精神疲惫、形体消瘦等，即

Excessive intake of uncooked and cold food will impair yang-qi in the spleen and the stomach, leading to endogenous cold-dampness and causing abdominal pain and diarrhea. Partiality to warm and spicy food or excessive intake of hot food may accumulate heat in the stomach and the intestines, leading to thirst, constipation or even hemorrhoids,etc.

The five flavors and five zang-organs have their own binding affinity respectively: the sour flavor enters the liver, the bitter flavor enters the heart, the sweet flavor enters the spleen, the acid flavor enters the lung and salty flavor enters the kidney. A long-term preference for a certain flavor will cause a certain organ's function to be abnormally exuberant or debilitated, damaging other zang-organs over time and leading to diseases. Only by keeping balance in five flavors can one keep fit and long-lived.

5.3　Insanitary Diet

Insanitary food intake may cause kinds of gastrointestinal diseases, manifesting as abdominal pain, vomiting, diarrhea and dysentery. Or it may trigger parasitic diseases, including ascarid, pinworm and proglottid of tapeworm. If people take decayed or toxic food, they will get food poisoned, leading to abdominal pain, vomiting and diarrhea. In severe cases they may go into comma or die. In modern ages, though the incidence of infectious diseases and parasitic diseases have greatly reduced, food safety is still Chinese peoples's major concern.

6　Maladjustment of Work and Leisure

Appropriate work and suitable rest are the essential prerequisites for a healthy body.

6.1　Over-work

Physical over-strain mainly refers to unsuitable activities beyond physical strength, manifesting as lack of energy and strength, fatigued cumbersome limbs, mental exhaustion and body emaciation. Over-strain leads to qi consumption. TCM has the saying that protracted use of eyes impairs blood,

所谓"劳则气耗"。中医有久视伤血、久卧伤气、久坐伤肉、久立伤骨、久行伤筋之说。

劳神过度：劳神过度指思虑劳神过度。劳神过度可耗伤心血，损伤脾气，出现心悸、健忘、失眠、多梦及纳呆、腹胀、便溏等症。

房劳过度：房劳是指房事过度。房劳过度会耗伤肾精，可致腰膝酸软、眩晕耳鸣、精神萎靡，或男子遗精滑泄、性功能减退，甚或阳痿。

6.2 过逸

过逸是使人体气血运行不畅，脾胃呆滞，或体虚发胖等。过度安逸，阳气不振，神倦，乏力，筋骨柔脆甚或继发他病。

 其他病因

7.1 外伤

外伤指因受扑击、跌仆、利器等外力所致，以及虫兽咬伤、烧烫伤、冻伤等而致形体组织的损伤。外伤一般有明显的外伤史。外伤的致病特点如下：

外力损伤：因暴力引起的创伤，包括枪炮、金刃、持重、跌打损伤等。这些外伤，可引起皮肤肌肉瘀血肿痛、出血，或筋伤骨折、脱臼。重则损伤内脏，甚至危及生命。

烧烫伤：烧烫伤多由沸水（油）、蒸汽、高温物品、火焰、雷电等灼伤人体而造成。烧烫伤火毒为患，轻者损伤肌肤，出现红、肿、

protracted lying in bed damages qi, protracted sedentariness injures the muscles, protracted standing injures the bones and protracted walking injures the joints.

Mental over-strain refers to over-thought. Over-strain may cause the exhaustion of heart blood and injury of spleen qi, manifesting as palpitation, amnesia, insomnia, dreaminess, anorexia, abdominal distention and loose stool.

Sexual over-strain may cause the consumption of kidney-essence, triggering soreness and weakness of waist and knees, dizziness and tinnitus, and listlessness, or nocturnal emission, hypogonadism, and even impotence.

6.2 Over-ease

Over-ease brings the disorder of qi and blood, stagnation of spleen and stomach or weakness and obesity. Over-ease can cause inactivation of yang qi, lassitude of the spirit, lack of strength, fragile muscles and bones and other diseases.

 Other pathogens

7.1 Traumatic Injuries

Traumatic injuries refer to body tissues damaged by insects or animals, burns and scalds and frostbite or by external forces, such as pounces, falls or sharp weapons. The pathogenic characteristics of traumatic injuries are as follows.

Traumatic injuries, caused by violence, includes guns, knives, holding heavy things and injuries from falls. All these may cause thrombotic pain and hemorrhage of the skin, or damage of tendons, fractures and dislocation. In severe cases they may injure the viscera, even cost lives.

Burns and scalds are ambustions mainly caused by boiled water (oil), steamed gas, things with high temperature, fire and thunder, etc. They pertain to the attack by fire-toxin. The light victims may get skin damaged, being red, swollen,

热、痛，表面干燥或起水泡，甚者火热内攻，出现烦躁不安、尿少尿闭等，及至亡阴亡阳而死亡。

冻伤：冻伤是低温所引起的全身或局部损伤。冻伤在我国北方冬季常见。局部性冻伤常常发生在指、趾、耳、鼻等易受寒冷影响暴露部位，出现紫斑、水肿等，甚至组织坏死。寒冷是造成冻伤的重要条件。冻伤一般有全身冻伤和局部冻伤之分。全身性冻伤可出现寒战、体温下降、面色苍白、唇舌、指甲青紫、感觉麻木、反应迟钝，甚至呼吸微弱、脉微欲绝、昏迷直至死亡。

虫兽伤：虫兽伤包括疯狗、野兽等猛兽咬伤或毒蛇、蝎子、蜈蚣、蜂等蜇伤。猛兽所伤轻则局部肿疼、出血，重可损伤内脏，或出血过多，或毒邪内陷而死亡。蝎、蜂蜇伤或毒蛇、蜈蚣咬伤，多局部肿痛，有时会出现头晕、心悸、恶心、呕吐等中毒症状，甚至昏迷，导致死亡。

7.2　药邪

医师聚毒药以供医事。所有药物都有偏性，包括四气、五味、升降浮沉、有毒无毒等。药物治病就是利用这一偏性，以偏纠偏。如果不问机体偏胜情况，也不问药物的偏性如何，滥用药物，或者不适当地多服、久服，都会有损于机体的健康。《礼记·曲礼》有云："君有疾饮药，臣先尝之。

painful, dry or blistering, while the serious patients would be attacked by inside heat, demonstrating as restlessness, oliguria and anuresis, and even death as the depletion of yin and yang.

Frostbite refers to whole or partial body injuries caused by low temperature. It is common in the winter of northern China. Partial frostbite usually happens in the exposed parts of the body influenced by coldness, such as fingers, toes, ears and nose, manifesting as purple plaque, edema and even tissue necrosis. Cold is the important premise for frostbite, which is generally divided into whole and partial body cases. The former one may cause many symptoms, including chill, decline of body temperature, pale face, greenish purple lips and tongue and nails, stolidity, slowness in reaction and even faint breath, barely palpable pulse, coma, or even death.

People are bitten by fierce beasts including rabid dogs, wild animals, or serpents, scorpions, centipedes and bees. The light injuries caused by animals can be partially swollen, painful and bleeding, while the severe ones can be damage of viscera, over-hemorrhage or evil pathogen invagination, even death. People stung by scorpions and bees or bitten by serpents and centipedes mostly suffer from partial swell and pain, sometimes may have toxic symptoms such as dizziness, palpitation, disgusting, vomiting, and even coma leading to death.

7.2　Toxic Medicinals

Physicians collect medicinals to carry out clinical operation. All medicinals have deflections, including four natures, five flavors, four directions of lifting, lowering, floating and sinking, and toxicity. Medicinal deflection is used to correct the pathological deflection. Medicinal abuse, or inappropriate over-dosage and long-time dosage without considering medicinal and pathological deflection will damage health. In the *Book of Rites* (*LiJi*): *Quli*, there is the saying, "If the emperor takes medicine, the minister

亲有疾饮药,子先尝之。医不三世,不服其药。"可见,服药是件很危险的事。

will take it for him firstly; if the parents take medicine, the children will take it for them at first; if the physician has not studied through the classics of TCM, his prescription can not be taken. Therefore, it is obvious that taking medicinals is very dangerous.

中医理论

Basic Theory of Traditional Chinese Medicine

第六章 望闻问切

Chapter 6 Four Examinations

望、闻、问、切四诊,是诊察疾病的四种基本方法。望诊,是对患者全身或局部进行有目的的观察以了解病情,测知脏腑病变。闻诊,是通过听声音、嗅气味以辨别患者内在的病情。问诊,是通过对患者或陪诊者的询问以了解病情及有关情况。切诊,是诊察患者的脉候和身体其他部位,以测知体内、体外一切变化的情况。

Four examinations are the basic methods of disease diagnosis, including observing, listening and smelling, inquiring, pulse examination and palpation. Observing refers to purposely looking at the patient's whole body or parts of it to learn the patient's condition and viscera lesions. Listening and smelling refers to identifying the patient's diseases through listening to sound and smelling. Inquiring refers to asking the patient or his companion to learn his condition. Pulse examination and palpation refers to feeling the patient's pulse or the other parts of his body to know all the changes in vivo and vitro.

1 中医诊断学原理及原则

诊断即对人体健康状态和病症所提出的概括性判断。正确的诊断来源于对患者临床症状和体征的周密观察和精确的辨证分析。诊断在防治疾病中是极为重要的一环。

1 Theory and Principle of TCM Diagnosis

Diagnosis is the general judgment on human health and diseases. The correct diagnosis comes from careful observation and accurate analysis of the clinical symptoms and signs of the patients. Diagnosis is a very important part in the disease prevention and treatment.

1.1 诊断原理

"视其外应,测知其内","有诸内者,必形诸外",这是前人认识客观事物的重要方法。通过观察外在表现的症状和体征,可以了解人体内部脏腑的变化;脏腑内部的病理变化必然会表现在外。疾病的发生和发展,一定有

1.1 Theory of Diagnosis

"Observing the outside to know the inside" and "the inside deciding the outside" are the important ways for TCM practiconers to understand the objective things. By observing the external manifestations of the symptoms and signs, physicians can understand the changes of viscera; pathological changes of viscera will be reflected in the external. The occurrence and development of diseases

相应的症状、体征、舌象和脉象。因此,可以运用望、闻、问、切等手段,把这些表现于外的症状、体征、舌象、脉象等有关资料收集起来,然后分析其脏腑病机及病邪的性质,以判断疾病的本质和证候类型,从而做出诊断,这就是中医诊断的原理:"司外揣内"(《灵枢·外揣》)。

1.2 诊断原则

诊断是对于疾病的一个认识过程,对疾病有所认识,才能对疾病进行防治。要正确认识疾病,必须遵循四诊合参。

人体是一个有机的整体,内在脏腑与外在四肢、百骸是统一的;而整个机体与外界环境也是统一的。人体一旦发生病变,局部可以影响全身,全身病变也可反映于某一局部;外部有病可以内传入里,内脏有病也可以反映于外;精神刺激可以影响脏腑功能活动,脏腑有病也可以造成精神活动的异常。同时,疾病的发生、发展变化也与气候及外在环境密切相关。因此,在诊察疾病时,首先要有整体观念,既要重视局部表现,也要观察全身症状;既要观察其外,又要审察其内,还要把患者与自然环境结合起来加以审察,才能做出正确的诊断。所以对患者做全面详细的检查和了解,必须四诊合参。

四诊合参,并不等于面面俱

must have the corresponding symptoms, signs, tongue and pulse condition. Therefore, through observing, hearing and smelling, asking, pulse examination and palpation, the external symptoms, signs, tongue and pulse condition and other relevant information are collected to analyze the nature of viscera pathogenesis and pathogenic factors for judging the nature of the disease and syndrome types. That's the theory of TCM diagnosis—"governing exterior to infer interior". (*Spiritual Pivot: Diagnosing the Interior to Examine the Exterior*)

1.2 Principle of Diagnosis

Diagnosis is a process of knowing the disease which can be prevented when people have some knowledge on it. To have a correct understanding of the disease one must apply the correlation of all four examinations.

The human body is an organic whole in which the internal organs and external limbs and bones are unified; the whole body and the external environment are also unified. Once pathological changes occur, the local lesion can affect the whole body, while the whole body's lesion can also be reflected in a local part; the external diseases can be transmitted into the internal, while visceral diseases can also reflect on the outside; mental stimulation can affect the functions of viscera, while viscera diseases can also cause abnormal mental activities. At the same time, the occurrence and development of diseases are closely related to climate and the external environment. Therefore, in the diagnosis of diseases, the first and foremost is to have the holism concept. The physician should not only pay attention to the local symptoms, but also observe the systemic symptoms. It is necessary to observe the inner and examine the outer, but also to investigate the patients against natural environment in order to make the correct diagnosis. So the overall and detailed examination and understanding of the patient must be based on the correlation of four examinations.

The correlation of all four examinations does not

中医理论

Basic Theory of Traditional Chinese Medicine

到。只有抓住主要矛盾,四诊并重,有目的、系统地收集临床资料,才能全面了解病情,辨证准确。疾病是复杂多变的,证候的表现有真象,也有假象,脉证不一,故有"舍脉从症"和"舍症从脉"现象的出现。

2 望诊

医生运用视觉对人体全身和局部、排出物以及舌象等进行有目的地观察,以了解健康或疾病状态,称为望诊。

望诊的内容主要包括:观察人的神、色、形、态、舌象、脉络、皮肤、五官九窍等情况以及排泄物、分泌物的形、色、质量等,其中舌诊和面部色诊虽属头面五官,但因舌象、面色反映内脏病变较为准确,实用价值较高,因而形成了面色诊、舌诊两项独特的中医传统诊法。

2.1 望神

望神就是观察人体生命活动的外在表现,即观察人的精神状态和机能状态。

望神重点在于观察病人的精神、意识、面目表情、形体动作、反应能力等,尤应重视眼神的变化。望神主要有以下几种情况:得神、失神、假神、神气不足、神志异常等。

mean covering everything. Only when the doctor seizes the main information, combines the four examinations and collects clinical data purposefully and systematically, can he get a comprehensive understanding of the disease and to differentiate accurately. Diseases are complex and changeable, the symptoms of which can be real or false, reflecting as different pulse conditions, so there appears the phenomenon "precedence of symptoms over pulse manifestation" and "precedence of pulse manifestation over symptoms".

2 Observing

By using vision, doctors purposefully observe the whole body and local parts, discharge and tongue in order to know the health or disease state which is called observing.

The doctors mainly observe the spirit, color, shape, form, tongue, meridian, skin, facial features and nine orifices and excreta, secretions including their shape, color and quality. Tongue and facial color diagnoses belong to facial features diagnosis, and they have high practical value because of their accurate reflection of visceral lesions. Therefore, tongue and facial color diagnoses form a unique traditional diagnostic method.

2.1 Observing Spirit

Observing spirit refers to looking at the external manifestation of life activity—observing the state of mind and function of the body.

The key of observing spirit is to observe the patient's spirit, consciousness, facial expressions, body movements, response ability and so on, especially changes in the eyes. Observing spirit is mainly to judge whether a patient has the following situations: fullness of vitality, loss of vitality, false manifestation of vitality, lack of vitality and mental abnormity etc.

2.1.1 得神

得神又称有神,是精充气足神旺的表现。得神的表现是:神志清楚、语言清晰、面色红润光泽、表情自然;目光明亮、精彩内含;反应灵敏、动作灵活、体态自如;呼吸平稳、肌肉不削。得神是健康的表现,若患病而有神,则表示虽病而正气未伤,是病轻浅的表现,往往预后良好。

2.1.2 失神

失神又称无神,是精气亏损的表现。失神的表现是:精神萎靡不振、言语不清,或神昏谵语,或猝然晕倒而目闭口开;面色晦暗、表情淡漠或呆板;目光呆滞;反应迟钝、动作僵硬、强迫体位;呼吸气微或喘;周身大肉已脱。病至此,已属重笃,预后不良。

2.1.3 假神

假神是垂危患者出现的暂时好转的假象,俗称"回光返照"、"残灯复明"。假神的表现是:久病重病之人,突然精神转佳,目光明亮,言语洪亮、清晰;或原来面色晦暗,突然颧赤如妆;或原来毫无食欲,忽然食欲大增。假神说明脏腑精气极度衰竭,阴阳即将离决,常为临终前的预兆。

2.1.4 神气不足

神气不足,介于有神和无神之间,属于轻度失神。其临床表现是:精神不振、健忘多梦、倦怠乏力、声低懒言、动作迟缓等,

2.1.1 Fullness of vitality

Its manifestations are clear consciousness, clear language, ruddy and lustrous complexion, natural facial expression; bright eyes containing spirit; sensitive reaction, flexible movement, free posture; smooth breathing and strong muscles. Fullness of vitality is a sign of health. Getting sick but full of vitality shows that one's vital qi is not injured and the disease is not serious, which often has a good prognosis.

2.1.2 Loss of vitality

Loss of vitality is the reflection of essence-qi deficiency. Its manifestations are low spirit, slurred speech, coma and delirium, or sudden faint with closed eyes, open mouth, dim complexion, indifferent or dull expression, dull eyes, lag in response, stiff movements, forced posture, shallow or heavy breath and emaciation. These symptoms are mainly seen in patients with serious illness and the prognosis is normally poor.

2.1.3 False manifestation of vitality

False manifestation of vitality is a false temporary improvement in dying patients, which is commonly compared as "the last radiance of the setting sun" and "the reviving flicker of an expiring lamp". Its manifestations are that the very sick man with chronic disease suddenly has good spirit, bright eyes, loud and clear speech; or the patient with dark complexion suddenly has flushed cheeks as makeup; or the patient with no appetite suddenly has increased appetite. False manifestation of vitality shows the exhaustion of essence-qi, which is often a harbinger of dying.

2.1.4 Lack of vitality

Lack of vitality, somewhat between full of vitality and loss of vitality, is light weakness in vitality. The clinical manifestations are dizziness, forgetfulness and dreaminess, lassitude, low sound and lazy words, slow movement etc. It

常见于虚证患者,所以临床更为多见。

2.1.5 神志异常

神志异常主要包括癫、狂、痫病等,是以精神失常为主要临床表现的疾病。

癫病表现为神志痴呆、表情淡漠、喃喃自语,或哭笑无常,多由先天禀赋或忧思郁结所致痰气郁结,阻蔽神明。

狂病多表现为神志昏狂、呼笑怒骂、打人毁物、妄行不休、少卧不饥、甚则登高而歌、弃衣而走,多由痰火上扰神明所致。

痫病表现为突然昏倒、不省人事、口吐涎沫、发有异声、或如猪、羊叫声,四肢抽搐、醒后如常,多由肝风挟痰,蒙蔽清窍。

2.2 望色

望色是通过观察患者的颜色与光泽以诊断疾病的方法。颜色就是色调变化,光泽则是明度变化。颜色主要分为青、赤、黄、白、黑五种,称为五色诊。由于五色的变化,在面部表现最明显,因此,常以望面色来阐述五色诊的内容。望面色要注意识别常色与病色。

2.2.1 常色

常色是人在正常生理状态时的面部色泽。常色又有主色、客色之分。

主色:所谓主色,是指人终生不改变的基本肤色、面色。由

is mainly seen in patients with deficiency syndrome, so it is clinically more common.

2.1.5 Mental abnormity

Mental abnormity includes depressive psychosis, mania and epilepsy which are the diseases with mental disorders as the main clinical manifestations.

Depressive psychosis manifests itself as dementia, apathy, muttering, or weeping and laughing hysterically. It is mainly due to stagnation of phlegm and qi caused by natural endowment or depression shading the spirit.

Mania mainly manifests itself as madness, fury, violent behavior, restless ness, less sleep with no appetite, even singing songs atop a high place and walking naked. It is mainly caused by phlegm fire disturbing the spirit.

Epilepsy manifests itself as sudden collapse, unconsciousness, foam around the mouth, queer cries like pigs' and sheep's, and twitching limbs. The patients would recover and look normal after their consciousness is regained. The condition is mainly caused by liver wind combined with phlegm misting the mind.

2.2 Observing Complexion

Observing complexion is a method of diagnosing a disease by observing the patient's color and luster. Color is the change of hue, luster and brightness. The color is divided into green, red, yellow, white and black, which is called five-colored examination. The change of color is most obvious on the face, so observing complexion is always used to elaborate the content of five-colored examination in which the recognition of healthy complexion and sick complexion should be emphasized.

2.2.1 Healthy complexion

Healthy complexion is the facial color in normal physiological state, including the chief and secondary color.

The so-called chief color is a person's basic skin color which does not change in his life. Because of different races,

于民族、禀赋、体质不同，每个人的肤色不完全一致。中国属于黄色人种，一般肤色都呈微黄，在此基础上，有些人可有略白、较黑、稍红等差异。

客色：人与自然环境相适应。随着季节、气候的变化，人的肤色也相应变化，所以客色也称为应时之色，即春青、夏赤、长夏黄、秋白、冬黑。年龄、饮食、起居、寒暖、情绪等变化，也可引起面色变化，也属于客色。

总之，常色有主色、客色之分，其共同特征是：红黄隐隐，明润含蓄。

2.2.2　病色

人体在疾病状态时的面部颜色与光泽主要有青、黄、赤、白、黑五种。

青色：主寒证、痛证、瘀血证、惊风证及肝病，为经脉阻滞，气血不通之象。

如面色青黑或苍白淡青，多属阴寒内盛；面色青灰，口唇青紫，多属心血痹阻；小儿高热，鼻柱、两眉间及口唇四周青紫色明显，是惊风先兆。

黄色：主湿证、虚证，是脾虚湿蕴表现。

如面色萎黄，多属脾胃气虚，营血不能上荣于面部所致；面色黄胖，多属脾虚失运，湿邪内停所致；黄色鲜明如橘皮者，属阳黄，为湿热熏蒸所致；黄色晦

endowments and constitutions, each person's skin color is different from others, Chinese belong to the yellow race, so the general color is slightly yellow, on the basis of which some people show slight difference of redness, whiteness and blackness.

Human beings can adapt themselves to natural environment. With the change of seasons and climate, people's skin color changes correspondingly, so the secondary color is also known as the color of time: blue in spring, red in summer, yellow in long-summer, white in autumn and black in winter. The complexion change caused by differences in age, diet, daily routine, coldness and warmth, emotional change also belongs to the secondary color.

In short, healthy complexion includes the chief and secondary colors, the common characteristics of which are slightly red and yellow, lustrous and concealed.

2.2.2　Sick complexion

One's complexion and luster in sick state are blue, yellow, red, white and black.

Blue mainly manifests itself as cold syndrome, pain syndrome, blood stasis syndrome, convulsion and liver disease due to the blocked meridian and qi-blood.

Bluish black or pale and light blue complexion is due to yin-cold excess; bluish grey complexion and cyanotic lips are normally due to heart-blood stagnation. When the child has high fever, its nasal column and skin between the eyebrows and around the lips appear to be cyanotic. This is also the sign of infantile convulsion.

Yellow mainly manifests itself as dampness and deficiency syndrome due to deficiency of the spleen and excessive dampness.

Sallow complexion is due to deficiency of spleen and stomach-qi and nutritive blood not ascending to face; edema with yellow complexion is due to deficiency of the spleen and retention of dampness; bright yellow complexion like orange peel is due to yang jaundice resulting from fuming or steaming of damp-heat; dark yellow complexion like

暗如烟熏者,属阴黄,为寒湿郁阻所致。

赤色:主热证。实热证,满面通红;虚热证,仅两颧嫩红。

白色:主虚证、寒证、血虚、气亏等症。

面色㿠白(白而虚浮),多为阳气不足;面色苍白,多属阳气虚脱,或失血过多。

黑色:主肾虚证、寒证、痛症、水饮及瘀血证,为阴寒水盛之色。

阴寒内盛,血失温养,经脉挛急,气血不畅,面色黧黑;面黑而焦干,多为肾精久耗;眼眶周围色黑,多见于肾虚水泛的水饮证;面色青黑,且剧痛者,多为寒凝瘀阻。

2.3 望形体

望形体是观察人体外形的强弱胖瘦、体型特征、躯干四肢、皮肉筋骨等,来了解内脏精气的盛衰,从而判断疾病的虚实和预后的好坏。

凡骨骼粗大、肌肉强健、皮肤润泽、形体强壮者,说明脏腑精气充实。即使有病,但正气尚充,预后多佳。凡骨骼细小、肌肉消瘦、皮肤干涩、形体衰弱者,说明脏腑精气不足,体弱易病,若病则预后较差。

形体肥胖,伴神疲乏力、多汗畏寒等为阳虚气弱,称为"形盛而气衰"。肥胖常兼有头晕、胸闷、

smoke is due to yin jaundice resulting from blocked cold dampness.

Red manifests itself as heat syndrome. Solid heat syndrome manifests as a blush overspreading one's face; deficient heat syndrome manifests as two zygomatic in pink.

White manifests itself as deficiency syndrome, coldness syndrome, and blood deficiency and qi insufficiency syndrome.

Pallor complexion (white and floating) is due to yang deficiency; pale complexion is due to exhaustion of yang qi or excessive loss of blood.

Black manifests itself as kidney deficiency syndrome, coldness syndrome, pain syndrome, retention of fluid and blood stasis syndrome due to yin coldness and excessive fluid.

Blackish complexion is caused by excessive yin coldness, failure of blood to nourish vessels, contraction of vessels and unsmooth qi-blood; black and parched complexion is mainly due to exhaustion of kidney essence; black color around orbit is mainly due to kidney deficiency causing retention of fluid; bluish black complexion and sharp pain is normally due to coldness stagnation.

2.3 Observing Physique

Observing physique means looking at body shape, feature, trunk and limbs, skin, muscles, tendons and bones to learn the wax and wane of viscera essence-qi and judge the actual situation and prognosis of diseases.

The person with thick bones, strong muscles, lustrous skin and strong physique indicates full viscera essence-qi. If the person's vital qi is sufficient, his prognosis will be good. The person with tiny bones, lean muscles, illustrious skin, and weak physique lacks viscera-qi, and is easy to get illnesses and has poor prognosis.

Obesity along with general lassitude and sweat and chills is due to yang deficiency and qi weakness, which is called "fat body with qi deficiency". Obesity together with

肢体麻木者多为阳虚不运,痰浊内生,多易患胸痹、消渴、中风等症。形瘦食少伴面色萎黄多为脾胃虚弱;形瘦多食,为胃火亢盛;形体消瘦常伴有两颧发红、潮热盗汗、五心烦热等症者,多属阴虚火旺,易患痨病咳嗽、消渴等病;若形体消瘦若达到"大肉脱失"、卧床不起的程度,则是脏腑精气衰竭的危象。

2.4 望姿态

望姿态,主要是观察病人的动静姿态、异常动作及与疾病有关的体位变化。

正常的姿态是舒适自然、运动自如、反应灵敏,行止坐卧各随所愿,皆得其中。在疾病中,由于阴阳气血的盛衰,姿态也随之出现异常变化,不同的疾病产生不同的病态。

手足软弱无力,行动不灵而无痛,是为痿证;关节肿大或痛,以致肢体行动困难,是为痹证。

恶寒喜暖,多为寒证;常欲揭衣被,恶热喜冷,多为热证。

卧时常向外,身轻能自转侧,或仰面伸足而卧,为阳证、热证、实证;卧时喜向里,身重不能转侧,蜷卧成团者多为阴证、寒证、虚证;但坐不得卧,卧则气逆,多为咳喘肺胀。

dizziness, chest tightness, limb numbness is mainly due to yang deficiency and failure of carrying out transportation, and due to phlegm and the turbid generated inside the body, usually resulting in diseases as chest pain, diabetes and stroke. Thin physique and polyphagia is due to stomach hyperactivity; emaciation accompanied with two zygomatic redness, hot flashes, night sweats, vexing heat in the chest belongs to yin deficiency and excessive fire, normally resulting in phthisis cough and diabetes etc.; emaciation to an extent of being completely bedridden is a critical sign of exhaustion of viscera essence-qi.

2.4 Observing Patterns of Movement

Observing patterns of movement is mainly to observe the patient's static and dynamic posture, abnormal movements and position changes related to the diseases.

Normal patterns of movement are supposed to be comfortable, moving freely, reacting sensitively, or walking, stopping, sitting and lying at ease.While in sickness, patterns of movement show correspondingly abnormal changes due to ups and downs of yin-yang and qi-blood. Different diseases have different pathological postures.

Feeble hands and feet, being inflexible but painless, belong to flaccidity syndrome; swelling or painful joints causing movement difficulties belong to arthromyodynia syndrome.

Aversion to cold and preference for warm mainly belong to cold syndrome. Aversion to heat and preference for cold belong to hot syndrome, for which the patient dislikes thick clothes or quilt.

If the patient often lies outward, being able to toss about, or lies on the back with stretched feet, the pathema will be the yang syndrome. If the patient prefers lying inward in curled-up posture, being inflexible to toss about, the pathema will mainly be the yin, cold and deficiency syndrome. If the patient can only sit instead of lying or he/she will have inverse qi, the pathema will be mainly cough with asthma and lung inflation.

如病人眼睑、面、唇、指（趾）不时颤动，在内伤杂病中，多是血虚阴亏，经脉失养；在外感病中，多是发痉的预兆；四肢抽搐或拘挛，项背强直，角弓反张，属于痉病。

弯腰屈背，以手护腹，多为腹痛；腰背转动艰难，不得俯仰，多为腰腿痛；以手护心，不敢行动，多为真心痛；蹙额捧头，多为头痛。

2.5 望头颈肢体皮肤

2.5.1 望头颈部

头形过大或过小，多因先天不足，伴有智力低下。头形过大也可因脑积水引起。囟门高突，中医称为"自填"，多为热邪亢盛；若小儿囟门迟迟不能闭合，称为解颅，是为肾气不足、发育不良的表现。

发黄干枯稀少，多为精血不足。若突然出现片状脱发，为血虚受风所致。青少年落发，多因肾虚或血热。青年白发，伴有健忘、腰膝酸软者，属肾虚；若无其他病象者，不属病态。

痄腮：腮部一侧或两侧突然肿起，多兼咽喉肿痛，多属温毒。

口眼㖞斜，多属中风症。

瘿瘤：颈前结喉处有肿物凸起，可随吞咽移动。或因水土，或因情志不遂、肝气郁结、痰瘀互结所致。

If the patient's eyelid, face, lips and fingers (toes) are in fibrillation from time to time, the pathema will mainly be blood and yin deficiency and meridian dystrophy in miscellaneous internal damages; while in exogenous diseases, there will mainly be a sign of spasm; tetany or spasm, neck stiffness and opisthotonos belong to convulsive diseases.

If the patient bends with his hands covering abdomen, the pathema will be mainly abdominal pain. If the patient can hardly turn his back, nor bend forward or backward, the pathema will mainly be pain in waist and lower extremities. If the patient protects his heart with his hand daring not move, the pathema will mainly be angina. If the patient always frowns and holds head with both hands, the pathema will be mainly headache.

2.5 Observing Head, Neck, Limbs, Trunk and Skin

2.5.1 Observing head and neck

The head, too large or small, is due to congenital deficiency accompanied by mental retardation. Too large head can also be caused by hydrocephalus. The bulging fontanel in infant is called "self-filled" in TCM, which is mainly due to heat-evil hyperactivity; delayed closure of fontanel is known as metopism due to kidney-qi deficiency and dysplasia.

Yellow, dry and sparse hair is mainly due to blood deficiency. Sudden hair loss might be caused by blood deficiency and exposure to wind. Adolescent hair loss is mainly due to kidney deficiency or blood-heat. Young people with white hair accompanied with forgetfulness, sore waist and knees normally have kidney deficiency. If there are no other symptoms, they are not sick.

Mumps manifest as one side or both sides of cheeks companied with sore throat suddenly swell, it will mostly be warm poison.

Facial paralysis is mostly due to stoke syndrome.

Gall is the cervical tumor at the Adam's apple moving with swallowing is caused by acclimatization, or emotional upset, phlegm stagnation and blood stasis.

瘰疬：在颈部皮肉间可触及大小不等的核块，其小者为瘰，大者为疬，因其互相串连，连贯如串珠状，故称之为瘰疬，俗称"老鼠疮"，均指淋巴结核。

2.5.2　望躯体

鸡胸：胸廓向前向外突起，多因先天不足，后天失调，骨骼失于充养。

龟背：脊骨后突，背部凸起，常因先天不足，后天失养，骨骼失于充养。

肋部硬块突起，连如串珠，是佝偻病，因肾精不足，骨质不坚，骨软变形。

胸似桶状，咳喘、羸瘦者，是肺气壅滞之肺胀。

肋间饱胀，咳则隐痛，常见于饮停胸胁之悬饮证。

腹皮绷紧、胀大如鼓者，称为膨胀。

婴幼儿脐中有包块突出，皮色光亮者谓之脐突，又称脐疝。

胸、腰、腹部皮肤生有水疱，如带状簇生，累累如珠者，为缠腰火丹。

2.5.3　望二阴：前阴包括外生殖器及尿道。

阴囊肿大不痒不痛，皮泽透明的，是水疝。

阴囊肿大，疼痛不硬的是㿗疝。

阴囊内有肿物，卧则入腹，起则下坠，名为狐疝。

阴茎萎软，缩入小腹的是阴缩，是内因阳气亏虚、外感寒凝经

Scrofolosis appears as palpable lumps with different sizes in the flesh of the neck—the small ones are called *luo* and large ones are called *li* in Chinese—connecting with each other like a string of beads, or commonly known as "rat sore", both referring to the lymph node tuberculosis.

2.5.2　Observing trunk

Pectus carinatum, or the chest bulging forward and outward, is mainly due to congenital deficiency and acquired disorders leading to the failure of skeleton to be nourished.

Spine kyphosis and back bulge is often caused by innate deficiency and acquired dystrophy leading to the failure of skeleton to be nourished.

Rib lumps bumping and connecting with each other like a string of beads are rickets caused by kidney deficiency, weak bones and soft bones leading to deformation.

The thin person with a barrel-like chest, cough and asthma gets lung swelling caused by qi stagnation of lungs.

Intercostal fullness and cough-induced pain is commonly caused by pleural effusion.

Tense abdomen swelling like a drum is known as expansion.

Enclosed mass with bright color sticking out of belly button is known as umbilical hernia.

Water sores on chest, waist and abdomen clustering like a ribbon or beads is known as girdling fire cinnabar.

2.5.3　Observing external genitals, urethra and anus

Swelling of scrotum, which is not itchy and painful, and is enclosed by lustrous and hyaline skin belongs to edema of scrotum.

Swelling of scrotum which is painful but not hard belongs to decadent hernia.

The lump in scrotum entering abdomen while lying and falling while getting up is called fox edema.

Flaccid penis retracting into abdomen known as retraction of the penis is caused by yang deficiency inside

中医理论

Basic Theory of Traditional Chinese Medicine

脉而成。

妇女阴中突物如梨状,称阴挺,或因中气不足,或因产后劳累,升提乏力,致胞宫下坠所致。

肛门上段直肠脱出肛外,名为脱肛。

肛门内外之周围有物突出,肛周疼痛,甚至便时出血者,是为痔疮,其生于肛门之外者,称外痔;生于肛门之内者,叫内痔;内外皆有,叫混合痔。

在肛周发生瘘管,管道或长或短,或有分支或通入直肠,叫肛瘘。

肛门有裂口,疼痛,便时流血,称为肛裂。

2.5.4　望四肢

掌心皮肤燥裂,疼痛,迭起脱屑,称鹅掌风。

手足拘急,屈伸不利者,多因寒凝经脉。

伸而不屈的,是关节强直。

手足抽搐常见于邪热亢盛,肝风内动之痉病。

手足振摇不定,是肝筋失养,虚风内动的表现。

四肢肌肉萎缩,多因脾气亏虚、四肢失荣之故。

半身不遂是瘫痪病。

胫肿或跗肿指压留痕,是水肿。

足膝肿大而股胫瘦削,是鹤膝风。

指趾关节肿大变形,屈伸不便,多系风湿久凝、肝肾亏虚

and exogenous cold coagulating in meridians outside.

The pear-like lump in the vagina is caused by the lack of vital qi, or lifting weakness after partum resulting in prolapse of the uterus.

The upper anal rectum prolapsing out of anus is known as archoptosis.

When a lump grows inside and (or) outside the anus and even bleeds when discharging, a hemorrhoid occurs. If the lump grows outside the pectinate line, it is external hemorrhoid; if the lump grows inside the pectinate line, it is internal hemorrhoid; if the lump grows both inside and outside the pectinate line, it is mixed hemorrhoid.

Fistulas forming around the ulcerous area are known as anal fistulas, which vary in length and some have branches or enter the rectum.

Opening in the skin of the anus with pain and bleeding on defecation is known as anal fissure.

2.5.4　Observing limbs

The dry cracked palm skin resulting in pain and frequent desquamation is called tinea unguium.

Hands and feet contract with difficulty in inflexion and extension is mainly due to accumulated coldness in meridian.

That the limbs can stretch and cannot bend is joint stiffness.

Tetany belongs to convulsive disease which is usually caused by excess heat and internal stirring of liver wind.

Vibrating hands and feet are caused by liver tendons dystrophy and endogenous deficient wind.

Limbs dystrophy is mainly caused by limbs failure resulting from spleen-qi deficiency.

Hemiplegia belongs to paralysis disease.

Swollen legs and spavin which have marks on pressing are edema.

If feet and knees are swollen while the legs and thighs are emaciated, it is called arthroncus of knee.

If finger or toe joints are swollen and deformed and hard to move, it is mainly caused by accumulated wind-

所致。

足趾皮肤紫黑，溃流败水，肉色不鲜，味臭痛剧，为脱疽。

2.5.5 望皮肤

望皮肤要注意皮肤的色泽及形态改变。

色泽：皮肤忽然变红，如染脂涂丹，名曰"丹毒"。可发于全身任何部位，初起鲜红如云片，往往游走不定，甚者遍身。发于头面者称"抱头火丹"，发于躯干者称"丹毒"，发于胫踝者称"流火"。总属心火偏旺、又遇风热恶毒所致。

皮肤发黄，皮肤、面目、爪甲皆黄，是黄疸病。其中黄色鲜明如橘子色，为阳黄，多因脾胃或肝胆湿热所致。黄色晦暗如烟熏，是阴黄，多因脾胃为寒湿所困。

形态：皮肤虚浮肿胀，按有压痕，多属水湿泛滥。

皮肤干瘪枯燥，多为津液耗伤或精血亏损；皮肤干燥粗糙，状如鳞甲称肌肤甲错，多因瘀血阻滞、肌失所养而致。

色红，点大成片，平摊于皮肤下，摸不应手称为斑；形如粟粒，色红而高起，摸之碍手称为疹。由于病因不同可分为麻疹、风疹、隐疹等等。

白㾦与水泡都是高出皮肤的病疹，内为水液，白㾦是细小的丘疱疹，而水泡则泛指大小不一的同类疱疹。

发病局部范围较大，红肿热痛、根盘紧束的为痈；漫肿无头、

dampness and liver and spleen deficiency.

When skin of toes gets dark purple, festered, smelly and painful, it is sphacelus.

2.5.5 Observing skin

The key of observing skin is to pay attention to the change of skin color and shape.

If the skin suddenly turns red as wearing blusher, it is called "erysipelas", which can appear in any part of the body. It is like red clouds at the beginning, and then often spreads randomly all over the body. It is called "erysipelas hugging head" when it appears on the head; it is called "erysipelas" when on the trunk; it is called "flowing fire" on malleolus tibiae. All of them are caused by flourishing heart-fire and wind and toxic heat.

If skin, face, eyes, fingers and fingernails turn yellow, it is jaundice. If the color is bright yellow like orange, it is yang yellow caused by dampness and heat in spleen and stomach, or in liver and gallbladder. When the color is dark as smoked, it is yin yellow, mainly caused by coldness and dampness in spleen and stomach.

If a mark is left on swollen skin on pressing, it is edema.

Dry and withered skin is mainly caused by fluid or essence and blood deficiency; dry and withered skin like scales is mainly due to blood stasis and malnutrition of the skin.

If red spots or patches on the skin are smooth, they are called maculae; millet-like red spots which are higher above the skin and unsmooth are called papulae. Papulae can be further divided into measles, rubella, and implicit rash and so on based on different causes.

Miliaria crystallina and blisters are higher than the skin with fluid inside. The former are the tiny papulae and the latter refer to different sizes of papulae the of same kind.

Red spots which are painful and swelling are carbuncle; diffusive swelling spots with unchanged color and less pain

根脚平塌、肤色不变、不热少痛者为疽；范围较小、初起如粟、根脚坚硬较深、麻木或发痒，继则顶白而痛者为疔；起于浅表、形小而圆、红肿热痛不甚、容易化脓、脓溃即愈为疖。

are called gangrene; millet-like spots with deep and hard root, numbness or itching, and then with white top and pain are called nail-like furuncle; small and round spots on the surface of the skin which are swelling, painful and easy to fester and heal once the pus is out are called boil.

3　闻诊

3.1　听声音

主要是听患者呼吸、言语以及咳嗽、呕吐、呃逆、嗳气等气息的高低、强弱、清浊、缓急等变化，以分辨病情的寒热虚实。

3.1.1　正常声音

虽有性别、年龄、身体等形质禀赋之不同，声音亦各不相同，如男性多低浊，女性多高尖，儿童多清脆，老人多低沉，但发声自然、音调和畅、刚柔相济，是正常声音的共同特点。

3.1.2　病变声音

语声高亢洪亮，多言而躁动，多属实证、热证。语声低微无力，少言而沉静，多属虚证、寒证。

音哑与失声：语声低而嘶哑称音哑，发音不出称失声。二者病因病机基本相同，当先辨虚实。新病多属实证，多因外感风寒或风热袭肺、肺失清肃所致。久病多属虚证，因精气内伤、肺肾阴虚所致。

鼻鼾：鼻鼾是指气道不利时发出的异常呼吸声。若鼾声不绝，可致昏睡不醒，甚或痴呆、中风入

3　Listening and Smelling

3.1　Listening to the Voice

Listening to the voice is to discern the pitch, strength, voice, speed and other changes of the patient's breath, speech, cough, hiccupping, belching and so on to distinguish between cold and heat, deficiency and excess.

3.1.1　Normal voice

Although people's voices vary according to their genders, ages and figures, such as men's voice is low and unclear, women's is high and sharp, children's is crisp and clear, the elderly's is low and deep, the normal voice is characterized with natural voicing, harmonic tone with flexibility.

3.1.2　Pathological voice

If the person has high pitched and loud voice, and is too talkative and restless, it is mostly due to heat syndrome. If the person has low and weak voice, and is very quiet, it is mostly due to deficiency and cold syndrome.

The etiology and pathogenesis of hoarseness and aphonia are basically the same, but deficiency and excess should be distinguished. The new disease normally belongs to excess syndrome resulting from exogenous wind-cold or wind heat attacking the lung to lose its function of clearing and dispersing. The chronic disease belongs to deficiency syndrome resulting from essence-qi deficiency and lung- and kidney-yin deficiency.

Snoring is abnormal breathing when the airway is unsmooth. It can cause lethargy, even dementia, stroke or

中医理论　Basic Theory of Traditional Chinese Medicine

脏等危症。

呻吟是因痛苦而发出的声音。由于出乎意料的刺激而突然发出喊叫声,称惊呼。骤发剧痛或惊恐常令人发出惊呼。

3.1.3 语言异常

一般来说,沉默寡言者多属虚证、寒证;烦躁多言者,多属实证、热证。语声低微,时断时续者,多属虚证;语声高亢有力者多属实证。

狂言:喜笑无常,胡言乱语,喧扰妄动,烦躁不安等,主要见于狂症。多因痰火扰心、肝胆郁火所致。

癫语:语无伦次,自言自语或默默不语,精神恍惚,不欲见人。主要见于癫症。多因痰浊郁闭或心脾两虚所致。

独语:独自说话,喃喃不休,见人便止。多因心之气血不足,心神失养所致。

错语:语言颠倒错乱,或言后自知说错,不能自主。多因肝郁气滞、痰浊内阻、心脾两虚所致。

谵语:神志不清,胡言乱语,声高有力等,以外感热病多见。

郑声:言语重复,低微无力,时断时续。多因心气大伤、神无所依而致。

3.1.4 呼吸异常与咳嗽

喘:指呼吸急促困难,甚至张口抬肩、鼻翼翕动、端坐呼吸、

中医理论 Basic Theory of Traditional Chinese Medicine

other dangerous illnesses.

Groan is the painful voice. Suddenly hooting due to unexpected stimuli is called exclamation. A sudden severe pain or fear often makes people exclaim.

3.1.3 Abnormal speech

Generally speaking, the person remaining silent tends to have deficiency and cold syndrome; the person who is always restless and talkative usually has excess and heat syndrome. The person with low and intermittent voice mainly has deficiency syndrome; the person with high-pitched and powerful voice mostly has excess syndrome.

Raving is mainly seen in mania, including abnormal laughter, talking nonsense, irritability and restlessness. It is mainly due to mental agitation from phlegm-fire and stagnated fire of liver and gallbladder.

The symptoms of epilepsy are mainly incoherent and automatic speaking or silence, trance and not wanting to meet people. It is mainly phlegm stagnation or heart and spleen deficiency.

Soliloquy, with symptoms of muttering endlessly, sudden stop when seeing people is mainly due to heart-qi and blood deficiency and malnutrition of heart-spirit.

If the person with incoherent talk then realizes what has happened, but loses self-control, it is due to liver-qi stagnation, phlegm stagnation and deficiency in the heart and spleen.

Delirious speech is characterized by a confused mind, incoherent speech and sonorous sound of voice. It is mainly seen in exogenous fever.

Muttering is characterized by repeated and intermittent speech in a feeble voice. It is mostly caused by severe injury to heart qi and derangement.

3.1.4 Abnormal breathing and coughing

It refers to syndromes such as dyspnea, even breathing with open mouth and raised shoulder, fierce flaring of nasal

不能平卧的现象,可见于多种急慢性肺脏疾病。喘分虚实。实喘的特点是声高气粗,唯以呼出为快,甚则仰首目突,脉数有力,多因外邪袭肺或痰浊阻肺所致。虚喘的特点是呼吸短促,似不相接续,但得引一长息为快,活动后喘促更甚、气怯声低、倦怠乏力、脉微弱,多因肺之气阴两虚,或肾不纳气所致。

哮:以呼吸急促、喉中痰鸣如哨为特征。多反复发作,不易痊愈。往往在季节转换、气候变动突然时复发。哮分寒热,寒哮多在冬春季节,遇冷而作,因阳虚痰饮内停,或寒饮阻肺所致。热哮则常在夏秋季节、气候燥热时发作,因阴虚火旺或热痰阻肺所致。

上气:以呼吸气急、呼多吸少为特点,可兼有气息短促,面目浮肿,为肺气不利、气逆于喉间所致,有虚实之分。实证:以痰饮阻肺或外邪袭肺多见;虚证以阴虚火旺多见。

咳嗽是肺病中最常见的症状,是肺失肃降、肺气上逆的表现。"咳"是指有声无痰,"嗽"是指有痰无声,"咳嗽"为有声有痰。咳嗽首当区分外感内伤。一般说来,外感咳嗽,起病较急,病程较短,必兼表证;内伤咳嗽,起病缓慢,病程较长或反复发作。

咳嗽之辨证,要注意咳声的

wings and discomfort of lying on one's back. It is mainly seen in a variety of acute and chronic lung diseases. It is divided into asthma and asthenia. Asthma is characterized by loud and harsh breathing, even head elevation and protrusion of eyes and strong pulse, which is mainly caused by pathogenic factors attacking the lung or phlegm blocking the lung. Asthenia is characterized by dyspnea, qi deficiency and low voice, lassitude, weak pulse, which is mainly caused by lung-qi and yin deficiency and kidney not containing qi.

It is characterized by dyspnea and sputum rumbling in the throat like whistle. It breaks out repeatedly and is not easy to heal, especially reoccurs in the seasonal and sudden climate change. It is divided into cold and heat syndrome. Cold wheezing mainly happens in the cold winter and spring due to yang deficiency and phlegm retention, or cold drink obstructing the lung. Heat wheezing often happens in the dry and hot summer due to yin deficiency and fire hyperactivity or phlegm obstructing the lung.

Abnormal rising of qi is characterized by dyspnea of exhaling a lot and inhaling little, or is accompanied with shortness of breath and edema of the face, which is caused by unsmooth lung-qi blocking in the throat. It can be divided into deficiency and excess syndromes. The former is mainly due to phlegm blocking the lung or exogenous evil attacking the lung; the latter is mainly due to yin deficiency and fire hyperactivity.

Coughing is the most common symptom of lung disease due to the failure of the lung in descending and dispersing, making lung-qi rise adversely. Coughing can be divided into three kinds: the first is coughing with sound but no phlegm; the second is coughing with phlegm but no sound; the third is coughing with sound and phlegm. Coughing can also be divided into exogenous and internal ones. Generally speaking, exogenous cough is characterized by acute onset and short course accompanied with superficial syndrome; internal cough is characterized by slow onset and long course or recurrent attacks.

Syndrome differentiation in coughing should be

特点,如咳声紧闷,多属寒湿,咳
声清脆多属燥热等。咳声低微者,
多属肺气虚。此外,对咳嗽的诊
断,还须参考痰的色、量等不同表
现和兼见症状以鉴别寒热虚实。

3.1.5 呕吐嗳气与呃逆

呕吐、嗳气与呃逆均属胃气
上逆所致,因病邪影响的部位不
同,而见呕吐、嗳气与呃逆等不同
表现。

呕吐:有声有物称为呕;有
物无声称为吐,如吐酸水、吐苦水
等;干呕是指欲吐而无物有声,
或仅呕出少量涎沫,临床统称为
呕吐。

吐势徐缓、声音微弱者,属
虚寒呕吐,多因脾胃阳虚和胃阴
不足所致;而吐势较急、声音响
亮者,为实热呕吐,多见于食滞胃
脘、外邪犯胃、痰饮内阻、肝气犯
胃等症。

嗳气:俗称"打饱嗝",是气
从胃中上逆出咽喉时发出的声
音。饱食之后,偶有嗳气不属病
态。嗳气声低弱无力,多因脾胃
虚弱所致虚证嗳气。其声高亢有
力,嗳后腹满得减,多为食滞胃
脘、肝气犯胃、寒邪客胃而致实证
嗳气。

呃逆:是胃气上逆,从咽部
冲出、发出的一种不由自主的冲
击声,为胃气上逆、横膈痉挛所
致。呃逆分虚、实、寒、热。一般呃
声高亢、音响有力的多属实、属

focused on the characteristics of cough, such as coughing with tight and low sound mainly belongs to cold-dampness, coughing with clear sound belongs to dryness-heat, coughing with low and weak sound belongs to lung-qi deficiency. In addition, the diagnosis of cough should also consider the color and amount of sputum and concurrent symptoms to differentiate cold and heat, deficiency and excess.

3.1.5 Vomiting, belching and hiccuping

Vomiting, belching and hiccuping are caused by adverse flow of stomach-qi. The pathogenic factor attacks different parts, reflecting as the different symptoms like vomiting, belching and hiccupping.

There are three Kinds of vomiting: vomiting with sound and vomitus; silent vomiting with vomitus such as acid and bitter water; retching, or vomiting aloud without vomitus, or only with a small amount of saliva. Clinically all of them are called vomiting.

A slow vomiting with a weak sound belongs to deficiency syndrome mainly caused by spleen and stomach-yang and stomach-yin deficiency. A rapid and loud vomiting belongs to excess syndrome mainly seen in the retention of food in the stomach, exogenous pathogen attacking the stomach, phlegm stagnation, liver-qi attacking the stomach.

Belching is commonly known as "burp", which is the voice from the throat when qi flows adversely from the stomach. It is normal when it occasionally occurs after eating too much. Belching with a low and tiny sound belongs to deficiency syndrome caused by spleen and stomach deficiency. Abdominal fullness being alleviated after belching with loud and powerful sound belongs to excess syndrome caused by food retention in the stomach, liver-qi attacking the stomach and cold invading the stomach.

Hiccupping is a shock sound beyond one's control caused by adverse flow of stomach-qi out of the throat and diaphragmatic spasm. It is divided into deficiency, excess, cold and heat syndrome. Usually, hiccupping with a loud and powerful sound belongs to excess and heat syndrome;

热；呃声低沉、气弱无力的多属虚、属寒。

叹息：又称"太息"，是指自觉胸中憋闷而长嘘气的一种表现，以肝气郁结多见。

3.2　嗅气味

主要是嗅患者病体、排出物、病室等的异常气味，以了解病情，判断疾病的寒热虚实。

3.2.1　病体气味

口臭：是指患者张口时，口中发出臭秽之气，多见于牙疳、龋齿或口腔不洁等口腔本身的病变或胃火上炎、宿食内停或脾胃湿热等症。

汗气：汗出量多而有酸腐之气多为气分实热壅盛或久病阴虚火旺之人；汗出色黄而带有特殊的臭气多为风湿久羁肌表化热之痹症；若汗出伴有"尿臊气"则是病情转危的险候。

鼻臭：鼻流黄浊黏稠腥臭之涕、缠绵难愈、反复发作，是鼻渊；呼出之气带有"烂苹果味"，是消渴病之重证。若呼气带有"尿臊气"，则多见于阴水患者、病情垂危的险症。

身臭：疮疡溃烂或有狐臭等均可致身臭。

3.2.2　排出物气味

排出物如痰涎、大小便、妇人经带等的异常气味，通过问诊，可以得知。一般而言，排出物混浊而有臭秽、难闻的气味多属湿热或热邪致病；排出物清稀而无特

hiccupping with a low and feeble sound belongs to deficiency and cold syndrome.

Deep sighing refers to a long breath due to the feeling of chest stiffness, which is mainly caused by stagnation of liver qi.

3.2　Smelling the Odor

This method is to smell the abnormal odor of the patient, his discharge and the ward to learn the disease and judge the cold, heat, deficiency and excess of the disease.

3.2.1　Odor of the patient

Odor from the mouth refers to the foul breath coming from the patient's open mouth. It is mainly caused by ulcerative gingivitis, decayed teeth and filthy mouth and other oral diseases or stomach inflammation, indigestion or damp and heat in the spleen and stomach and other syndromes.

Profuse sweat with decaying and sour odor from a patient suggests solid heat or chronic disease with yin deficiency and excess heat; sweat with yellow color and offensive odor mainly belongs to arthromyodynia caused by rheumatism. Sweat with urine smell suggests a critical condition.

A turbid, thick and foul nasal discharge suggests ozaena which is difficult to cure and attacks repeatedly. A rotten apple-like breath indicates diabetes; a urine breath is more commonly seen in patients with edema and suggests a critical condition.

Sore and fester or hircismus can produce body odor.

3.2.2　Odor from the excretions

The abnormal smell of excretions such as phlegm, urine, menstruation and leucorrhea, etc. can be learned through asking the patients. In general, turbid excretions with foul odor suggest damp-heat or heat pathogen; clear and thin excretions without odor indicate cold pathogen or

中医理论

Basic Theory of Traditional Chinese Medicine

殊气味是寒邪或寒湿邪气致病。

呕吐物气味臭秽,多因胃热炽盛。若呕吐物气味酸腐,多为宿食内停;呕吐物腥臭,挟有脓血,多见于胃痈;若呕吐物为清稀痰涎,无明显气味者为脾胃有寒。

小便臊臭,色黄混浊,属实热证。若小便清长,无特殊气味,属虚证、寒证。

大便恶臭,黄色稀便或赤白脓血,为大肠湿热。小儿大便酸臭,伴有不消化食物,为食积内停。大便溏泻,气味不重者多为脾胃虚寒。

矢气如败卵味,多是食滞中焦或肠中有宿屎内停所致。矢气连连,声响不臭,多属肝郁气滞,腑气不畅。

月经或产后恶露臭秽,因热邪侵袭胞宫。带下气臭秽,色黄,为湿热下注。带下气腥,色白,为寒湿下注。

4 问诊

问诊,是医者通过询问患者或陪诊者,了解疾病的发生、发展、治疗经过以及现在症状和其他与疾病有关的情况,以诊察疾病的方法。

4.1 问诊原则

问诊时要做到恰当准确,简要而无遗漏,应当遵循以下原则:

确定主诉:首先明确病人感受最明显或最痛苦的主要症状及其持续的时间是什么,围绕主

cold-damp.

Vomitus with foul odor mainly indicates excessive heat of stomach. Vomitus with sour and decaying odor indicates indigestion. Vomitus with fishy odor and pus and blood suggests gastric ulcer. If the vomitus is clear and thin phlegm without odor, it suggests cold invades the spleen and stomach.

Yellow and turbid urine with foul odor indicates excessive heat syndrome. Clear and profuse urine without odor indicates deficiency and cold syndrome. Fetid stools, loose stools or stools with white pus and blood suggest damp-heat. Children having foul stools and indigestion suggest food retention. Loose stools with light smell indicate spleen and stomach deficiency.

Flatus with rotten egg-like smell is mainly caused by food retention in middle-energizer and stools in the large intestines. Constant flatus with loud noise and no odor mainly indicates liver-qi stagnation and unsmooth fu-qi.

Menstruation and postpartum with foul odor is caused by heat invading the uterus. Foul and yellow leucorrhea is caused by damp-heat flowing downward. Leucorrhea with fishy odor and white color is caused by cold-damp flowing downward.

4 Inquiry

Inquiry is the disease diagnosis method of asking the patient or his companions to know the disease occurrence, development, treatment, and present symptoms and other related information.

4.1 Principle of Inquiry

Inquiry will be done appropriately and accurately, briefly and thoroughly, if only the following principles are complied with.

Identifying the chief complaint should focus on the patient's most obvious and painful symptoms and their dura-

诉进行询问。

问辨结合：问诊时要对病人或陪诊者的回答加以分析辨证，缺少哪些情况的证据就再进一步询问那些方面，可以使问诊的目的明确，做到详而不繁，简而不漏，搜集的资料全面准确。

4.2　问诊内容

问诊的主要内容包括：一般项目、主诉和病史、现在症状等。

一般项目：包括姓名、性别、年龄、民族、职业、婚否、籍贯、现单位、现住址等。

主诉：主诉是患者就诊时感受最明显或最痛苦的主要症状及其持续的时间，通常是患者就诊的主要原因，也是疾病的主要矛盾。

现病史：包括疾病（主诉所述的疾病）从起病之初到就诊时病情演变与诊察治疗的全部过程，以及就诊时的全部自觉症状。

既往史：既往史包括既往健康状况，曾患病，是否痊愈，或留有后遗症，是否患过传染病。药物或其他过敏史。对小儿还应注意询问既往预防接种情况。

生活史：生活史包括患者的生活习惯、经历、饮食嗜好、劳逸起居、工作情况等。生活经历，应询问出生地、居住地及时间较长的生活地区，尤其是注意有地方病或传染病流行的地区。

家族病史：家族病史，是指患者直系亲属或者血缘关系较近的旁系亲属有否传染性疾病或遗传性疾病。

现在症状：问现在症状，是指询问患者就诊时的全部症状。这是问诊的主要内容。

tion, and then inquire the patient about the chief complaint.

To inquire should also analyze and differentiate the patient's or his companion's answer and further inquire about the aspects without enough proof in order to make the purpose clear and get the detailed, brief, comprehensive and accurate information.

4.2　Content of Inquiry

The main contents of inquiry include: general condition, chief complaints, history of illness and present symptoms.

General condition includes name, gender, age, nationality, occupation, marital status, native place, current employed institution and address etc.

Chief complaints are the most obvious and painful symptoms and their duration, usually the main reason for seeing a doctor and the main part of the disease.

History of recent illness refers to the onset, progress and change of the disease, treatment and all the present symptoms.

Anamnesis refers to the health condition, past illness condition including its recovery or squealer, infectious diseases, history of drug or other allergies, and past vaccination for children.

Life experience includes the patient's life habits, experience, eating and drinking, working and resting etc.; it also covers birth place, home place, and long-term residential place, especially the areas where endemics and infectious diseases occur.

Family history refers to whether the patient's immediate family members or collateral relatives have infectious disease or hereditary disease.

Present symptoms refer to all the symptoms on the consultation which are the main contents of inquiry.

中医理论

Basic Theory of Traditional Chinese Medicine

症状是疾病的反映,是临床辨证的主要根据。通过问诊掌握患者的现在症状,可以了解疾病目前的主要矛盾,并围绕主要矛盾进行辨证,从而揭示疾病的本质,对疾病作出确切的判断。因此,问现在症状是问诊中重要的一环,为求问得全面准确,无遗漏,后世医家将张景岳"十问歌"略加修改补充成为:"一问寒热二问汗,三问头身四问便,五问饮食六问胸,七聋八渴俱当辨,九问旧病十问因,再兼服药参机变;妇女尤必问经期,迟速闭崩皆可见;再添片语告儿科,天花麻疹全占验。"下面分而述之。

4.2.1　问寒热

问寒热是询问患者有无冷与热的感觉。二者是单独存在还是同时并见,还要注意询问寒热症状的轻重程度、出现的时间、持续时间的长短、临床表现特点及其兼症等。临床常见的寒热症状有以下几种情况:

但寒不热:患者只有怕冷的感觉而无发热者,即为但寒不热,可见于外感病初起尚未发热之时,或者寒邪直中脏腑经络,以及内伤虚证等。根据患者怕冷感觉的不同特点,临床又分别称为恶风、恶寒、寒战、畏寒等。

但热不寒:患者但觉发热而无怕冷的感觉者,称为但热不寒。可见于里热证,根据热势轻重、时间长短及其变化规律的不同,临床上有壮热、潮热、微热之分。

恶寒发热:恶寒与发热感觉

Symptoms reflect the illness, which is the main evidence for clinical differentiation. Through inquiry, the doctor can know the patient's present symptoms and the main paradox around which differentiation is carried out in order to uncover the nature of the disease and make an accurate diagnosis. Therefore, asking the present symptoms is the key part in order to get accurate and thorough information. Later doctors modified and supplemented Zhang Jingyue's *The song of Inquiry* as: "Ask about cold and feverish sensation, sweating, head and body, defecation and urination, diet, chest, blindness, thirst, anamnesis and causes of illness, and then give a prescription based on the ten items and differentiation; for females, ask about menstruation including delayed and proceeded menstruation, amenorrhea, metrorrhagia; for children, ask about smallpox and measles."

4.2.1　Inquiring about cold and heat

It refers to inquiring the patient's subjective sensation of cold and heat. Doctors should ask whether the two types of sensations occur alone or co-occur, and also pay attention to severity, time, duration, clinical characteristics and complication of the symptoms. Common clinical symptoms of cold and feverish sensations are as the following.

If the patients only have the sensation of chills but no fever, suggests the exogenous disease stays at the first stage and fever does not appear or cold pathogen directly attacks zang-fu organs and meridians, and it also indicates internal injuries and deficiency syndrome. According to the different characteristics of cold sensation, there are aversion to wind, aversion to cold, chills and fear of cold.

Fever without chills means patients have the sensation of fever but no chills. It indicates heat syndrome. According to the severity, duration and different change rules, there are high fever, hectic fever and low fever.

Chills and fever refers to the coexistence of chills and fever. It is one of the main symptoms of exterior syndrome. At

并存称恶寒发热。它是外感表证的主要症状之一。在表证初起,外邪束表,郁遏卫阳,肌表失煦故恶寒。卫阳失宣,郁而发热。

询问寒热的轻重不同表现,常可推断感受外邪的性质。如恶寒重,发热轻,多属外感风寒的表寒证。发热重,恶寒轻,多属外感风热的表热证。

寒热往来:指患者恶寒与发热交替发作,或一日一发或一日数发,可见于少阳病、温病及疟疾,是因外邪侵人体,在由表入里的过程中,邪气停留于半表半里之间,既不能完全入里,又不能外出,此时邪气不太盛,正气亦未衰,正邪相争处于相持阶段,正胜邪弱则热,邪胜正衰则寒,一胜一负,一进一退,故见寒热往来。

4.2.2 问汗

正常人在过劳、运动剧烈、环境或饮食过热、情绪紧张等情况下皆可以出汗,这属于正常现象。发生疾病时,各种因素影响了汗的生成与调节,可引起异常出汗。发病时出汗也有两重性,一方面出汗可以排出致病的邪气,促进机体恢复健康。另一方面汗为津液所化生,过度地出汗可以耗伤津液,导致阴阳失衡。问汗时要询问病人有无出汗,出汗的时间、部位,汗量有多少,出汗的特点、主要兼症以及出汗后症状的变化。常见有以下几种情况:

无汗:外感内伤,新病久病都可见有全身无汗。外感病中,

the beginning of exterior syndrome, the exterior is tightened by exogenous pathogens. Defensive yang is restricted and the texture and interstitial spaces of the muscles cannot be warmed, thus resulting in chills. The defensive yang fails to spread, thus resulting in fever.

Doctors inquire the different degrees of cold and heat sensation to infer the nature of exogenous evils. Such as, heavy chills and low fever suggest the exterior cold syndrome. High fever and light chills indicate the exterior heat syndromes.

Chills alternating with fever refers to alternate attack of chills and fever once a day or several times a day, suggesting shaoyang disease, epidemic febrile disease and malaria due to exogenous evil invading the human body in the process of which exogenous evil lingers between the exterior and interior. At the time, exogenous evil is not very abundant and vital qi is not deficient, so they are at a stalemate. If the vital qi defeats exogenous evil, there will appear fever; if exogenous evil defeats vital qi, there will appear chills. Therefore, there are chills alternating with fever.

4.2.2 Inquiring about sweating

Normally, people perspire when they are overworked, in hot environment and under emotional stress and take strenuous exercise and hot food. When a disease occurs, a variety of factors affect the generation and regulation of sweating, even cause abnormal sweating. Sweating also has a dual nature. On the one hand, sweating can discharge pathogenic evil and promote recovery of body. On the other hand, sweat is generated from fluid, so excessive sweating can over-consume fluid, resulting in the imbalance of yin and yang. Inquiring about perspiration is to ask the patient whether sweating or not, time, position, characteristics of sweat, main accompanied symptoms and change of symptoms after sweating. Common situations are as the following.

Absence of sweating can occur both in exogenous and internal injuries, new and chronic diseases. For exogenous

邪郁肌表、气不得宣、汗不能达，故无汗，属于卫气的调节功能失常。当邪气入里，耗伤营阴，亦无汗，属于津亏。内伤久病无汗，病机复杂，或为肺气失于宣达或为血少津亏、汗失生化之源。

汗出伴有发热恶风等症状，属太阳中风表虚证，是外感风邪所致。

若大汗不已，伴有高热、面赤、口渴饮冷，属实热证，是里热炽盛、蒸津外泄。

若冷汗淋漓，或汗出如油，伴有呼吸喘促、面色苍白、四肢厥冷、脉微欲绝，此时汗出常称为"脱汗"、"绝汗"，是久病重病正气大伤、津液大泄、阳亡阴竭的危候，预后不良。

白天经常汗出不止，活动后尤甚，常伴有神疲乏力、气短懒言或畏寒肢冷等症状，称为自汗。多因阳虚或气虚不能固护肌表，使腠理疏松，津液外泄。

睡则汗出，醒则汗止，称为盗汗，伴有潮热、颧红、五心烦热、舌红脉细数等症。睡时卫阳入里、肌表不密、虚热蒸津外泄，故盗汗出。醒后卫阳出表，故汗止。

先恶寒战栗，继而汗出者，称为战汗。战汗的转归，一为汗出病退，脉静身凉，烦渴顿除，此

diseases, evil lingers in the texture and interstitial spaces of the muscles, qi cannot disperse and sweat cannot arrive, so there is absence of sweating. This is caused by the disorder of defensive qi's regulation function. When evil comes inside and consumes nutritive yin, there will also be absence of sweating due to fluid deficiency. Internal injuries without sweating are complicated in pathogenesis, which indicates dispersing deficiency of lung-qi or blood and fluid deficiency, resulting in the loss of generation source.

Sweating accompanied with aversion to hot and wind and other symptoms indicates deficiency syndrome of taiyang wind stroke and exogenous pathogenic wind.

Profuse sweating along with high fever, flushing face, thirst for cold dink indicates heat syndrome manifesting as internal excessive heat steaming fluid to leak outside.

Profuse sweating with oil-like sweat, rapid or short breath, pale complexion, cold limbs and very weak pulse is called "sweating exhaustion", which is a sign of deterioration of protracted or severe illness injuring vital qi, severe release of fluid and collapse of yin and yang. This usually signifies severe condition and poor prognosis.

Spontaneous sweating is often characterized by constant sweating during the day intensified when active, which is accompanied by fatigue, shortness of breath or aversion to cold and cold limbs. It is mainly caused by yang or qi deficiency manifesting as not supporting the muscle and skin, resulting in loose textual and interstitial spaces of muscles and release of body fluid.

Sweating during sleep and no sweating when awakes is called night sweating. It indicates yin deficiency manifesting as hot flashes, red face, vexing heat in the chest, palms and soles, red tongue, weak pulse and so on. During sleep, defensive yang comes into the interior, makes the muscle and skin loose and deficiency-heat evaporate the fluid to dive out. When one awakes defensive yang comes out of the interior, so sweating stops.

Aversion to cold and shivers followed by sweating is called shiver sweating. On the one hand, after sweating, if high fever fades, the pulse calms down and thirst and

中医理论 Basic Theory of Traditional Chinese Medicine

为正气胜于邪气,病渐转愈,属佳象;一为战汗之后热势不退,症见烦躁,脉来急疾。此为正气虚弱,不能胜邪,而热复内陷,疾病恶化,属危象。

仅头部或头颈部出汗较多,叫头汗,多因上焦邪热或中焦湿热上蒸,逼津外泄;或病危虚阳浮越于上所致。

半身汗:指半侧身体有汗,或半侧身体经常无汗,或上或下,或左或右,可见于中风先兆、中风症、痿证、截瘫等病,多因患侧经络闭阻、气血运行不调所致。

手足汗:指手心、足心出汗较多。多因热邪郁于内或阴虚阳亢,逼津外出而达于四肢所致。

4.2.3 问周身

就是询问患者周身有无疼痛与其他不适。临床可按从头至足的顺序,逐一进行询问。

疼痛是临床常见的一种自觉症状,各科均可见到。问诊时,应问清疼痛产生的原因、性质、部位、时间、喜恶等。

胀痛:痛且有胀感,为胀痛。多因气机郁滞所致,在身体各部位都会出现,但以胸胁、胃脘、腹部较为多见。

刺痛:疼痛如针刺,称为刺痛。其特点是疼痛的范围较小,部位固定不移,多因瘀血所致,全身各处均可出现,但以胸胁、胃脘、小腹、少腹部最为多见。

绞痛:痛势剧烈如绞割者,称为绞痛。其特点是疼痛有剜、割、绞结之感,疼痛难以忍受,多见于

irritability disappears, it indicates the righteous qi defeats the evil and the disease is gradually cured; on the other hand, if fever does not subside after sweating, irritability still remains and pulse is acute, it indicates weak righteous qi cannot defeat the evil, resulting in heat invagination and disease deterioration, which would be a dangerous signal.

Sweating only on the head and neck is mainly due to the fluid driven out by heat in the upper-energizer and damp-heat in the middle-energizer, or by deficiency-yang floating upward.

Sweating on half of the body or no sweating on the other half—which can be the upper or the lower, the left or the right—is usually seen in the aura of stroke, stroke, paraplegia and flaccidity and other diseases caused by meridian obstruction, qi and blood disharmony of the diseased area.

Sweating on palms and soles is mainly caused by lingering heat in the interior or deficient yin and hyperactive yang which forces fluid out to the limbs.

4.2.3 Inquiring about the whole body

It refers to asking the patient whether there is pain or other discomfort. Clinically, the docotor should ask about the condition head to toe in sequence.

Clinically, pain is one of the common subjective symptoms, occurring in any diseases. Inquiry should cover cause, nature, location, time of the disease, likes and dislikes of the patients.

Distending pain is mainly caused by qi stagnation. It occurs in any part of the body, especially in the chest, stomach and abdomen.

Stabbing pain is characterized by small range and stable position. It is mainly caused by blood stasis. It occurs in any part of the body, especially in the chest, stomach, abdomen, and lower abdomen.

Gripping pain is the intolerable sensation of great pain, as if being scooped, cut, and twisted, mainly seen in cardiac pain caused by heart-blood stagnation, ascaris going

中医理论 Basic Theory of Traditional Chinese Medicine

心血瘀阻的心痛，蛔虫上窜或寒邪内侵胃肠引起的脘腹痛等。

窜痛：疼痛部位游走不定或走窜攻痛称为窜痛。其特点是痛处不固定，或者感觉不到确切的疼痛部位，多为风邪留着机体的经络关节，阻滞气机，产生疼痛。

掣痛：痛处有抽掣感或同时牵引他处而痛，称为掣痛。其特点是疼痛多呈条状或放射状，或有起止点，有牵扯感多由筋脉失养或经络阻滞不通所致。

灼痛：痛处有烧灼感，称灼痛，多由火热之邪串入经络，或阴虚阳亢、虚热灼于经络所致，可见于肝火犯络两胁灼痛，胃阴不足脘部灼痛及外科疮疡等症。

隐痛：痛而隐隐，绵绵不休，称隐痛，多因气血不足，或阳气虚弱，导致经脉气血运行滞涩所致。

不同部位的头部疼痛，一般与经络分布有关，如头颈痛属太阳经病，前额痛属阳明经病，头侧部痛属少阳经病，头顶痛属厥阴经病，头痛连齿属少阴经病。

胸痛憋闷，痛引肩臂者，为胸痹。闷痛，多为痰浊内阻或气虚血瘀等症。胸痛彻背、疼痛剧烈、面色青灰者，为真心痛。

胸痛、潮热盗汗、咳痰带血者，属肺阴虚证，因虚火灼伤肺络所致。

胸胁胀痛、走窜、太息易怒者，属肝气郁滞。

胃脘冷痛、疼势较剧、得热

upward or abdominal pain caused by cold-evil invading stomach and intestines.

Scurrying pain means the position of pain migrates from time to time, characterized by unfixed site of pain. It is mostly caused by wind-evil in the channels and collaterals and joints obstructing qi dynamic and causing pain.

Pulling pain is characterized by pain in strip and radial pattern, or having the starting and ending points and the sensation of pulling. It's mainly caused by tendons losing nourishment and meridians obstruction.

Scorching pain is mainly caused by heat-evil coming into meridians or yin deficiency and yang hyperactivity resulting in deficiency heat burning meridians. It can be seen in costal regions caused by liver-heat invading meridians and in gastral cavity caused by stomach-yin deficiency and ulcers.

Dull pain is a faint but lingering pain, caused by qi-blood deficiency or yang-qi deficiency resulting in obstruction of meridians and qi-blood.

Headache in different parts generally is associated with the meridian distribution, such as, pain at the back of head and nape indicates disease of taiyang channels; pain in the forehead indicates disease of shaoyang channels; pain on the top of the head indicates disease of jueyin channels; headache along with toothache indicates disease of shaoyin channels.

Choking chest pain radiating to shoulders and arms is known as thoracic obstruction, caused by phlegm resistance or qi deficiency and blood stasis. Severe chest pain radiating to the back accompanied with livid complexion is angina pectoris.

Chest pain, tidal fever and night sweating, blood sputum suggest lung-yin deficiency syndrome caused by deficient fire burning lung collaterals.

Hypochondriac pain migrating from place to place with deep sigh and irritability indicates liver-qi obstruction.

Epigastric severe pain with a cold sensation alleviated

中医理论 Basic Theory of Traditional Chinese Medicine

痛减,属寒邪犯胃。胃脘灼痛、多食善饥、口臭便秘者,属胃火炽盛。胃脘胀痛、嗳气不舒,属胃腑气滞,多是肝气犯胃所致。胃脘刺痛、固定不移,属瘀血胃痛。胃脘胀痛、嗳腐吞酸、厌食为食滞胃脘。胃脘隐痛、呕吐清水,属胃阳虚。胃脘灼痛嘈杂、饥不欲食,属胃阴虚。

腹痛:大腹隐痛、便溏、喜温喜按,属脾胃虚寒。小腹胀痛,小便不利多为癃闭,病在膀胱少腹冷痛,牵引阴部,为寒凝肝脉。凡腹痛徐缓、隐痛、喜按、得食痛减者,多属虚证。凡腹痛得热痛减者,多属寒证。凡腹痛、痛而喜冷者,多属热证。

腰脊骨痛,多病在骨;如腰痛以两侧为主,多病在肾;如腰脊痛连及下肢者,多病在下肢经脉。

四肢痛:四肢痛,多由风寒湿邪侵犯经络、肌肉、关节阻碍其气血运行所致,亦有因脾虚、肾虚者。如四肢关节疼痛不定,多为风痹;四肢关节困重多为湿痹;四肢关节疼痛剧烈,得热痛减为寒痹。四肢关节灼痛,喜冷,或有红肿,多为热痹;如足跟或胫膝隐隐而痛,多为肾气不足。

头晕:是指患者自觉视物昏花旋转,轻者闭目可缓解,重者感

in warmth indicates cold evil invading the stomach. Epigastric pain with a burning sensation, large food intake with rapid hunger, bad breath and constipation is mainly caused by excessive stomach-fire. Epigastric pain with a swelling sensation, belching and discomfort of stomach, qi stagnation is caused by liver-qi invading the stomach. Epigastric pain with a stabbing sensation migrating from place to place indicates blood stasis. Epigastric pain with a swelling sensation, putrid belching and acid swallowing and anorexia indicates retention of food in the stomach. Epigastric pain with a dull sensation and vomitus of clear water indicates stomach-yang deficiency. Epigastric pain with burning sensation and anorexia indicates stomach-yin deficiency.

Dull abdominal pain along with loose stool, predilection for warmth and pressure indicates deficiency and cold in the spleen and stomach. Abdominal pain with a swelling sensation and difficulty in urination indicates urinary retention, bladder disease and cold pain in the abdomen radiating to genitals, caused by cold lingering in hepatic veins. All the dull abdominal pain along with predilection for pressure alleviated when taking food indicates deficiency syndrome. All the abdominal pain alleviated by warmth indicates cold deficiency. All the abdominal pain alleviated by cold indicates heat syndrome.

Backache and spine pain mainly indicates bone disease; the pain on both sides of the back indicates kidney disease; the pain on the spine radiating to lower limbs indicates disease of meridians on lower limbs.

Limb pain is mainly caused by wind, cold and dampness invading meridians, muscles, and joints and hindering their qi and blood circulation or by spleen and kidney deficiency. Migrating pain indicates wandering arthritis; tired and heavy joints and limbs indicate warm arthritis; severe pain on joints alleviated in warmth indicates cold arthritis. If joints with a burning pain alleviate with cold or appear red and swollen, it indicates heat arthritis. A dull pain in heels or in legs and knees indicates kidney-qi deficiency.

Dizziness means the patient has a whirling sensation. In mild cases, it alleviates when the patient closes his/her

觉天旋地转,不能站立,闭目亦不能缓解。临床常见风火上扰、阴虚阳亢、心脾血虚、中气不足、肾精不足、痰浊中阻等症型。

目痛而赤,属肝火上炎;目赤肿痛、羞明多眵,多属风热;目痛较剧,伴头痛、恶心呕吐、瞳孔散大,多是青光眼。

患者自觉耳内鸣响,如闻蝉鸣或潮水声,或左或右,或两侧同时鸣响,或时发时止,或持续不停,称为耳鸣,临床有虚实之分。若暴起耳鸣声大,用手按而鸣声不减,属实证,多因肝胆火盛所致;渐觉耳鸣,声音细小,以手按之,鸣声减轻,属虚证,多由肾虚精亏、髓海不充、耳失所养而成。

新病突发耳聋多属实证,因邪气蒙蔽清窍,清窍失养所致,渐聋多属虚证,多因脏腑虚损而成。一般而言,虚证多而实证少,实证易治,虚证难治。

在正常的条件下,患者即自觉心跳异常,心慌不安,不能自主,称为心悸。若因惊而悸称为惊悸。引起心悸的原因很多,如心阳亏虚、鼓动乏力;气血不足、心失所养;阴虚火旺、心神被扰;水饮内停,上犯凌心;痰浊阻滞、心气不调。

腹胀有虚、有实、有寒、有热,其病机却总以气机不畅为主。

eyes; in severe cases, the patient is unable to stand, feeling things go round and the symptom does not alleviate by closing eyes. Clinically, it is seen as wind-fire disturbance, yin deficiency and yang hyperactivity, blood deficiency of heart and spleen, kidney essence deficiency, stagnation of turbid phlegm in middle-energizer and other syndromes.

Red and painful eyes indicate liver-fire inflammation; red and swollen eyes with photophobia and much eye excretion indicate wind-heat; severely painful eyes with headache, vomiting and mydriasis indicate glaucoma.

If the patient feels ringing in his ears like sound of cicadas and tide on one side or both sides, sounding from time to time or continuously, it indicates tinnitus which can be divided into deficiency and excess syndromes. If a sudden attack of tinnitus cannot be reduced by pressing the ears, it indicates excess syndrome caused by abundant fire in the liver and gallbladder. If a gradual attack of tinnitus with a tiny sound can be reduced by pressing the ears, it indicates deficiency syndrome caused by kidney and essence deficiency, lack of marrow and malnutrition of ears.

A sudden attack of deafness in a recent disease suggests excess syndrome which is caused by evil blinding orifices resulting in malnutrition of orifices. A gradual attack of deafness indicates deficiency syndrome caused by viscera deficiency. Generally speaking, deficiency syndromes are prone to occur compared with excess syndromes. The former is easy to be cured and the latter is difficult to be cured.

Normally, if patients feel the heartbeat is abnormal but nervous, and restless, it is known as palpitation. Palpitation is due to many causes such as, heart-yang deficiency leads to weak agitation; qi and blood deficiency is unable to nourish heart; yin deficiency and excessive heat disturb heart-spirit; fluid retention invades heart; phlegm blocking leads to malfunction of heart-qi.

Abdominal distension can be divided into deficiency, excess, cold and heat. Its pathogenesis is mainly dominated by unsmooth qi-dynamic.

中医理论

Basic Theory of Traditional Chinese Medicine

麻木多见于头面四肢部，可因气血不足或风痰湿邪阻络、气滞血瘀等导致经脉失去气血营养所致。

4.2.4 问二便

询问患者大小便的有关情况，如大小便的性状、颜色、气味、便量多少、排便的时间、两次排便的间隔时间、排便时的感觉及排便时伴随症状等，可以判断机体消化功能的强弱，津液代谢的状况，同时也是辨别疾病的寒热虚实性质的重要依据。

健康人一般一日或两日大便一次，为黄色成形软便，排便顺利通畅。

便秘：即大便秘结，指粪便在肠内滞留过久，排便间隔时间延长，便次减少，称为便秘。其病机总由大肠传导功能失常所致，可见于胃肠积热、气机郁滞、气血津亏、阴寒凝结等症。

溏泻：又称便溏或泄泻，即大便稀软不成形，甚则呈水样，排便间隔时间缩短，便次增多，日三、四次以上，总由脾胃功能失调、大肠传导亢进所致。可见于脾虚、肾阳虚、肝郁乘脾、伤食、湿热蕴结大肠、感受外邪等症。

健康人在一般情况下，一昼夜排尿量约为1000～1800毫升，尿次白天3～5次，夜间0～1次。

尿量减少：可见于实热证、汗吐下证、水肿病及癃闭、淋证等病症。

Numbness mainly occurs on head, face and limbs , and is caused by qi-blood deficiency or wind, phlegm and dampness obstructing collaterals, qi stagnation and blood stasis, leading to malnutrition of channels.

4.2.4 Inquiring about defecation and urination

This is to inquire about their shape, properties, color, odor, amount, time, interval, sensation and associated symptoms when defecating and urinating etc., based on which the digestive function and the metabolism of body fluid can be judged and at the same time the nature of disease, including cold, heat, deficiency and excess can be identified.

Healthy people generally have bowls once a day or every other day. The stools are yellow, shaped, soft and smoothly discharged.

Constipation means that stools stay in the intestines for a long time, the interval of discharge prolongs and the frequency of discharge is reduced. Its pathogenesis is caused by the abnormal conductive function of the large intestine, which is seen in the heat accumulation in the intestines and stomach, qi stagnation, qi, blood and fluid deficiency, yin-cold coagulation and other syndromes.

Diarrhea refers to loose, water-like, frequent discharge of stools which are discharged more than three or four times a day. It is caused by the abnormal function of the spleen and stomach and conductive hyperactivity of large intestine, which is seen in the spleen and kidney-yang deficiency, liver depression impairing spleen, dyspepsia, accumulation of damp-heat in the large intestine, invasion of exogenous pathogen and other syndromes.

Healthy people generally urinate 1000-1800ml, 3-5 times in daytime and 0-1 at night.

Decreased amount of urine is seen in excessive heat, profuse perspiration, vomiting and diarrhea, edema, retention of urine, stranguria and other symptoms.

中医理论

Basic Theory of Traditional Chinese Medicine

排尿次数增多,又叫小便频数,总由膀胱气化功能失职而致,多见于下焦湿热、下焦虚寒、肾气不固等症。

排尿不畅,且伴有急迫灼热疼痛感,多为湿热流入膀胱、灼伤经脉、气机不畅而致,可见于淋证。

小便不畅,点滴而出为癃,小便不通,点滴不出为闭,一般多统称为癃闭。病机有虚有实。实者多为湿热蕴结、肝气郁结或瘀血、结石阻塞尿道而致。虚者多为年老气虚、肾阳虚衰、膀胱气化不利而致。

小便失禁:多为肾气不足,下元不固;下焦虚寒,膀胱失煦,不能制约水液而致。睡眠中小便自行排出,俗称尿床,多见于儿童。

4.2.5 问饮食与口味

口不渴:为津液未伤,见于寒证或无明显热邪之证。

口渴多饮是津液大伤的表现,多见于实热证、消渴病及汗吐下后。

渴不多饮是津液轻度损伤或津液输布障碍的表现,可见于阴虚、湿热、痰饮、瘀血等症。

食欲减退,又称"纳呆"、"纳少",即病人不思进食。不思饮食与厌食,大体上有两种情况,一是不知饥饿不欲食,二是虽饥亦不欲食或厌恶食物。二者病机均属脾胃不和消化吸收功能减弱所致。

饥不欲食,是患者感觉饥饿而

Frequent urine is caused by disturbed water metabolism of the bladder due to damp-heat and deficiency cold in lower-energizer and insecurity of kidney-qi.

Difficulty in urination accompanied by an urgent and burning sensation is due to damp-heat in the bladder impairing meridians, and unsmooth qi which are seen in stranguria.

Pathogenesis means little or no urine. It can be divided into excess and deficiency syndrome. The excess syndrome is caused by accumulation of damp-heat, liver qi stagnation or blood stasis, urethral obstruction caused by gallstone. The deficiency syndrome is caused by qi deficiency for the elderly, kidney-yang deficiency and the failure of bladder gasification.

Incontinence of urine is caused by kidney-qi deficiency or deficiency-cold in the lower-energizer which cannot warm the bladder and control urination. Urine is expelled when people, especially children, fall in asleep, which is commonly known as bedwetting.

4.2.5 Inquiring about diet and taste

No feeling of thirst indicates body fluid is not impaired, which is seen in cold syndrome or syndrome without evident heat.

Thirst and drinking a lot of water indicates body fluid is impaired seriously, which is seen in excess-heat syndrome, diabetes and vomiting, sweating and discharging.

Thirst without drinking much water indicates a mild impairment of body fluid or dysfunction of body fluid distribution, which is seen in yin deficiency, damp-heat and phlegm retention.

Declined appetite refers to reduction of repast. There are two cases for declined appetite and anorexia. One is the loss of appetite; the other is no demand for food even when hungry. Both of them are caused by disharmony of spleen and stomach and impaired digestion and absorption.

Hunger with no desire to eat means the patient feels

中医理论

Basic Theory of Traditional Chinese Medicine

中医理论

Basic Theory of Traditional Chinese Medicine

又不想进食,或进食很少,亦属食欲减退范畴,多见于胃阴不足症。

多食易饥,中医称为"消谷善饥",可见于胃火亢盛、胃强脾弱等症,亦可见于消渴病。

偏嗜,是指嗜食某种食物或某种异物。其中偏嗜异物者,又称异嗜,若小儿异嗜,喜吃泥土、生米等异物,多属虫积。若妇女已婚停经而嗜食酸味,多为妊娠。

询问食欲与食量时,还应注意进食情况如何。如病人喜进热食,多属寒证;喜进冷食多属热证。进食后稍安,多属虚证;进食后加重,多属实证或虚中夹实证。疾病过程中,食欲渐复,表示胃气渐复,预后良好;反之,食欲渐退,食量渐减,表示胃气渐衰,预后多不良。若病重不能食,突然暴食,食量较多,是脾胃之气将绝的危象,称"除中",实际上是中气衰败、死亡前兆,属"回光反照"的一种表现。

口淡乏味,多因脾胃气虚而致。口甜,多见于脾胃湿热证。口粘腻,多属湿困脾胃。口中泛酸,可见于肝胆蕴热证。若口中酸腐,多见于伤食症。口苦,属热证的表现,可见于火邪为病和肝胆郁热之证。口咸,多属肾病及寒证。

4.2.6　问睡眠

失眠又称"不寐"、"不得眠",是指经常不易入睡,或睡而

hungry, but he does not want to eat or eats little, which is seen in stomach-yin deficiency.

Excessive eating and frequent hunger is seen in exuberance of stomach fire, hyperfunction of stomach and spleen and also diabetes.

Addiction eating refers to preference for some food or inedible things. Children's preference for inedible things such as dirt and raw rice indicates vermination. That Married females have menopause and prefer sour food indicates pregnancy.

The condition of food intake should also be asked about. If the patient prefers to eat hot food, it indicates cold syndrome, while preference for cold food indicates hot syndrome. If the illness is alleviated after eating, it indicates deficiency syndrome; if the illness is aggravated after eating, it indicates excess syndrome or deficiency syndrome accompanied with excess syndrome. In the course of illness, gradual recovery of appetite indicates gradual recovery of stomach-qi and prognosis is good; by the contrast, gradual decrease of appetite indicates gradual decrease of stomach-qi and prognosis is not good. If the patient suffering from serious illness suddenly eats a lot, it indicates the exhaustion of spleen and stomach-qi. In fact, it is the manifestation of vital-qi declination and death.

Bland taste in the mouth is caused by spleen and stomach-qi deficiency. Sweet taste in the mouth is caused by damp-heat in the spleen and stomach. Sticky and greasy taste in the mouth is caused by damp in the spleen and stomach. Sour taste in the mouth is caused by heat retention in the liver and gallbladder. Sour and decaying taste in the mouth is caused by improper diet. Bitter taste in the mouth is caused by heat syndrome and heat retention in the liver and gallbladder. Salty taste in the mouth is caused by kidney disease and cold syndrome.

4.2.6　Inquiring about sleep

Insomnia refers to being difficult to fall asleep or easy to wake up but difficult to return to sleep or difficult to

易醒、不易再睡，或睡而不酣、易于惊醒，甚至有彻夜不眠的表现。其病机是阳不入阴、神不守舍：气血不足、神失所养；阴虚阳亢、虚热内生；肾水不足、心火亢盛等，皆可扰动心神、导致失眠，属虚。痰火、食积、瘀血等邪火上扰，心神不宁，亦可出现失眠，属实。

嗜睡称为"但欲寐"，如日夜沉睡、呼应可醒、神志朦胧、偶可对答，称为"昏睡"。湿邪困阻、清阳不升、脾气虚弱、中气不足、不能上荣、心肾阳衰、阴寒内盛、神气不振、邪扰清窍、热蔽心神、中风病等皆可出现嗜睡。大病之后，精神疲惫而嗜睡，是正气未复的表现。

4.2.7　问经带

正常经期约为28～32天，每次5～7天。应注意询问月经的周期，行经的天数，月经的量、色、质、有无闭经或行经腹痛等表现。

月经先期：月经周期提前八、九天以上，称为月经先期，多因血热妄行，或气虚不摄而致。

月经后期：月经周期错后八、九天以上，称月经后期，多因血寒、血虚、血瘀而致。

月经先后不定期：月经超前与错后不定，相差时间多在八、九天以上者，称为月经先后不定期，又称月经紊乱，多因情志不舒、肝气郁结、失于条达、气机逆乱，或者脾肾虚衰、气血不足、冲任失调，或瘀血内阻、气血不畅、经期

have deep sleep and easy to wake up, even staying awake the whole night. It is caused by deficiency syndrome such as yang failing to enter yin and mental derangement, qi-blood deficiency and malnutrition of spirit, yin deficiency and yang hyperactivity and deficiency heat, deficiency of kidney yin and heart-fire hyperactivity. Evil fire, such as, phlegm-fire, food retention and blood stasis disturbing heart and spirit, can also lead to insomnia, which is excess syndrome.

Lethargy refers to sleeping day and night. The patient can wake up when called, and respond at questions from time to time in confused state of mind, which is also known as "hypnody" caused by dampness obstruction and lucid yang failing to rise, spleen-qi deficiency, deficiency of qi in middle-energizer, yang deficiency of heart and kidney, excessive yin-cold, evil disturbing clear orifices and heat covering heart-spirit and stroke. Lassitude after recovery from serious illness is a sign of vital qi deficiency.

4.2.7　Inquiring about menstruation

The normal menstrual cycle is about 28~32 days and the menorrhea period is about 5~7 days. Inquiry about menstruation should involve menstrual cycle, period, amount, color, quality, whether there is amenorrhea or abdominal pain and other syndromes.

Proceeded menstrual cycle means menstruation occurs more than 8 or 9 days earlier. It is caused by blood heat and qi deficiency.

Delayed menstrual cycle means menstruation occurs more than 8 or 9 days later. It is caused by blood-cold, blood deficiency and blood stasis.

Irregular menstrual cycle means menstruation occurs earlier or later more than 8 or 9 days,which is also known as menstrual disorder. It is caused by emotional discomfort and liver-qi stagnation or deficiency of spleen, kidney and qi-blood or blood stasis, unsmooth qi-blood.

错乱,故月经先后不定期。

崩漏:指妇女不规则的阴道出血,临床以血热、气虚最为多见。瘀血也可致崩漏。

成熟女性,月经未潮,或来而中止,停经三月以上,又未妊娠者,称闭经或经闭,可见于肝气郁结、瘀血、湿盛痰阻、阴虚、脾虚等症。闭经应注意与妊娠期、哺乳期、绝经期等生理性闭经,或者青春期、更年期,因情绪、环境改变而致一时性闭经及暗经加以区别。

经行腹痛是在月经期,或行经前后出现小腹部疼痛的症状,亦称痛经。得热痛减为寒,得热痛不减或益甚为热;绞痛为寒,刺痛、钝痛、闷痛为血瘀;隐隐作痛为血虚;持续作痛为血滞;时痛时止为气滞;胀痛为气滞血瘀。气滞为主则胀甚于痛;瘀血为主则痛甚于胀。

凡带下色白而清稀、无臭,多属虚证、寒证。带下色黄或赤、稠粘臭秽,多属实证、热证。若带下色白量多、淋漓不绝、清稀如涕,多属寒湿下注。带下色黄、黏稠臭秽,多属湿热下注。若白带中混有血液,为赤白带,多属肝经郁热。

4.2.8　问小儿

小儿科古称"哑科",不仅问诊困难,而且不一定准确。问小

Metrorrhagia and metrostaxis refer to irregular vaginal bleeding in large amount, which is usually caused by blood heat, qi deficiency or blood stasis.

For mature women, no menstruation or cessation of menstruation for more than three months without pregnancy is called amenorrhea. It is caused by liver-qi stagnation, blood stasis, excessive heat and phlegm obstruction, yin deficiency and spleen deficiency and other syndromes. Amenorrhea should be differentiated from temporary cessation of menstruation or latent menstruation during pregnancy, lactation, cessation of menstruation or temporary amenorrhea caused by mood and environment during puberty and menopause.

Dysmenorrhea refers to abdominal pain during, before or after menstruation. Abdominal pain is alleviated with warmth indicates cold syndrome and otherwise indicates heat syndrome. Colic pain indicates cold syndrome; stabbing pain, blunt pain and stuffy pain indicate blood stasis; dull pain suggests blood deficiency; continuous pain suggests blood stasis; pain from time to time suggests qi stagnation; distending pain indicates qi stagnation and blood stasis. When the pain is caused by qi stagnation, the sensation of swelling is keener than pain. When the pain is caused by blood stasis, the sensation of pain is keener than swelling.

Clear leucorrhea without foul odor mainly belongs to deficiency and cold syndrome. Yellowish or red, thick and sticky leucorrhea belongs to heat and excess syndrome. A large amount of whitish, clear and thin leucorrhea indicates pouring down of cold-dampness. Yellowish, thick, sticky and viscous leucorrhea indicates pouring down of damp-heat. Discharge mingled with blood, or red leucorrhea is mostly caused by heat stagnation of liver meridian.

4.2.8　Inquiring about children's condition

Pediatrics was called "dumb department" in ancient times since inquiry is difficult and not accurate. When

中医理论

Basic Theory of Traditional Chinese Medicine

儿,除了一般的问诊内容外,还要注意询问出生前后情况、喂养情况、生长发育情况及预防接种情况,传染病史及传染病接触史。

asking about children's condition, besides the common items, the condition before and after birth, of feeding, growth and development, preventive inoculation and history and contact history of infectious diseases should also be covered.

5 切诊

切诊包括脉诊和按诊两部分内容,脉诊是按脉搏,按诊是在患者身躯上一定的部位进行触、摸、按压,以了解疾病的内在变化或体表反应,从而获得辨证资料的一种诊断方法。

5.1 脉诊

诊脉的部位,有遍诊法、三部诊法和寸口诊法。前两种诊脉的部位,后世已少采用,自晋以来,普遍选用的切脉部位是寸口。

寸口又称脉口、气口,其位置在腕后桡动脉搏动处,寸口分寸、关、尺三部,以高骨(桡骨茎突)为标志,其稍内方的部位为关,关前(腕端)为寸,关后(肘端)为尺。两手各分寸、关、尺三部,共六部脉。寸、关、尺三部可分浮、中、沉三候,是寸口诊法的三部九候。

寸关尺分候脏腑,历代医家说法不一,目前多以下列为准:

左寸:心与膻中;右寸:肺与胸中;左关:肝胆与膈,右关:脾与胃;左右尺:肾与膀胱。

5 Pulse Examination and Palpation

Pulse examination refers to pressing a patient's pulse; palpation refers to diagnostic methods through touching and pressing certain parts of a patient's body to know the internal change and external reaction of a disease to get data of syndrome differentiation.

5.1 Pulse Examination

There are three methods of pulse examination according to the examination positions: general diagnostic method, three-portion diagnostic method and cunkou diagnostic method. The first two methods are rarely used in the later generation and the last one is generally used since Jin dynasty.

Cunkou is also known as maikou and qikou. It is located at the posterocarpal radial artery. Cunkou is divided into three portions: cun, guan and chi. The inner side of prominent bone (the styloid process of the radius) marks the guan. In front of the guan (at the wrist joint) is cun, and behind the guan is chi. There are six portions of cunkou pulse on two hands. Each portion is divided into three readings: the light reading, medium reading and heavy reading. There are nine readings on three portions in cunkou diagnostic method.

Three portions correspond to different zang-fu organs. However, doctors in past dynasties have different versions. The frequently used version is as follows:

cun on the left hand: heart and danzhong; cun on the right hand: lung and chest; guan on the left hand: liver, gallbladder and diaphragm; guan on the right hand: spleen and stomach; chi on both hands: kidneys and bladder.

中医理论 Basic Theory of Traditional Chinese Medicine

正常脉象称为平脉。脉象从容和缓、柔和有力、节律一致、不浮不沉、不大不小。一息四～五至，相当于72～80次／分），并随生理活动和气候环境的不同而有相应的正常变化。中医脉象特别讲究有胃气。

正常脉象不浮不沉、不快不慢、从容和缓、节律一致便是有胃气。即使是病脉，无论浮沉迟数，但有徐和之象者，便是有胃气。脉少胃气，则为病变，脉无胃气，则属真脏脉，或为难治或不治之征象，故脉有无胃气对判断疾病凶吉预后有重要的意义。

个别人脉不见于寸口，而从尺部斜向手背，称斜飞脉；若脉出现于寸口的背侧，则称反关脉，还有出现于腕部其他位置者，都是生理特异脉位，不属病脉。

临床上有时须辨明脉证的真假以决定从舍，或舍脉从症，或舍症从脉。如症见腹胀满、疼痛拒按、大便燥结、舌红苔黄厚焦燥，而脉迟细者，此时当舍脉从症；而如伤寒、热闭于内，症见四肢厥冷，而脉滑数，此时当舍症从脉。

不同的病理脉象，反映了不同的病症，我国最早的脉学专书

The normal pulse is stable with regular rhythms, neither floating nor deep, neither too big nor small with a frequency of about 4~5 beats per breath (72~80 times per minute). It has corresponding change according to physiological and climatic conditions. Stomach-qi is especially emphasized in pulse taking in TCM.

The normal pulse which is neither floating nor deep, neither quick nor slow, stable with regular rhythms means stomach-qi is sufficient. Even the abnormal pulse, though being floating, deep, slow or rapid, indicates the existence of stomach-qi as long as it's harmonious. If the pulse lacks stomach-qi, it indicates pathological changes. Absence of stomach-qi belongs to critical pulse condition, indicating syndromes of serious or incurable diseases. Therefore, whether the pulse has stomach-qi or not plays a significant role in diagnosing the disease.

Some individual's pulse is not seen at cunkou, but it slants from chi to the back of the hand, which is known as oblique flying pulse. If the pulse appears at the back of cunkou, it is called reverse pulse. If the pulse appears at the wrist joint or other positions, it is specific pulse position physiologically rather than sick one.

Clinically, sometimes it is imperative to tell the true pulses and symptoms from the false ones and decide to make diagnosis based on symptoms and signs rather than pulse conditions, or make diagnosis based on pulse conditions rather than symptoms and signs. For example, if there are symptoms and signs like abdominal distention and pain which is aggravated by pressure, constipation, red tongue with yellowish thick and dry coating and a slow thready pulse, diagnosis should be made according to symptoms and signs rather than pulse conditions; if there are symptoms and signs like cold limbs, slippery and rapid pulse which is seen in cold and interior heat, diagnosis should be made according to pulse conditions rather than symptoms and signs.

Different abnormal pulses reflect different symptoms. The first book about pulse study in China, *The Pulse*

《脉经》提出二十四种脉象,《濒湖脉诀》有二十七种,李士材的《诊家正眼》又增加疾脉,故近代多从二十八脉论述。下面介绍一些常见脉象分类与主病:

Classic (*Maijing*), puts forward twenty-four kinds of pulses and there are twenty-seven in *Binhu's Sphygmology* (*Binhu Maijue*). In addition, *Key to Physicians* written by Li Shicai (*Zhenjia Zhengyan*) adds the racing pulse. So, now there are twenty-eight pulses to be discussed. The following are the classification of common pulses and their suggestion of problems.

5.1.1 浮脉

脉象:轻取即得,重按稍减而不空,举之泛泛而有余,如水上漂木。

主病:表证、虚证。

脉理:浮脉主表,反映病邪在经络肌表部位,邪袭肌腠,卫阳奋起抵抗,脉气鼓动于外,脉应指而浮,故浮而有力。内伤久病体虚,阳气不能潜藏而浮越于外,亦有见浮脉者,必浮大而无力。

5.1.1 Floating pulse

Pulse condition The pulse is easily felt when pressed gently but it is felt a little weaker when pressed heavily. This pulse condition is just like the condition of a floating wood.

Main disease It indicates the exterior and deficiency syndrome.

Clinical significance It suggests that pathogenic factors attack the superficial part of the body. Defensive yang-qi rises up fighting against them; vessel qi comes to the surface and then the floating and powerful pulse appears. Because of the weakness after protracted disease, instead of hiding, yang-qi floats outside leading to floating and weak pulse.

5.1.2 沉脉

脉象:轻取不应,重按乃得。

主病:里证。

脉理:病邪在里,邪正相搏,气血内困,故脉沉而有力,为里实证;若脏腑虚弱、阳气衰微、气血不足、无力统运营气于表,则脉沉而无力,为里虚证。

5.1.2 Deep pulse

Pulse condition It is only felt when pressed heavily.

Main disease It indicates interior syndrome.

Clinical significance The healthy qi and pathogenic factors fight against each other, qi and blood is blocked inside, so the pulse is deep and forceful, which suggests interior excessive syndrome; if weak zang-fu organs, faint yang-qi, deficient qi and blood cannot carry nutritive qi to the exterior, the pulse will be deep and weak, suggesting interior deficient syndrome.

5.1.3 迟脉

脉象:脉来迟慢,一息不足四至(相当于每分钟脉搏60次以下)。

主病:寒证。

脉理:阳气不足,鼓动血行

5.1.3 Slow pulse

Pulse condition It beats less than 4 times per breath (less than 60 per minute).

Main disease It indicates cold syndrome.

Clinical significance Deficient yang qi leads to weak

中医理论 Basic Theory of Traditional Chinese Medicine

无力,故脉来一息不足四至。阴寒冷积阻滞、阳失健运、血行不畅、脉迟而有力;阳虚而寒者,脉多迟而无力;邪热结聚、阻滞气血运行,也见迟脉,但必迟而有力、按之必实;久经锻炼的运动员,脉迟而有力,则不属病脉。

5.1.4 数脉

脉象:一息脉来五至以上。

主病:热证。有力为实热,无力为虚热。

脉理:邪热内盛,气血运行加速,故见数脉。邪热炽盛、正气不虚、正邪交争剧烈,故脉数而有力,主实热证;久病阴精耗伤、虚热内生,则脉虽数而无力;若脉浮数、重按无根,是虚阳外越之危候。

5.1.5 缓脉

脉象:一息四至,来去怠缓。

主病:湿证,脾胃虚弱。

脉理:湿邪黏滞,气机为湿邪所困;脾胃虚弱、气血乏源,气血不足以充盈鼓动,故见缓脉。

5.1.6 洪脉

脉象:脉形极大,状若波涛汹涌,来盛去衰。

主病:里热证。

脉理:阳气有余、气盛血涌,致使脉道扩张,故脉见洪象;若久病气虚或虚劳、失血、久泄等病

blood circulation, so there is less than 4 beats per breath. Blocked cold yin, stagnated yang-qi, impeded flow of qi and blood lead to slow and forceful pulse; yang deficiency and cold syndrome always lead to slow and forceless pulse; heat accumulation blocking qi and blood circulation also lead to slow but forceful pulse; the slow and forceful pulse felt on the athletes is not a disease pulse.

5.1.4 Rapid pulse

Pulse condition It beats more than 5 times per breath.

Main disease It indicates heat syndrome. The forceful pulse is excessive heat and the forceless is deficient.

Clinical significance The rampancy of heat accelerates qi and blood circulation leading to the rapid pulse. Heat prevails inside, vital qi is not deficient, the healthy qi and pathogenic factors fight against each other fiercely, so the pulse is rapid and forceful, suggesting excessive heat syndrome; a protracted disease leads to yin deficiency and deficiency heat, so the pulse is rapid but forceless; if the pulse is floating, rapid and rootless when pressed, it indicates deficiency yang escaping outside and a critical disease.

5.1.5 Moderate pulse

Pulse condition It beats 4 times per breath, which is moderate and slack.

Main disease It indicates damp syndrome, spleen and stomach deficiency.

Clinical significance Sticky dampness impedes qi flow; spleen and stomach deficiency together with exhausted qi and blood fails to push the pulse, so it gets moderate.

5.1.6 Surging pulse

Pulse condition It is characterized by wide size, beating like roaring waves in huge coming and sudden declining.

Main disease It indicates interior heat syndrome.

Clinical significance Abundant yang-qi and hyperfunction of qi and blood cause vessels to dilate leading to surging pulse; a protracted disease, qi deficiency, a

症而出现洪脉,是正虚邪盛的危险证候或为阴液枯竭,孤阳独亢或虚阳亡脱。

consumptive disease, blood loss, long-time diarrhea result in surging pulse, which is a critical condition of deficient healthy qi and excessive pathogenic factors or body fluid deficiency, hyperfunction of yang or exhausted deficient yang.

5.1.7　濡脉

脉象:浮而细软,如帛在水中。

主病:虚证,湿证。

脉理:精血两伤、阴虚不能维阳,故脉浮软、精血不充,则脉细;湿邪阻压脉道,亦见濡脉。

5.1.8　散脉

脉象:浮散无根,至数不齐,如杨花散漫之象。

主病:元气离散。

脉理:心力衰竭、阴阳不敛,阳气离散,故脉来浮散而不紧,稍用重力则按不着,漫无根蒂;阴衰阳消、心气不能维系血液运行,故脉来时快时慢,至数不齐。

5.1.9　芤脉

脉象:浮大中空,如按葱管。

主病:失血,伤阴。

脉理:突然失血过多、血量骤然减少、营血不足、无以充脉,或津液大伤、血不得充、血失阴伤则阳气无所附而浮越于外,因而形成浮大中空之芤脉。

5.1.7　Soggy pulse

Pulse condition　It is floating and soft, like silk in the water.

Main disease　It indicates deficiency and damp syndrome.

Clinical significance　Injury to essence and blood, and yin deficiency failing to maintain yang leads to soggy pulse. When the essence and blood are not sufficient, the pulse would be fine and small; when the pathogenic dampness blocks and presses the vessels, there will also appear soggy pulse.

5.1.8　Scattered pulse

Pulse condition　It is rootless and arrhythmic, like scattered poplar filaments.

Main disease　It indicates depletion of original qi.

Clinical significance　Heart failure, the dissipation of yin and yang leads to scattered pulse which is rootless under heavy pressure; weakness of yin and yang and heart-qi failing to maintain blood circulation leads to rootless and arrhythmic pulse.

5.1.9　Hollow pulse

Pulse condition　It is floating, large and hollow like a scallion when pressed.

Main disease　It indicates blood loss and injury to yin.

Clinical significance　It is caused by sudden loss of large amount of blood and insufficient nutritive blood failing to fill the pulse, injury to body fluid leading to failure of reproducing blood, rootless yang-qi floating outside.

中医理论　Basic Theory of Traditional Chinese Medicine

161

5.1.10　涩脉

脉象：迟细而短、往来艰涩、极不流利，如轻刀刮竹。

主病：精血亏少、气滞血瘀，挟痰，挟食。

脉理：精伤血少津亏、不能濡养经脉、血行不畅、脉气往来艰涩，故脉涩而无力；气滞血瘀、痰食胶固、气机不畅、血行受阻，则脉涩而有力。

5.1.11　结脉

脉象：脉来缓、时而一止、止无定数。

主病：阴盛气结、寒痰血瘀、症瘕积聚。

脉理：阴盛气机郁结、阳气受阻、血行瘀滞，故脉来缓急、脉气不相顺接、时一止、止后复来、止无定数，常见于寒痰血瘀所致的心脉瘀阻症。

5.1.12　促脉

脉象：脉来数、时而一止、止无定数。

主病：阳热亢盛、气血痰食郁滞。

脉理：阳热盛极，或气血痰饮、宿食郁滞化热、正邪相搏、血行急速，故脉来急数。邪气阻滞、阴不和阳、脉气不续、故时一止、止后复来、指下有力、止无定数。

5.1.13　虚脉

脉象：三部脉举之无力，按之空虚。

5.1.10　Rough pulse

Pulse condition　It is slow, thin and short with unsmooth coming and going, like lightly cutting bamboo.

Main disease　It indicates essence and blood deficiency, qi stagnation and blood stasis, phlegm and food retention.

Clinical significance　Injury to essence, blood and body fluid deficiency fail to nourish vessels leading to unsmooth circulation of pulse-qi, so the pulse is rough and forceless; qi stagnation and blood stasis, phlegm and food retention, impeded qi and blood circulation leads to rough and forceful pulse.

5.1.11　Knotted pulse

Pulse condition　It is slow with irregular intermittence.

Main disease　It indicates yin excess, qi stagnation, cold phlegm, blood stasis and accumulation of abdominal mass.

Clinical significance　Yin excess, qi stagnation, impeded yang-qi and blood stasis lead to knotted pulse with irregular intermittence which is seen in the syndrome of heart and vessel stasis caused by cold phlegm and blood stasis.

5.1.12　Hasty pulse

Pulse condition　It is rapid with irregular intermittence.

Main disease　It indicates yang and heat predominance, qi stagnation, blood stasis, phlegm and food retention.

Clinical significance　Yang and heat predominance, retained heat turned from retained qi, blood, phlegm and food, struggle between healthy qi and pathogenic factors and rapid blood circulation result in hasty pulse. Pathogenic qi stagnation and disharmony between yin and yang lead to irregular, intermittent and forceful pulse which stops sometimes and returns after a while, being forceful under pressure with regular intermittence.

5.1.13　Deficient pulse

Pulse condition　It is featured with weak beating at cun, guan and chi portions, and felt feeble and deficient

中医理论　Basic Theory of Traditional Chinese Medicine

主病：虚证。

脉理：气虚不足以运其血，故脉来无力，血虚不足充盈脉道，故按之空虚。

5.1.14　细脉

脉象：脉细如线，但应指明显。

主病：气血两虚、诸虚劳损。

脉理：气血亏虚不能充盈脉道，故脉体细小。

5.1.15　代脉

脉象：脉来时见一止、止有定数、良久方来。

主病：脏气衰微，风证，痛证。

脉理：脏气衰微、气血亏损、以致脉气不能衔接而歇止、不能自还、良久复动；风证、痛证见代脉，因邪气所犯、阻于经脉，致脉气阻滞、不相衔接。

5.1.16　实脉

脉象：三部脉举按均有力。

主病：实证。

脉理：邪气亢盛而正气不虚、邪正相搏、气血壅盛、脉道紧满，故脉来应指坚实有力。

5.1.17　滑脉

脉象：往来流利，如珠走盘，应指圆滑。

主病：痰饮、食积、实热。

脉理：邪气壅盛于内、正气

when pressed.

Main disease　It indicates deficiency syndrome.

Clinical significance　Qi deficiency cannot circulate blood, so the pulse is forceless. Blood deficiency cannot fill vessels, so the pulse is feeble and deficient.

5.1.14　Thready pulse

Pulse condition　It is fine like thread, but clearly perceptible by the finger.

Main disease　It indicates qi and blood deficiency and other deficiencies and injuries.

Clinical significance　Deficiency of qi and blood cannot fill the vessels, so the pulse is fine and small.

5.1.15　Intermittent pulse

Pulse condition　It beats with regular intermittence.

Main disease　It indicates zang-qi exhaustion, wind and pain syndrome.

Clinical significance　Zang-qi exhaustion, qi and blood deficiency lead to disconnection of vessel qi; wind and pain syndrome seen in intermittent pulse is caused by pathogenic qi blocking in the vessels, vessel qi stagnation and disconnection.

5.1.16　Excess pulse

Pulse condition　It beats forcefully at all the three portions.

Main disease　It indicates excess syndrome.

Clinical significance　The evil qi is sufficient yet the healthy qi is not deficient, leading to the fight between them, filling and tightening the vessels, therefore the pulse feels forceful and excessive.

5.1.17　Slippery pulse

Pulse condition　It comes and goes freely just like beads rolling on a plate and feels smooth.

Main disease　It indicates phlegm and food retention and excessive heat.

Clinical significance　The pathogenic factors are

中医理论

Basic Theory of Traditional Chinese Medicine

不衰、气实血涌,故脉往来甚为流利、应指圆滑。妇女妊娠见滑脉,是气血充盛而调和的表现。

5.1.18　弦脉

脉象:端直以长,如按琴弦。

主病:肝胆病,痰饮,痛证,疟疾。

脉理:弦是脉气紧张的表现。邪气滞肝、疏泄失常、气郁不利则见弦脉。诸痛、痰饮、气机阻滞、阴阳不和,脉气因而紧张,故脉弦。疟邪为病,伏于半表半里,少阳枢机不利而见弦脉。

5.1.19　紧脉

脉象:脉来绷急,状若牵绳转索。

主病:寒证、痛证。

脉理:寒邪侵袭人体,与正气相搏,以致脉道紧张而拘急,故见紧脉。

一般来说,脉见洪、数、滑、实,表示邪实正盛,正气足以抗邪;脉见沉、细、微、弱,说明正气已衰。

临床还多见数种脉象并见的相兼脉。相兼脉象的主病,往往等于各个脉所主病的总和,如浮为表,数为热,浮数主表热,依此类推。

浮紧:表寒,风痹。

浮缓:伤寒表虚证。

prosperous yet the healthy qi is not deficient, leading to abundant qi and surging blood, so the pulse comes and goes freely and smoothly. Slippery pulse seen in pregnant women indicates abundant and harmonious qi and blood.

5.1.18　Wiry pulse

Pulse condition　It is straight and long like pressing on the string.

Main disease　It indicates liver or gallbladder diseases, phlegm retention, pains and malaria.

Clinical significance　It indicates tense vessel qi. Pathogenic factors retained in the liver cause dysfunction of the liver and qi stagnation, leading to wiry pulse. Pains, phlegm retention, qi stagnation, disharmony between yin and yang result in tense vessel qi and wiry pulse. Malaria pathogen, being semi-exterior-interior, and dysfunction of shaoyang leads to wiry pulse.

5.1.19　Tight pulse

Pulse condition　It is tight, like a stretched cord.

Main disease　It indicates cold syndrome and pain.

Clinical significance　When pathogenic cold attacks the body, it combats with healthy qi leading to tense vessels and tight pulse. Generally speaking, if the pulse is large, rapid, slippery and excessive, it indicates pathogenic excess is predominant and healthy qi can resist pathogenic factors; if the pulse is deep, tiny and feeble, it indicates healthy qi has been exhausted.

Clinically, there is multi-feature pulse which is compounded by several single pulses. The main disease of the multi-feature pulse is compounded by the main diseases of the other pulses: the floating pulse indicates exterior syndrome and the rapid pulse indicates heat syndrome, so the floating and rapid pulse indicates exterior and heat syndrome and so on.

Floating and tight pulse suggests cold syndrome and wandering arthritis.

Floating and slow pulse suggests exterior deficiency

中医理论

Basic Theory of Traditional Chinese Medicine

沉迟：里寒。

弦数：肝热，肝火。

滑数：痰热，内热食积。

弦细：肝肾阴虚，肝郁脾虚。

沉细：阴虚，血虚。

5.2 按诊

按诊，就是医者用手直接触摸、按压患者体表某些部位，以了解局部的异常变化，从而推断疾病的部位、性质和病情的轻重等情况的一种诊病方法。

按诊的手法大致可分触、摸、推、按四类。触是以手指或手掌轻轻接触患者局部，以了解凉、热、润、燥等情况。在临床上，常常是先触摸、后推按、由轻到重、由浅入深，各种手法综合运用。

按诊时，医者要体贴患者，手法要轻巧，要避免突然暴力，冷天要事先把手暖和后再行检查。同时病人要主动配合，随时反映自己的感觉，还要边检查边观察病人的表情变化了解其痛苦所在。

按诊的应用范围较广。临床上以按肌肤、按手足、按胸腹、按腧穴等为常用。

5.2.1 按肌肤

凡身热初按甚热，久按热反减轻的，是热在表；若久按其热反甚，热自内向外蒸发者，为热

syndrome seen in exogenous febrile disease.

Deep and slow pulse indicates interior cold.

Wiry and rapid pulse indicates liver-heat and liver-fire.

Slippery and rapid pulse indicates phlegm heat, interior heat and food retention.

Wiry and thready pulse suggests yin deficiency of liver and kidney, liver-qi stagnation and spleen deficiency.

Deep and thready pulse suggests yin deficiency and blood deficiency.

5.2 Palpation

Palpation is a diagnostic method used by doctors to touch and press a certain part of a patient's body to know its abnormal changes and infer the portion, nature and severity of a disease.

Diagnostic methods include touching, stroking, percussion and pressing. Touching is to touch a certain part of a patient's body to know its conditions, such as, coldness, heat, moist, dryness and so on. Clinically, touching and stroking are followed by percussion and pressing, with a degree from light to heavy, from superficial to deep and a comprehensive use of four methods.

In palpation, the doctor should be considerate of the patient with slight pressure. The doctor should avoid sudden heavy pressure and perform with warm hands in winter. At the same time, the patient should take the initiative to cooperate with the doctor and express their feelings at any time. When performing, the doctor should also pay attention to the patient's facial expression change and know the location of the pain.

Palpation is widely used. Clinically, there is palpation of skin, hands and feet, chest and abdomen, and points.

5.2.1 Palpation of skin

If the patient with a burning heat feels hotter after palpation and then the heat is alleviated after a long-time pressure, it indicates exterior heat; if the heat is aggravated

在里。

肌肤濡软而喜按者,为虚证;患处硬痛拒按者,为实证。

轻按即痛者,病在表浅;重按方痛者,病在深部。

按之凹陷,放手即留手印、不能即起的,为水肿;按之凹陷、举手即起的,为气肿。

5.2.2 按手足

凡疾病初起、手足俱冷的,是阳虚寒盛,属寒证。手足俱热的,多为阳盛热炽,属热证。

手足的背部较热的,为外感发热,手足心较热的,为内伤发热。

额上热甚于手心热的,为表热;手心热甚于额上热的,为里热。

5.2.3 按胸腹

按虚里:虚里位于左乳下心尖搏动处,虚里按之应手、动而不紧、缓而不急,为健康之征。其动微弱无力,为不及,是宗气内虚。若动而应手,为太过,是宗气外泄之象。若按之弹手,洪大而博,属于危重的证候。

按胸胁:前胸高起、按之气喘者,为肺胀病。胸胁按之胀痛者,可能是痰热气结或水饮内停。

若扪及右胁内肿大之肝脏、

after long-time pressure and evaporates from the interior to the exterior, it indicates interior heat.

Moist and soft skin with preference for pressure indicates deficiency syndrome; the painful and hard portion with aversion to pressure indicates excess syndrome.

If pains can be felt by light pressure, the disease is in the superficial area; if pains are felt by heavy pressure, the disease is in the deeper area.

If skin appears sunken by light pressure and does not return to normal soon, it indicates edema; if skin appears sunken by light pressure and returns to normal soon, it indicates edema because of disorder of qi.

5.2.2 Palpation of hands and feet

If both hands and feet are cold at the beginning of the disease, it indicates yang deficiency and cold excess. If both hands and feet are hot, it indicates yang and heat excess and heat syndrome.

Heat on the back of hands and feet indicates fever caused by exogenous pathogens; heat on palms and soles indicates fever due to internal injury.

When the forehead is hotter than palms, it indicates exterior heat; when the palms are hotter than forehead, it indicates interior heat.

5.2.3 Palpation of chest and abdomen

Xuli is under the left nipple and at the pulsation point of the cardiac apex. If it quickly responds to fingers with vigor but is not tense, gentle but not rapid, that is the sign of fitness. The weak pulsation of this area indicates deficiency of pectoral qi. The strong pulse indicates leaking of the pectoral qi. If it rebounds by pressure and is vigorous and large, it indicates a critical syndrome.

A high chest and shortness of breath by pressure indicates lung distention. Swelling pain of the hypochondrium by pressure indicates phlegm-heat, qi stagnation and fluid retention.

Lumps either soft or hard on the right hypochondrium

中医理论

Basic Theory of Traditional Chinese Medicine

或软或硬,多属气滞血瘀,若表面凹凸不平,则要警惕肝癌。

按腹部:腹壁冷、喜暖手按放者,属虚寒证;腹壁灼热、喜冷物按放者,属实热证。

凡腹痛、喜按者属虚,拒按者属实;按之局部灼热、痛不可忍者,为内痛。

腹部胀满、按之有充实感觉、有压痛、叩之声音重浊者,为实满;腹部膨满,但按之不实、无压痛、叩之作空声的,为气胀,多属虚满。腹部高度胀大、如鼓之状者,称为膨胀。

积聚是指腹内的结块或胀或痛的一种病症,但积和聚不同。痛有定处、按之有形而不移的为积,病属血分;痛无定处、按之无形聚散不定的为聚,病属气分。

左小腹作痛、按之累累有硬块者,肠中有宿粪。右小腹作痛、按之疼痛、有包块应手者,为肠痈。

5.2.4　按腧穴

按压身体上某些特定穴位,通过这些穴位的变化与反应,来推断内脏的某些疾病。肺病患者,有些可在肺俞穴摸到结节,有些在中府穴出现压痛。肝病患者可出现肝俞或期门穴压痛;胃病在胃俞和足三里有压痛;肠痈在阑尾穴有压痛。

indicate qi stagnation and blood stasis; uneven lumps indicate potential liver cancer.

Cold abdomen with preference for pressure of warm hands indicates cold syndrome; hot abdomen with preference for cold indicates heat syndrome.

Painful abdomen alleviated by pressure indicates deficiency syndrome and aggravated by pressure indicates excess syndrome; painful abdomen with burning part and great pain by pressure suggests abscess of internal organs.

Distending abdomen with fullness and pain by pressure with deep and turbid sound by knocking indicates fullness sensation due to excess; distending abdomen without fullness and pain by pressure with hollow sound by knocking indicates flatulence and fullness sensation due to deficiency. A great distention in the abdomen like a drum is tympanites.

Accumulation refers to lumps either soft or hard in the abdomen. A stable pain and immovable lump indicate the disease of blood system; pain of unfixed location and movable lump indicates the disease of qi system.

Feeling pain in the left abdomen with lumps when touching indicates remained feces in the intestine. Feeling pain in the right abdomen aggravated by pressure with lumps when touching indicates periappendicular abscess.

5.2.4　Palpation of points

It refers to pressing certain points and inferring the disease of internal organs through the change and response on pressing. For some patients suffering from lung disease, nodules can be felt on lung-shu point; for some others, there is pain on pressing in zhongfu point. Patients suffering from liver disease will be painful when pressing on ganshu or qimen point. Pains by pressure on weishu and zusanli indicate stomach disease. Pains by pressure on lanwei indicate periappendicular abscess.

第七章 中药理论

Chapter 7 Chinese Materia Medica

中医理论

Basic Theory of Traditional Chinese Medicine

中药有植物药、动物和矿物药,其中以植物药占绝大多数,使用也更普遍,所以古代相沿把药学叫做"本草"学。这些药物的应用与中国历史、文化等方面关系密切,是中医理论体系的有机组成和应用形式,所以又称为"中药",而"本草"学也相应地称为"中药学"或"中草药学"。"中草药学"就是专门介绍各种中药的采制、性能、功效及应用方法等知识的一门学科。

几千年来,中草药一直是防治疾病的主要工具,中医学家日渐积累宝贵的用药知识,并形成了一整套中药理论体系。在先秦时期,已有不少关于药物的文字记载。东汉末期(公元二世纪),《神农本草经》载药365种,是汉以前药学知识和经验的总结。书中还简要记述了药学的基本理论。李时珍(公元1518—1593年)的《本草纲目》载药1892种,按药物的自然属性,分为十六纲、六十类。中草药学历代相承,各个时代都有它的成就和特色,日渐繁富。到了现代,常用中草药已达

Chinese medicinals include plants, animals and minerals, among which, the first one is used widely with an overwhelming majority. That's why pharmaceutical in China has been passed down as "herbalism" since ancient time. These drugs are also called "Chinese herbs", since they are an essential part and application form of the TCM theory and their application closely correlates with Chinese history and culture. Accordingly, "herbalism" is also called "Chinese materia medica" or "Chinese herbology". The latter is a discipline dealing with the collection, processing, property, efficacy, and application methods of Chinese materia medica.

For thousands of years, Chinese herbal medicine has been used as the dominant way for prevention and treatment of diseases, thus it has formed a set of traditional Chinese medicinal theory system through accumulating valuable medication knowledge. Many records on drug use already appeared in pre-Qin period. *Shen Nong's Herbal* in Later Eastern Han Dynasty (the second century AD) records 365 kinds of medicine, which is a summary of pharmaceutical knowledge and experience of pre-Han period. This book briefly describes the basic theory of Pharmacy. *Compendium of Materia Medica* by Li Shizhen (1518—1593 AD) contains 1892 kinds of drugs. It is divided into sixteen headings and sixty categories according to the natural properties of the drugs. Chinese herbology has been inherited generation by generation and increasingly become more complex and rich, with each era having its own characteristics and achievements. In modern times, Chinese Herbal Medicine

5000种左右。

1 中药名称、采集、贮存与炮制

1.1 中药的名称

中药的来源广泛,品种繁多,其名称也较复杂,但也有一定的规律可循。中药的名称往往反映了它的某些特征,对于掌握中药知识有一定帮助。中药的命名法则,概括起来有以下几种:

1.1.1 按药用部分命名

以入药部位命名的中药最为广泛。如以根命名的葛根、芦根、山豆根等;而枇杷叶、桑叶、侧柏叶、荷叶、淡竹叶、艾叶、紫苏叶等则是以叶命名;以花命名的有金银花、菊花等;车前子、白芥子、苏子以种子、种仁命名;以种皮、茎皮及根皮命名的有大腹皮、陈皮、桂皮等;以藤茎命名的有石楠藤、青风藤、海风藤、络石藤、鸡血藤等。动物药中有以入药器官、组织命名的,如鸡内金、鹿茸、鹿角、熊胆汁、猪胆汁、海狗肾、黄狗肾等;阳起石、花蕊石、海浮石、寒水石、滑石、磁石、代赭石、炉甘石等,则是以矿石得名的。

1 Naming, Collection, Storage and Processing of Chinese Medicinals

1.1 Names of Chinese Medicinals

Chinese medicinals have a wide range of sources, a wide variety, and their names are also quite complex, but there are certain rules to follow. The names of Chinese medicinals often reflect some of their characteristics which are helpful for people to master the knowledge of them. The naming rules can be summed up as the following:

1.1.1 Naming according to the used part

Most Chinese medicinals are named according to the used parts, such as, kudzuvine root (gegen), reed rhizome (lugen) and vietnamese sophora root (shandougen) are named after their roots; loquat leaf (pibaye), mulberry leaf (sangye), Chinese arborvitae twig and leaf (cebaiye), lotus leaf (heye), lophatherum herb (danzhuye), argy wormwood leaf (aiye) and perilla leaf (zisuye) are named according to their leaves; honeysuckle bud and flower (jinyinhua) and chrysanthemum flower (juhua) are named according to their flowers; plantain seed (cheqianzi), white mustard seed (baijiezi) and perilla (suzi) are named according to their seeds; areca peel (dafupi), dried tangerine peel (chenpi) and cinnamon bark (guipi) are named according to their seed bark, stem bark and root bark; piper wallichii (shinanteng), orientvine vine (qingfengteng), kadsura pepper stem (haifengteng), Chinese starjasmine stem (luoshiteng) and suberect spatholobus stem (jixieteng) are named according to their rattans. Chinese medicinals originating from animals are named according to their organs and tissues, such as, inner membrane of chicken gizzard (jineijin), pilose antler (lurong), antler (lujiao), bear bile (xiongdanzhi), pig bile (zhudanzhi), urine seal testes and penis (haigoushen) and dog penis (huanggoushen) etc; actinolite (yangqishi), ophicalcitum (huaruishi), pumice stone (haifushi), glauberitum (hanshuishi), talc (huashi), magnetite (cishi), haematitum (daizheshi) and calamine

1.1.2 按药物产地命名

按药物产地命名的多为道地药材。有按古代当时的国名来命名的：如秦艽、秦椒、吴茱萸等；有以当时的行政区来命名：如四川产的川乌、川芎、川贝母、川楝子、川牛膝等，东北产的北细辛、北口芪、关防风、关木通、辽五味等；浙江的杭白芍、杭菊花等；河南怀庆府(今焦作市)产的"四大怀药"(怀生地、怀牛膝、怀山药、怀菊花)等。从国外进口的则多冠以胡、番之名：如胡椒、胡麻仁、胡桃仁、胡黄连、番木鳖、番泻叶等。

1.1.3 按药物气味命名

麝香、丁香、木香、沉香、松香、乳香、檀香、苏合香等，都是以其具有特异香气而得名的；又如有鱼腥气的鱼腥草、败酱气的败酱草等；而龙胆草、苦参、苦楝皮等以苦有名，甜味的甘草、甜杏仁等，多味的五味子，则均以其药味作为命名的依据。

(luganshi) are named after ores.

1.1.2 Naming according to place of origin

Chinese medicinals named after the place of origin are mainly original materia medica. Some of them are named according to ancient states, such as, largeleaf gentian root (qinjiao), xanthoxylum piperitum (qinjiao) and medicinal evodia fruit (wuzhuyu); some of them are named according to ancient administrative regions, such as, common monkshood mother root (chuanwu), sichuan lovage rhizome (chuanxiong), tendrilleaf fritillary bulb (chuanbeimu), szechwan chinaberry fruit (chuanlianzi) and medicinal cyathula root (chuanniuxi) from Sichuan, manchurian wildginger (beixixin), stilbene of Northeast China (beikouqi), divaricate saposhnikovia root (guanfangfeng), akebia stem (guanmutong) and schisandra chinensis (liaowuwei) from Northeast of China, and debark peony root (hangbaishao) and chrysanthemum flower (hangjuhua) from Zhejiang, "four major medicinals", rehmanniae radix (huaishengdi), twotoothed achyranthes root (huainiuxi), common yam rhizome (huaishanyao) and chrysanthemum flower (huaijuhua) from Huaiqing (today's Jiaozuo city) Henan etc. Medicinals imported from abroad are always added with "hu" or "fan": pepper fruit (hujiao), sesame seed (humaren), walnut meat (hutaoren), figwortflower picrorhiza rhizome (huhuanglian), nux vomica (fanmubie) and senna leaf (fanxieye) etc.

1.1.3 Naming according to odor

Musk (shexiang), clove (dingxiang), common aucklandia root (muxiang), Chinese eaglewood (chenxiang), rosin (songxiang), frankincense (ruxiang), sandalwood (tanxiang) and storax (suhexiang) are named according to their specific aroma; heartleaf houttuynia herb (yuxingcao) is named based on its fishy smell and atrina glass (baijiangcao) on its sauce smell; Chinese gentian (longdancao), light yellow sophora root (kushen), Sichuan chinaberry bark (kulianpi) are famous with their bitter taste, and liquorice root (gancao) and dessert almond (tianxingren), with their sweet taste, Chinese magnoliavine fruit (wuweizi), with its multi smell. All of them are named according to their odor.

1.1.4　按性能命名

活血调经的益母草,清肝明目的决明子、石决明,治创伤骨折的续断、骨碎补,舒筋通络的伸筋草,泻热导滞的番泻叶,用治疮疡的蚤休,治风通用的防风,乌须黑发的何首乌,益智安神的远志等都是按药物性能命名。

1.1.5　按药物颜色命名

白芷、白芍、白菊花、白及、白附子、紫草、红花、红藤、鸡血藤、青黛、青蒿、黄连、黄柏、黄芩、大黄等都是按药物颜色命名。

1.1.6　按采药季节命名

迎春花、半夏、夏枯草、冬虫夏草、款冬花、忍冬藤等,都是以其采收时节而命名的。

1.1.7　按药物形态命名

典型的有七叶一枝花、半边莲、垂盆草、紫花地丁、桑寄生等,其他如人参形如人体,钩藤节上对生两个向下弯曲的钩,乌头形似乌鸦之头,木蝴蝶形似白色蝶翅,猫爪草为数个呈纺锤形的块

1.1.4　Naming according to function

Motherwort herb (yimucao) is able to activate blood circulation to dissipate blood stasis; cassia seed (juemingzi) and abalone shell (shijueming) are able to clear liver to improve vision; himalayan teasel root (xuduan) and fortune's drynaria rhizome (gusuibu) are able to treat traumatic fracture; common clubmoss herb (shenjincao) is able to relax muscle and tendons; senna leaf (fanxieye) is able to purge heat and dredge stagnation; Paris polyphylla (zaoxiu) is able to cure sore; divaricate saposhnikovia root (fangfeng) is able to expel pathogenic wind from the body surface; fleeceflower root (heshouwu) is able to prevent early graying of hair; milkwort root (yuanzhi) is able to soothe the nerves.

1.1.5　Naming according to color

Dahurian angelica root (baizhi), debark peony root (baishao), chrysanthemum (baijuhua), common bletilla rubber (baiji), giant typhonium rhizome (baifuzi), arnebia root (zicao), safflower (honghua), sargentgloryvine stem (hongteng), suberect spatholobus stem (jixieteng), natural indigo (qingdai), sweet wormwood herb (qinghao), golden thread (huanglian), amur cork-tree (huangbai), baical skullcap root (huangqin), rhubarb (dahuang) and other medicinals are named according to their colors.

1.1.6　Naming according to collection season

Winter jasmine (yingchunhua), pinellia tuber (banxia), common selfheal fruit-spike (xiakucao), Chinese caterpillar fungus (dongchongxiacao), common coltsfoot flower (kuandonghua) and honeysuckle stem (rendongteng) are named according to their collection and harvest seasons.

1.1.7　Naming according to shape

Some medicinals are named after their shapes such as Paris polyphylla (qiyeyizhihua), Chinese lobelia herb (banbianlian), stringy stonecrop herb (chuipencao), Tokyo violet herb (zihuadiding), Chinese taxillus herb (sangjisheng). There are many other examples, too: the shape of ginseng (renshen) is like the shape of a human; on uncaria root, there are twin hooks bending downward; the shape of aconite (wutou) is like a crow head; the shape of Indian trumpet flower seed (muhudie) is like white butterfly wings; catclaw

根簇生形似猫爪，金银花因其一蒂二花、黄白相映等，都是按药物形态命名的。

1.1.8　按人名命名

以最早发现和应用该药的人来命名，带有纪念性质。如徐长卿、使君子、杜仲、刘寄奴等。

1.1.9　按进口地命名

如番红花主产于西班牙、希腊、伊朗等国家，过去多经西藏输入内地又名藏红花、西红花；高丽参产于朝鲜(古代称高丽)，西洋参主产于美国等。

1.1.10　按译音命名

以翻译后的中文音而命名。如诃黎勒即诃子、曼陀罗等。

1.2　中药的采集

中草药的采收季节、时间、方法和贮藏等与中草药的品质好坏有着密切的关系，是保证药物质量的重要环节。因此，采药要根据不同的药用部分(如植物的根、茎、叶、花、果实、种子或全草都有一定的生长成熟时期，动物亦有一定的捕捉与加工时期)，有计划地进行采制和贮藏，才能得到较高的产量和品质较好的药物，以保证药物的供应和疗效。除某些药物所含的有效成分在采制和贮藏方面有特殊要求外，一

buttercup root (maozhuacao) clusters in fusiform like cats' paws; each honeysuckle bud and flower (jinyinhua) has one stalk and a yellow and white flower. All of them are named according to their shapes.

1.1.8　Naming after person

Some of the medicinals are named after the persons who first discovered and used them, such as paniculate swallowwort root (xuchangqing), rangooncreeper fruit (shijunzi), eucommia bark (duzhong), diverse wormwood herb (liujinu) and so on.

1.1.9　Naming according to imported places

Saffron (fanhonghua) mainly originates from Spain, Greece, Iran and other countries and it was taken into the mainland via Tibet (xizang), so it is also called as zanghonghua or xihonghua; Korean ginseng originates from Korea; American ginseng originates from the United States.

1.1.10　Naming according to transliteration

Some of the herbs are named according to their Chinese transliteration, such as, terminalia (heliliejikezi) and datura stramonium (mantuoluo).

1.2　Collection of Chinese Medicinals

The harvest season, time, method and storage of Chinese medicinals have a close relationship with their medicinal quality, and they are important aspects of ensuring the quality. Therefore, well-planned collection and storage according to their different medicinal parts guarantee higher yield and better quality to ensure supply and curative effect. Therefore roots, stems, leaves, flowers, fruits, seeds or whole plants have a certain growth and mature period, and animals are captured and processed due to a certain period of time. In addition to effective ingredients contained in some herbs needing special requirements in processing and storage, the collection principles for common herbs should

中医理论

Basic Theory of Traditional Chinese Medicine

般植物类药物的采收原则如下：

1.2.1全草、茎枝及叶类药物大多在夏秋季节植株充分成长、茎叶茂盛的花前期或初见花时采集，但有些植物的叶亦有在秋冬时采收的。多年生草本常割取地上部分，如益母草、薄荷等；一些必须带根用的药物则连根拔起，如蒲公英、紫花地丁等。茵陈以幼嫩全草入药。

1.2.2根和根茎类药物一般是在秋季植物地上部分开始枯萎或早春植物抽苗时采集，这时植物的养分多贮藏在根或根茎部，所采的药物产量高，质量好，如天麻、大黄、苍术、葛根等。但也有些根及根茎如孩儿参、半夏、延胡索等则在夏天采收。多数的根及根茎类药物需生长一年或二年以上才能采收供药用。

1.2.3花类药物多在花未开放的花蕾时期或刚开时候采集，以免香味失散、花瓣散落、影响质量，如金银花、月季花等。由于植物的花期一般很短，有的要分次及时采集，如红花要采花冠由黄变红的花瓣，花粉粒需盛开时采收，如松花粉、蒲黄等。采花最好在晴天早晨，以便采后迅速晾晒干燥。

1.2.4果实类药物除少数采用未成熟果实如青皮、桑槐等外，

also be paid attention to.

1.2.1 The entire plants, stems and leaves of most herbs are collected in summer and autumn when they are in full growth before blooming or in the early stage of blooming, but some leaves are collected in autumn and winter. For perennial herbs, the parts above the ground are usually cut and collected, such as, motherwort herb (yimucao), peppermint (bohe) and so on; plants with their roots for medicinal use are uprooted, such as, dandelion (pugongying), Tokyo violet herb and so on. The entire tender plant of virgate wormwood herb (yinchen) is for medicinal use.

1.2.2 Root and rhizome are collected in autumn when the parts above the ground begin to wither or in spring when early-spring plants are in seedling, because at the time, their nutrients mainly stored in roots and rhizomes are collected with high yield and good quality, such as, tall gastrodia tuber (tianma), rhubarb (dahuang), atractylodes rhizome (cangshu) and kudzuvine root (gegen) etc. However, some root and rhizome, such as, radix pseudostell (haiershen), pinellia tuber (banxia), and rhizoma corydalis (yanhusuo) etc. are collected in summer. Most of the root and rhizome herbs have to grow for one year or more than two years to be harvested for medicinal use.

1.2.3 Flowers such as honeysuckle bud and flower, Chinese rose flower (yuejihua) etc. for medicinal use are mainly collected in buds before bloom or in the early stage of bloom so as not to lose flavor and petals to affect quality. Because of the short blooming period, some flowers should be collected in time, such as, the petals of safflower (honghua) should be collected when they are turning from yellow to red; pollen should be collected when flowers are in full blossom, such as, pine pollen and cattail pollen etc. The best time for collection is in the sunny morning so that they can be dried rapidly.

1.2.4 Fruits for medicinal use, except for few immature ones such as immature tangerine peel (qingpi) and mulberry

一般应在果实成熟时采集。

1.2.5种子通常在完全成熟后采集。有些种子成熟后容易散落,如牵牛子、急性子(凤仙花子)等,则在果实成熟而未开裂时采集。有些既用全草、又用种子的药物,则可在种子成熟时割取全草,将种子打下后分别晒干贮藏,如车前子、紫苏子等。

1.2.6树皮和根皮类药物通常是在春夏间剥取,这时正值植物生长旺盛期,浆液较多,容易剥离,如厚朴、黄柏、杜仲等,而肉桂多在十月含油多时剥离。剥树皮时应注意不能将树干整个一圈剥下,以免影响树干的输导系统,造成树木的死亡。

1.2.7动物药:潜藏在地下的小动物,宜在夏秋季捕捉,如蚯蚓、蟋蟀等;大动物虽然四季皆可捕捉,但一般宜在秋冬季猎取,不过鹿茸必须在雄鹿幼角未角化时采取。

此外,在采收药物时还须注意天气变化,如阴雨时采集,往往不能及时干燥,以致腐烂变质。采集药物时,还应重视保护药源,既要考虑当前的需要,又要考虑长远的利益。

1.3　中药的贮存

药物在采集后,应采取一定的加工处理,以便贮藏。

1.3.1植物类药品,采集后应先除去泥土杂质和非药用部分,

and sophora japonica (sanghuai), are generally collected when they are ripe.

1.2.5 Seeds are usually collected at full maturity. Some of the mature seeds are easily scattered, such as pharbitis seed (qianniuzi) and garden balsam seed (jixingzi) etc., so they should be collected without cracking. If both of the whole plants and seeds are for medicinal use, the whole plants should be collected when their seeds are mature, and then the collected seeds are stored after being dried up, such as, plantain seed (cheqianzi), perilla fruit (zisuzi) etc.

1.2.6 Rinds and root cortices are usually peeled in spring and summer when plants are in fastest growth period and there is so much nutrition fluid in the plant that rinds are easy to be peeled off, such as official magnolia bark (houpu), amur cork-tree (huangbai) and eucommia bark (duzhong); cassia bark (rougui) is peeled off in october when its oil is at the highest level. A whole lap of rinds should not be peeled off at all so as not to affect the transport system of the trunk, resulting in the death of trees.

1.2.7 Generally, small animals hidden below the ground should be captured in summer and autumn, such as, earthworms and crickets; though large animals can be captured in four seasons, the proper collection time is in autumn and winter, and antlers must be collected before the antlers of male deer keratinize.

In addition, weather changes need to be considered when collecting. For example, medicinal herbs collected in rainy day are not easy to dry up resulting in decay and deterioration. When collecting, we should also pay attention to the protection of drug sources, not only to consider the current needs, but also to consider the long-term interests.

1.3　Storage of Chinese Medicinals

After collection, Chinese medicinals should be processed before storage.

1.3.1 After collection, dirt, foreign matters and non-medicinal parts should be removed. In addition to some

洗净切断,除鲜用外,都应根据药物的性质,及时放在日光下晒干,或阴干,或烘干,分别保藏。

1.3.2五味子、女贞子、莱菔子、葶苈子、白芥子等植物的果实或种子须放在密封的容器内保存,以防虫鼠;植物的茎叶或根部没有芳香性的如益母草、木贼草、夏枯草、大青叶、板蓝根、首乌藤等可放在干燥阴凉处;芳香性药物及花类如菊花、金银花、月季花等,须放在干燥阴凉处,以防受潮霉烂变质;动物药及脏器组织如蕲蛇、乌梢蛇、蜈蚣、地鳖虫、胎盘等,在烘干后,应保持干燥,以防虫蛀或腐烂。

1.3.3矿物药如石膏、滑石、灵磁石等较易保存;但其中如芒硝、硼砂等须放在有盖子的容器内,以防受潮。

1.3.4剧毒药物要另行贮藏保管,防止发生事故。

贮藏药物的库房须经常保持清洁干燥和防虫、鼠的侵蚀;药物仍须勤加翻晒,对某些易生虫蛀或容易受潮发油的药物,如前胡、羌活、独活、甘遂、当归等,必须经常检查,以防霉蛀变质。

1.4 中药的炮制

炮制,又称炮炙,是药物在制成各种剂型之前对药材的整理

medicinal herbs for fresh use, the others should be washed clean and cut. Then according to their natures, they should be dried in the sun, in the shade or over the fire.

1.3.2 Chinese magnoliavine fruit (wuweizi), glossy privet fruit (nüzhenzi), radish seed (laifuzi) and white mustard seed (baijiezi) should be preserved in sealed containers away from pests and rats; stems, leaves and roots without fragrance, such as motherwort herb, common scouring rush herb (muzeicao), common selfheal fruit-spike (xiakucao), dyers woad leaf (daqingye), isatis root (banlangen) and tuber fleece flower stem (shouwuteng) should be placed in dry shade; aromatic herbs and flowers, such as chrysanthemum, honeysuckle bud and flower and Chinese rose flower should be placed in dry shade lest they may decay or deteriorate with dampness; medicinal animals or their organs and tissues, such as agkistrodon (qishe), black-tail snake (wushaoshe), centipede (wugong), eupolyphaga sinensis walker (dibiechong) and placenta (taipan), should remain dry after being dried to avoid being damaged by worms, or decay.

1.3.3 Medicinal minerals, such as gypsum (shigao), talc (huashi) and magnetite (lingcishi), are easy to preserve; crystallized sodium sulfate (mangxiao) and borax (pengsha) should be placed in a container with a lid to keep away from moisture.

1.3.4 Highly toxic drugs should be stored separately to prevent accidents.

Drug storage warehouse should always be kept clean and dry, and be prevent from worms and rats; medicinals should be frequently tedded. For some easy to be affected by worms and damp, such as hogfennel root (qianhu), incised notopterygium rhizome and root (qianghuo), pubescent angelica (duhuo), gansui root (gansui) and Chinese angelica (danggui) etc., they must be examined regularly to prevent decay and deterioration.

1.4 Processing of Chinese medicinals

Processing of Chinese medicinals is the processing method before they are made into various dosage forms

加工以及根据医疗需要而进行处理的一些方法。

1.4.1　炮制的目的

增效、减毒：在炮制过程中加一些酒、醋、姜、蜜等以增强药物作用、提高药物疗效，如酒川芎、蜜炙桑叶等。也可以通过特殊处理使毒性或副作用降低或消除，如马钱子砂烫；生半夏、生南星用生姜或明矾炮制；巴豆用霜等可解除毒性。

纠性：改变药物的性能功效，适应病情需要或扩大应用范围。如生地黄蒸制成熟地用，其性寒凉血变微温而补血；何首乌制熟由润肠通便、解疮毒而转为补肝肾、益精血等。

保质量：一些药物在采集后必须清除泥沙杂质和非药用的部分；植物类药物切制成一定规格的饮片，便于煎煮；某些生药在采集后必须烘焙，使药物充分干燥，以便贮藏。

矫臭味：有些海产品与动物类的药物需要漂去咸味及腥味等，便于服用。

1.4.2　炮制的方法

修制：通过簸、筛、刮、刷、拣等方法清除杂质；通过研磨、捣、挫等切制、粉碎药物，使药物便于贮存、调剂和制剂。

水制：通过洗、漂、泡、渍等方法将有腥气的龟板、鳖甲、乌贼骨等或有咸味的昆布、海藻或有

according to medical needs for treatment.

1.4.1　The purpose of processing

Increasing therapeutic effects and eliminating toxicity Some wine, vinegar, ginger and honey are added into the processed medicinals to enhance their effectiveness, such as stir-baking sichuan lovage rhizome (chuanxiong) with liquor and stir-baking mulberry leaf (sangye) with honey. Also, through special treatment, toxicity or side effects can be reduced or eliminated, such as, stir-baking nux vomica (maqianzi); stir-baking raw pinellia tuber (banxia) and dragon arum with ginger or alum; making croton fruit (badou) into frost-like powder can eliminate its toxicity.

Modifying nature The nature and efficacy of medicinals can be changed to adapt to the needs of the patient or to expand the scope of application. Rehmanniae radix (shengdihuang) is cold for cooling blood. After being steamed, it becomes prepared rehmannia root (shudihuang), and slightly warm to enrich blood. After being processed, the nature of fleeceflower root (heshouwu) is changed from relaxing bowel to tonifying the liver and kidney and nourishing essence-blood.

Assuring quality After collection, the foreign and non-pharmaceutical parts should be removed. Medicinal plants are cut into some certain size pieces for decoction. Some crude medicinals must be baked after collecting to make them fully dried for storage.

Correcting odor The salty or fishy smell of some seafood and animal medicinals needs to be rinsed for the convenience of in-taking.

1.4.2　Methods of processing

Purifying Impurities are removed through winnowing, sieving, scraping, brushing and selecting; medicinals are cut and powdered through grinding, pounding and grating in order for storage, dispensing and preparation.

Processing with water Through washing, bleaching and soaking, the fish-like odor of tortoise carapace and plastron (guiban), turtle shell (biejia) and cuttlefish bone

毒性的乌头、附子等药物,使用清水反复浸漂,可以漂去这些气味或减少毒性。其中水飞比较特殊,适用于矿石和贝壳类不易溶解于水的药物如朱砂、炉甘石等,放在研钵内和水同研,反复操作,研至细粉,目的是使药物粉碎得更加细腻,便于内服和外用,并可防止粉末在研磨时飞扬,以减少损耗。

火制:是最常用的炮制方法,将药物直接用火加热,或与辅料拌炒。

煅:将药物通过烈火直接或间接煅烧,使之质地松脆、易于粉碎、充分发挥药效。又分直接煅和间接煅:

直接煅,又叫明煅:适用于矿石和贝壳类不易碎裂的药物如磁石、牡蛎等。煅的程度视药物性质不同而定。矿石类药物必须煅至红色为度;贝壳类药物则煅至微红冷却后呈灰白色。

间接煅,又称为焖煅:少数体轻质松的药物如陈棕、人发等,即将药物放在耐高温的密闭容器中用火煅烧。

炒是将药物放于锅内加热,用铁铲不断铲动,炒至一定程度取出。炒的方法有清炒和辅料炒两种:

清炒:不加辅料进行炒制,根据火力和药材变色情况,又有炒黄、炒焦、炒碳之分。

辅料炒:将药物与固体辅料如米、砂、土、麸皮等拌炒,如麸炒枳壳,土炒白术等,一般以炒至微

(wuzeigu), and the saline taste of kelp (kunbu) and seaweed (haizao), or toxicity of aconite (wutou) and aconite, can be eliminated or reduced. Refining with water is a special method which is suitable for minerals and shells not easy to dissolve in water, such as, cinnabar (zhusha) and calamine (luganshi). Grind them with water in a mortar repeatedly until all of them are ground into fine powder for oral and external use and to avoid powder flying in grinding and minimizing their loss.

Processing with fire   It is the mostly used processing method that medicinals are put in a pan to be heated or stirred with other adjuvant medicinals.

Calcining   It is a method of heating medicinals directly or indirectly to make them crisp and easy to be powdered and give full play to efficacy. There are direct and indirect calcinings.

Direct calcining is suitable for minerals and shells not easy to crack, such as, magnetite (cishi) and oyster shell (muli). The degree of direct calcining is according to the different natures of the medicinals. Medicinal minerals should be calcined to turn red; medicinal shells should be calcined to turn light red and appear grey after cooling.

Indirect calcining is a method of putting some light medicinals, such as petiolo-nervus trachycarpi (chenzong) and human hair (renfa) into a sealed container with high temperature resistance to calcine with fire.

Stir-baking is a method of putting medicinals into a pan to heat and stir constantly to some extent and then get them out. There are single stir-baking and stir-baking with other adjuvant.

Single stir-baking is to stir-bake without other adjuvant. According to the fire and the changing colors of the medicinal materials, there are stir-baking to yellow, stir-baking to brown and stir-baking to charcoal.

Stir-baking with other adjuvant is to stir-bake medicinal materials with solid adjuvant like rice, sand, soil and bran, such as stir-baking orange fruit (zhike) with bran and stir-baking largehead atractylodes rhizome (baishu) with soil to

中医理论 Basic Theory of Traditional Chinese Medicine

黄色为度。

炙法：将药物与液体辅料如酒、蜂蜜、醋、盐水、姜汁等拌炒。按用药的不同要求有酒炒大黄、醋香附、蜜炙甘草、炙紫菀、炙兜铃等，山甲片、龟板、鳖甲等经过砂炙后变得松脆，利于研粉制药，有效成分易于吸收利用。

水火共制法：利用液体辅料与火共同对药材进行加工的方法，常见的有蒸、煮、淬等。如何首乌与生地黄蒸熟，生大黄经蒸制成为熟大黄；附子、川乌与豆腐同煮可减少毒性；灵磁石、代赭石用醋淬，除能使被淬的药物酥松易于粉碎外，还因药汁的吸收会改变其性能。

除上述炮制法外，还有一些特殊的方法。

制霜：将种子类药物压榨出油或将某些矿物质药材重新结晶，如西瓜霜是把芒硝放入西瓜内所析出的结晶；巴豆霜是由巴豆榨出的油脂制成。

发酵：如神曲、淡豆豉等。

发芽：如麦芽、谷芽等。

② 中药的性能

药性理论是认识和概括中药性质和功能的理论，是中药基本理论的核心部分。药性是药物共同具有的一些普遍特性，它既

light yellow.

Stir-baking with liquid adjuvant is to stir-bake medicinal materials with liquor, honey, vinegar, brine and ginger juice. There are stir-baking rhubarb (dahuang) with liquor, stir-baking liquorice root (gancao) with honey, stir-baking tatarian aster root (ziyuan) and stir-baking dutchmanspipe fruit (douling). Stir-baking pangolin scales (shanjiapian), tortoise carapace and plastron and turtle shell with sand will become so crisp that they are easy to be ground, and effective ingredients are easy to be taken in.

Processing with water and fire is to process medicinal materials with water, liquid adjuvant and fire like steaming, boiling and quenching. Rehmanniae radix steamed with fleeceflower root, it is transformed into prepared rehmannia root; boiling aconite, common monkshood mother root (chuanwu) with tofu can reduce toxicity; quenching magnetite (lingcishi) and haematitum (daizheshi) with vinegar can not only make them crisp and easy to be ground, but also change their nature because of absorbing the medicine juice.

In addition to the above processing methods, there are other special ones.

Making into frost-like powder is to process medicinal seeds out of oil or recrystallize medicinal minerals, such as, watermelon frost (xiguashuang) is the crystallization from purring precipitation in watermelon; defatted croton seed powder (badoushuang) is made from the oil squeezed from croton fruit (badou).

Fermenting Typical medicinals are medicated leaven (shenqu) and fermented soybean (dandouchi).

Germinating Typical medicinals are germinated barley (maiya) and millet sprout (guya).

② Characteristics of Chinese Medicinals

The theory of characteristics of Chinese medicinals is the theory of understanding and summarizing the nature and function of Chinese materia medica and it is also the core part of the basic theory of Chinese materia medica.

是中药功效的高度概括，也是认识中药功效和应用中药的理论基础。概括起来，主要有四气、五味、升降浮沉、补泻、归经、有毒无毒几个方面。

2.1　四气

四气，指寒、热、温、凉四种药性，可以调节机体寒热变化和纠正人体阴阳盛衰，是药物作用性质的重要药性理论。

药性的寒热温凉是由药物作用于人体所产生的不同反应和所获得的不同疗效而总结出来的，这与所治疗疾病的性质是相对而言的。能够减轻或消除热证的药物，一般属于寒性或凉性，如黄芩、板蓝根、生石膏等对于发热口渴、咽喉疼痛等热证有清热解毒作用，表明这两种药物具有寒凉性质；反之能够减轻或消除寒证的药物，一般属于温性或热性，如附子、肉桂、干姜等对于腹中冷痛、脉沉无力等寒证有温中散寒作用，表明这两种药物具有温热性质。

寒凉和温热是两种对立的药性，而寒与凉、热与温之间只是程度的不同。一般来讲，寒凉药分别具有清热泻火、凉血解毒、滋阴除蒸、泻热通便、清热利水、清化热痰、清心开窍、凉肝息风等作用；而温热药则分别具有温里散寒、暖肝散结、补火助阳、温阳利

The characteristics of Chinese medicinals are not only the high generalization of the efficacy of Chinese materia medica, but also the theoretical basis for understanding the efficacy and application of it. To sum up, it includes four natures, five flavors, four directions, reinforcing and reducing, meridian entry and toxicity.

2.1　Four Natures

The four natures refer to cold, hot, warm and cool, which can adjust the temperature of body and correct ups and downs of yin and yang, and is the important theory of functions and characteristics of Chinese medicinals.

The four natures are the summary of different reactions and effects caused by medicinals acting on human body, which is relative with the nature of treating diseases. Chinese medicinals reducing or eliminating heat syndromes generally belong to cold or cool, such as baical skullcap root (huangqin), isatis root (banlangen), raw gypsum (shigao) have the detoxification effect on fever with thirst, throat pain and other heat syndromes, which shows that they have cold nature. By contrast, medicinals reducing or eliminating cold syndromes generally are warm or hot, such as aconite, cassia bark (rougui) and dried ginger (ganjiang) have the effect of warming spleen and stomach for dispelling cold on cold pain in the abdomen and deep and weak pulse and other cold syndromes.

Cold and cool, warm and hot are the two opposite natures, while the difference between cold and cool, hot and warm is the difference of range. Generally speaking, cold and cool medicinals respectively have the effects of clearing heat and purging fire, detoxification, nourishing yin and removing steam purge, eliminating heat-phlegm, waking up unconscious patients by clearing away heart-fire, cooling the liver for calming endogenous wind; warm and hot medicinals respectively have the effects of warming the internal to dispel the cold, warming the liver to dispel knots, nourishing fire to assist yang, warming yang for dieresis,

中医理论

Basic Theory of Traditional Chinese Medicine

水、温经通络、引火归元、回阳救逆等作用。

《素问·至真要大论》里有"寒者热之、热者寒之"，指出了四气理论指导临床用药的原则。具体来说，温热药多用于治疗中寒腹痛、阴寒水肿、风寒痹证、寒疝作痛、阳痿不举、宫冷不孕、血寒经闭、亡阳虚脱等一系列阴寒证；而寒凉药主要用于实热烦渴、温毒发斑、血热吐衄、火毒疮疡、热结便秘、热淋涩痛、痰热喘咳、高热神昏、热极生风等一系列阳热证。如果阴寒证用寒凉药，阳热证用温热药必然导致病情恶化，甚至引起死亡。

2.2 五味

药性的五味，是指酸、苦、甘、辛、咸五种味道，具有不同的治疗作用。有些药物还具有淡味或涩味，但五味是最基本的五种滋味，所以仍然称为五味。

五味的含义既代表了药物味道的"味"，又包含了药物作用的"味"，而后者构成了五味理论的主要内容。

辛，具有发散、行气、行血等作用。一般来讲，解表药（麻黄、桂枝、薄荷等）、行气药（枳实、陈皮等）、活血化瘀药（川芎、郁金等）多具辛味。一些气味芳香辛辣的药物，具有芳香辟秽、芳香化湿、醒脾开胃、芳香开窍等作用，

warming channels and activating collaterals, letting the fire back to its origin and reviving yang for resuscitation.

In *Plain Questions: Discussion on the Most Important and Abstruse Theory*, there is the saying, "heating the cold and cooling the hot", which points out the theory of the four natures to guide the clinical medication. Specifically, warm and hot medicinals are mainly used for treating cold abdominal pain, yin-cold and edema, cold arthralgia, cold and painful hernia, impotence, uterine cold with infertility, cold blood causing amenorrhea and yang depletion and other cold syndromes; cold medicinals are mainly used for treating solid heat and polydipsia, warm toxicity for developing macules, hot blood causing spontaneous external bleeding, hot toxicity causing sores, hot obstruction causing constipation, heat astringent pain, phlegm-heat causing dyspnea with cough, high fever causing unconsciousness and extreme heat causing wind and other yang-heat syndromes. If yin-cold syndromes are treated with cold and cool medicinals and yang-heat syndromes are treated with warm and hot medicinals, it will inevitably lead to disease deterioration, even death.

2.2　Five Flavors

Five flavors refer to sour, bitter, sweet, pungent and salty, which have different therapeutic effects. Some medicinals also have bland or astringent flavor, but five flavors are the most basic ones.

The meaning of five flavors not only represents the "flavor" of medicinals, but also contains the "flavor" of medicinal effect, while the latter constitutes the main content of the theory of five flavors.

The pungent flavor has the function of dispelling, promoting qi and circulating blood. Generally speaking, medicinals for relieving exterior syndrome [(ephedra mahuang), cassia twig (guizhi), peppermint (bohe)], promoting qi [immature orange fruit (zhishi), dried tangerine peel (chenpi)], invigorating blood circulation and eliminating stasis [sichuan lovage rhizome, turmeric root tuber (yujin)] are pungent. Some fragrant and spicy medicinals have the

Basic Theory of Traditional Chinese Medicine

中医理论

也有能散、能行的特点,一般也标以辛味。

甘,具有补益、和中、调和药性和缓急止痛的作用,如人参大补元气,熟地、大枣滋补精血,甘草调和诸药并解药食中毒等。

酸,具有收敛、固涩的作用。一般固表止汗、敛肺止咳、涩肠止泻、固精缩尿、固崩止带的药物多具有酸味,如五味子固表止汗、石榴皮涩肠止泻、山茱萸涩精止遗等。涩,与酸味药的作用相似,多用于治疗虚汗、泄泻、尿频、遗精、滑精、出血等症,如莲子固精止带、禹余粮涩肠止泻、乌贼骨收涩止血等,故本草文献常有"涩附于酸"之说,常将两者并列。

苦,具有"泄"和"燥"的特点,可以清泄火热、泄降气逆、通泄大便、燥湿、坚阴(泻火存阴)等。如黄芩清热泻火、杏仁降气平喘、半夏降逆止呕、大黄泻热通便、龙胆草清热燥湿、苍术苦温燥湿等。

effect of dispelling filth, removing dampness, arousing the spleen and stimulating appetite and inducing resuscitation. Medicinals having the characteristics of dispelling and promoting generally are marked with pungency.

The sweet flavor can nourish, harmonize, regulate medicinal property and relieve pain. For example, ginseng (renshen) nourishes vital qi, prepared rehmannia root and Chinese date (dazao) nourish essence-blood, and liquorice root (gancao) harmonizes medicinals and detoxifies drugs and food poisoning.

The sour flavor has the function of absorbing and consolidating. The medicinals with the sour flavor have the function of strengthening exterior and reducing sweat, astringing the lung to stop cough, astringing intestinal and stopping diarrhea, securing essence and reducing urination, curing metrorrhagia and leukorrhagia. For instance, Chinese magnoliavine fruit (wuweizi) has the function of strengthening exterior and reducing sweat; pomegranate rind (shiliupi) has the function of astringing intestinal and stopping diarrhea; asiatic cornelian cherry fruit (shanzhuyu) has the function of arresting seminal emission. The astringent favor has the similar function with the sour flavor for treating abnormal sweating, diarrhea, frequent urination, spermatorrhea and bleeding. For example, lotus seed (lianzi) treats spontaneous emission and leukorrhagia; limonite (yuyuliang) astringes intestinal and stops diarrhea; cuttlefish bone (wuzeigu) induces astringency and stops bleeding. Therefore, the herbal literature often says, "the astringent flavor is attached to the sour flavor". The sour flavor is often compared to the astringent flavor.

The bitter flavor is purging and drying. It has the function of clearing heat, purging the adverse rising of qi, discharging stool, eliminating dampness, reinforcing yin (purging fire and storing yin). For example, baical skullcap root clears heat and purges fire; bitter apricot seed (xingren) descends qi and relieves asthma; pinellia tuber descends overflow and controls vomiting; rhubarb (dahuang) discharges fire and stool; Chinese gentian (longdancao) clears fire and eliminates dampness; atractylodes rhizome (cangshu) expels heat and dries dampness.

中医理论

Basic Theory of Traditional Chinese Medicine

咸,具有泻下通便、软坚散结的作用,多用于治疗大便燥结、瘰疬痰核、瘿瘤、癥瘕痞块等症,如芒硝泻热通便,海藻、牡蛎消瘰散瘿,鳖甲、土鳖虫软坚消癥等。此外,咸味药如紫河车、海狗肾、龟板等都具有良好的补肾作用。为了引药入肾增强补肾作用,不少药物如知母、杜仲、巴戟天等药用盐水炮制。

淡,具有渗湿利水的作用,多用治水肿、脚气、小便不利之症,如通草、灯心草、茯苓、猪苓、泽泻等。

药物的五味,只是药性的一个方面,对于药物性能的全面认识,必须结合其他特性,才能全面掌握药物功能。

2.3 升降浮沉

升降浮沉是指药物在体内的作用趋向。

升与降、浮与沉都是相对的。升是上升、升提,作用趋向于上;降是下降、降逆,作用趋向于下;浮是升浮、上行发散,作用趋向于外;沉是下沉、下行泄利,作用趋向于内。一般来讲,升浮药具有升阳举陷、发散表邪、宣毒透疹、涌吐开窍等作用;而沉降药具有清热泻下、潜阳息风、降逆止呕、止呃、利水渗湿、重镇安神、降气平喘等作用。

The salty flavor is purging and softening. The medicinals with salty flavor is used for treating dry feces, scrofula, phlegm nodule, goiter, abdominal mass. For example, crystallized sodium sulfate (mangxiao) purges fire and discharges stool; seaweed (haizao) and oyster shell (muli) dissipate scrofula and goiter; turtle shell (biejia) and ground beetle(tubiechong) soften hardness and dissipate abdominal mass. In addition, the medicinals with salty flavor, such as, human placenta (ziheche), urine seal testes and penis (haigoushen) and tortoise carapace and plastron, have the good effect of nourishing the kidney. In order to induce medicinals to nourish the kidney, a lot of them, such as common anemarrhena rhizome (zhimu), eucommia bark (duzhong) and morinda root (bajitian) are processed in salty water.

The bland flavor is draining and promoting and used for treating edema, beriberi, urination, such as, ricepaperplant pith (tongcao), common rush (dengxincao), Indian buead, polyporus (zhuling) and oriental waterplantain rhizome (zexie).

The five flavors are just one part of the characteristics of Medicinals. In order to get a comprehensive knowledge of them, other characteristics should be considered.

2.3 Ascending, Descending, Floating and Sinking

Ascending, descending, floating and sinking refer to the functional trend of Chinese medicinals on human body.

Ascending and descending, floating and sinking are relative pairs. Ascending is promoting; descending is calming the adverse; floating is dispelling outside; sinking is purging inside. Generally speaking, the medicinals with ascending and floating have the function of raising yang and lifting prolapsed zang-fu organs, dispersing superficial exopathogens, dissipating poison and promoting eruption, encouraging vomiting and regaining consciousness; the medicinals with descending and sinking has the function of clearing heat and draining precipitation, subduing yang and extinguishing wind, descending the adverse and checking vomiting, relieving hiccup, clearing damp and promoting dieresis, soothing the nerves and descending qi to relieve asthma.

Basic Theory of Traditional Chinese Medicine

中医理论

药物的升降浮沉性能，主要是以改善脏腑气机升降紊乱和病势顺逆的功效为依据，但与药物的四气五味、气味厚薄和其质地的轻重及药用部位等也有着密切联系，此外还受炮制和配伍的影响。

就药物的性味及厚薄而言，凡味属辛、甘(味之薄者)，气属温、热(气之厚者)的药物，大都属升浮药，如麻黄、升麻、黄芪等药；凡味属苦、酸、咸(味之厚者)，性属寒、凉(气之薄者)的药物，大都属沉降药，如大黄、芒硝、山楂等。

从药物的质地、部位与升降浮沉的关系来看，一般花、叶、皮、枝等质轻的药物大多为升浮药，如苏叶、菊花、蝉衣等；而种子、果实、矿物、贝壳及质重者大多属沉降药，如苏子、枳实、牡蛎、代赭石等，但某些药物也有特殊性，如旋覆花虽然是花，但能降气消痰、止呕止噫，药性沉降而不升浮；苍耳子虽然是果实，但功能通窍发汗、散风除湿、药性升浮而不沉降，故有"诸花皆升，旋覆独降；诸子皆降，苍耳独升"之说。

炮制与配伍也可以影响药

Ascending, descending, floating and sinking natures of Chinese medicinals mainly take the effect of improving zang-fu organs' abnormal movement of qi dynamics and upward and downward tendency of diseases as the basis, and they are also closely related with the four natures and five flavors, heaviness and lightness, texture and medicinal parts of the medicinals, and are also affected by processing and compatibility.

As to the natures and flavors, and their heaviness and lightness, medicinals with pungent and sweet flavor (light flavor), and warm and hot nature (heavy nature) pertain to ascending and floating medicinals, such as ephedra (mahuang), largetrifoliolious bugbane rhizome (shengma) and milkvetch root (huangqi); medicinals with bitter, sour and salty flavor (heavy flavor), and cold and cool nature (light nature) pertain to sinking and descending medicinals, such as rhubarb (dahuang), crystallized sodium sulfate and hawthorn fruit (shanzha).

As to the relationship between the texture, medicinal parts and ascending, descending, floating, sinking natures, generally speaking, flowers, leaves, rind and stems with light texture are ascending and floating, such as perilla leaf (suye), chrysanthemum and cicada slough (chanyi); seeds, fruits, minerals and shells with heavy texture are descending and sinking, such as perilla (suzi), immature orange fruit (zhishi), oyster shell (muli) and haematitum (daizheshi). However, some medicinals have their specialty. For example, though the flower of inula (xuanfu) is the medicinal part, it can descend qi and dissipate phlegm, stop vomiting, and its nature is sinking and descending, not floating and ascending; though the fruit of siberian cocklebur fruit (canger) is the medicinal part, it can arouse consciousness and induce perspiration, disperse wind and remove dampness, and its nature is ascending and floating, not sinking and descending. So, there is the saying "all the flowers have the nature of ascending except inula; all the fruits have the nature of descending except siberian cocklebur fruit."

Processing and compatibility can also affect ascending,

物的升降浮沉,如酒制则升、姜炒则散、醋炒收敛、盐炒下行。如大黄,属于沉降药,峻下热结、泻热通便,经酒炒后,大黄则可清上焦火热,以治目赤头痛。

2.4　归经

归是作用的归属,经是脏腑经络的概称。归经,就是指药物对于机体某部分的选择性作用,即主要对某经(脏腑或经络)或某几经发生明显的作用,而对其他经则作用较小,甚或无作用。也就是说,归经是说明某种药物对某些脏腑经络的病变起着主要或特殊的治疗作用,药物的归经不同,其治疗作用也就不同。药物的归经,还指明了药物治病的适用范围,也就说明了其药效之所在。

归经理论是以脏腑经络学说为基础,以所治疗的具体病症为依据总结出来的用药理论。朱砂、远志能治愈心悸失眠,说明它们归心经;桔梗、苏子能治愈喘咳胸闷,说明它们归肺经;白芍、钩藤能治愈胁痛抽搐则说明它们归肝经。

药物的归经,主要以其临床疗效为依据,但与药物自身的特性(即形、色、气味、禀赋等)也有一定联系,如味辛、色白入肺、大肠经;味苦、色赤入心、小肠经等都是以药物的色与味作归经的依

descending, floating, sinking. Medicinals stir-baked with liquor become ascending, stir-baked with ginger become scattering, stir-baked with vinegar become astringent and stir-baked with salt become descending. For example, rhubarb with sinking and descending nature can purge heat and relax bowels. Rhubarb stir-baked with liquor can purge fire-heat in upper-energizer to cure red eyes and headache.

2.4　Meridian Tropism

Meridian tropism refers to the selective effect of medicinals on some parts of the body, that is, evident effects on a certain meridian (internal organs or meridians) or some certain meridians, few or even no effects on the others. That is to say, meridian tropism explains some certain medicinal exerts a major or special therapeutic effect on pathological changes of some organs and meridians. The meridian tropism of medicinals is different, so their treatment effect is also different. Meridian tropism also points out the application scope of treatment, and expounds the effectiveness.

The theory of meridian tropism is based on the theory of zang-fu organs and meridians, which is the medication theory summed up on the basis of the specific syndromes. Cinnabar (zhusha) and milkwort root (yuanzhi) can cure palpitation and insomnia, indicating that they pertain to the heart meridian; platycodon root (jiegeng) and perilla can cure cough and chest tightness, suggesting that they pertain to the lung meridian; debark peony root (baishao) and gambir plant nod (gouteng) can cure pains in hypochondrium and twitch, suggesting that they pertain to the liver meridian.

Meridian tropism is mainly based on its clinical efficacy. However, there is also a certain link with the characteristics of the medicinals themselves (that is, shape, color, flavor, nature, etc.). The medicinals with pungent flavor and white color pertain to the lung and large intestine meridian and the medicinals with bitter flavor and red color, to the heart and small intestine meridian, which takes color and flavor as

据。再如麝香芳香开窍入心经；佩兰芳香醒脾入脾经；连翘状如心形而入心经清心降火等等，都是以形、气归经的例子。其中尤以五味与归经的关系最为密切。

掌握归经便于临床辨证用药，提高用药的针对性。根据疾病的临床表现，通过辨证审因，诊断出病变所在脏腑经络部位，按照归经来选择适当药物进行治疗。如热证，若肺热咳喘，当用桑白皮、地骨皮等归肺经药来泻肺平喘；若胃火牙痛当用石膏、黄连等归胃经药来清泻胃火；若心火亢盛心悸失眠，当用朱砂、丹参等归心经药以清心安神；若肝热目赤，当用夏枯草、龙胆草等归肝经药以清肝明目，可见归经理论为临床辨证用药提供了方便。

掌握归经理论还有助于区别功效相似的药物。如同为治头痛之药，但羌活善治太阳经头痛、

the basis for meridian tropism. Also, the fragrance of musk (shexiang) can regain consciousness, pertaining to the heart meridian; the fragrance of fortune eupatorium herb (peilan) can activate the spleen, pertaining to the spleen meridian; weeping forsythia capsule (lianqiao) with the heart-like shape can clear the heart and purge fire, pertaining to the heart meridian. All of them show examples about meridian tropism according to colors and shapes, among which the five flavors are closely related with meridian tropism.

To master meridian tropism is easy for clinical syndrome differentiation and medication to improve the use of targeted medicinals. According to the clinical manifestations of the disease, through syndrome differentiation and investigating etiology, the lesion location of the internal organs and meridians will be diagnosed and appropriate medicinals will be chosen for treatment. Take heat syndrome as an example, lung heat and cough with asthma can be treated with medicinals, such as white mulberry root-bark (sangbaipi) and Chinese wolfberry root-bark (digupi) pertaining to the lung meridian, to remove heat from the lung and relieve asthma; stomach fire and toothache can be treated with medicinals, such as gypsum (shigao) and golden thread (huanglian) pertaining to the stomach meridian, to clear and purge stomach fire; heart fire hyperactivity, palpitation and insomnia can be treated with medicinals, such as cinnabar (zhusha) and salvia (danshen) pertaining to the heart meridian, to clear away heart-fire and soothe the nerves; liver-fire and red eyes can be treated with medicinals, such as common selfheal fruit-spike (xiakucao) and Chinese gentian (longdancao) pertaining to the liver meridian, to clear the liver and improve vision. Therefore, the theory of meridian tropism provides convenience for clinical syndrome differentiation.

Mastering meridian tropism is conducive to distinguish the efficacy of similar medicinals. As medicinals for treating headache, incised notopterygium rhizome and root (qianghuo) is good at treating headache of the taiyang

中医理论 Basic Theory of Traditional Chinese Medicine

葛根善治阳明经头痛、柴胡善治少阳经头痛、吴茱萸善治厥阴经头痛、细辛善治少阴经头痛。

2.5 毒性

毒性是指药物对机体的伤害性,反映了药物安全性能。

历来对药物的毒性存在不同的认识。一种认为毒性是药物的偏性,我们用药物的偏性来纠治疾病的偏性;现代药物毒性是指毒物对机体组织器官的损害性。

在应用毒药时要针对体质的强弱、疾病部位的深浅,恰当选择药物并确定剂量,中病即止,不可过服,以防止过量和蓄积中毒,尤其砒霜、胆矾、马钱子、乌头等毒性较大的药物。同时要注意配伍禁忌,凡两药合用能产生剧烈毒副作用的禁止同用,如甘遂与甘草、乌头与瓜蒌等;严格毒药的炮制工艺,以降低毒性;对某些毒药还要采用适当的剂型和方式给药。此外,还要注意患者的个体差异,适当增减用量,并说服患者不可自行服药。同时要抓好药品鉴别,防止伪品混用;通过各个环节的把关,以确保用药安全、避免药物中毒的发生。

中医根据"以毒攻毒"的原则,在保证用药安全的前提下,经

meridian; kudzuvine root (gegen) is good at treating headache of the mingyang meridian; Chinese thorowax root (chaihu) is good at treating headache of the shaoyang meridian; medicinal evodia fruit (wuzhuyu) is good at treating headache of the jueyin meridian; manchurian wild ginger (xixin) is good at treating headache of shaoyin meridian.

2.5 Toxicity

Toxicity is the harm of medicinals to the body, which reflects the safety of medicinals.

There have always been different understandings of medicinal toxicity. One is that the toxicity is the medicinal deflection which is used to correct the pathological deflection; in modern times, medicinal toxicity refers to harmful effects on organism.

In the application of toxicant, according to physical strength and depth of pathological location, toxic medicinals should be chosen appropriately and the dose of them should be confirmed to avoid poisoning especially strongly toxic arsenic (pishuang), chalcanthite (danfan), nux vomica (maqianzi) and aconite (wutou). At the same time, take notice of medicinal combination rules. Any combination of two medicinals which can produce severe side effects should be prohibited, such as gansui root (gansui) and liquorice root (gancao), aconite and snakegourd fruit (gualou). Toxic medicinals should be processed strictly to reduce toxicity; for some toxic medicinals, the appropriate dosage and method should be applied. In addition, increase or decrease dosage appropriately according to individual differences, and persuade patients not to take medicinals by themselves. At the same time, medicinals identification and cheek should be emphasized to prevent counterfeit, ensuring medicinal safety and avoid poisoning.

According to the "combating poison with poison" principle in TCM and under the premise of ensuring safety,

中医理论

Basic Theory of Traditional Chinese Medicine

常采用某些毒药治疗某些疾病，以取得更好的临床疗效。如用大枫子治疗恶疮麻风、斑蝥治疗癌肿、砒霜治疗瘰疬等。

掌握药物的毒性及其中毒后的临床表现，便于诊断中毒原因，以便及时采取合理、有效的抢救治疗手段。

certain toxic medicinals are used to treat certain illnesses in order to achieve better clinical efficacy. For example, chaulmoogra seed (dafengzi) is used to treat malignant sores and lepra; blister beetle (banmao) is used to treat cancer; arsenic is used to treat scrofula etc.

Mastering medicinal toxicity and clinical manifestations is easy for finding poisoning causes in order to take reasonable and effective rescue treatment.

3 中药的应用

3.1 中药的配伍

配伍是指有目的地按病情需要和药性特点，有选择地将两味以上药物配合同用。药物通过配伍后，药和药之间会发生许多变化。这些变化在《神农本草经》中称为"七情"。七情是单行以及其他六种配伍关系的总称。

3.1.1 单行

单行就是指用单味药治病。病情比较单纯，选用一种针对性强的药物即能获得疗效，如黄芩治疗肺热咳血，鹤草芽驱除绦虫，以及许多行之有效的"单方"等。它符合简、便、廉、验的要求，便于使用和推广。

3.1.2 相须

即性能功效相类似的药物配合应用，可以增强某种或某几种治疗效应，如麻黄与桂枝配伍，能明显增强发散风寒的效果；石膏与知母配伍，能明显增强清热泻火的治疗效果；大黄与芒硝配

3 Application of Chinese Medicinals

3.1 Combination

The combination of Chinese medicinals means that two or more medicinals are selectively combined according to clinical application and characteristics of medicinals. There will be a lot of changes among medicinals after combination. These changes are called "seven groups", a general term including a single application and six combinations.

3.1.1 Single Application

It refers that one medicinal is used to treat an illness. When the condition is relatively simple, a strong targeted medicinal can obtain curative effect, such as baical skullcap root can treat lung-heat and hemoptysis, agrimony (hecaoya) can expel tapeworm and other effective single applications. It conforms to the requirements of briefness, convenience, inexpensiveness and examination and is easy to use and spread.

3.1.2 Mutual reinforcement

Medicinals with similar properties and efficacies can be combined together to reinforce one or several specific effects. For example, when combining ephedra (mahuang) and cassia twig (guizhi), the efficacy to dissipate wind-cold will be reinforced; when combining gypsum (shigao) and common anemarrhena rhizome (zhimu), the efficacy to clear heat and purge fire will be reinforced; when combining

合,能明显增强攻下泻热的治疗效果。

3.1.3 相使

即在性能功效方面有某种共性的药物配合应用,以一味药物为主,另一味药物为辅,辅药能提高主药物的疗效,如黄芪与茯苓配合,茯苓能提高黄芪补气利水的治疗效果;黄芩与大黄配合,大黄能提高黄芩清热泻火的治疗效果。

3.1.4 相畏

即一种药物的毒性反应或副作用,能被另一种药物减轻或消除,如生半夏和生南星的毒性能被生姜减轻和消除,所以说生半夏和生南星畏生姜。

3.1.5 相杀

即一种药物能减轻或消除另一种药物的毒性或副作用,如生姜能减轻或消除生半夏和生南星的毒副作用,所以说生姜杀生半夏和生南星的毒。

3.1.6 相恶

即一种药物某种治疗效果会被另一药物削弱或降低,甚至药效完全丧失,如人参恶莱菔子,因莱菔子能削弱人参的补气作用。

3.1.7 相反

即两种药物合用,能产生毒

rhubarb (dahuang) and crystallized sodium sulfate (mangxiao), the efficacy to purge heat will be reinforced.

3.1.3 Mutual assistance

It refers to combining medicinals with similar properties and efficacies, and with one medicinal taking the major role and the other as the assistant to the major medicinal, to improve efficacy of the major medicinal. For example, when milkvetch root (huangqi) is combined with Indian buead, Indian buead can improve the efficacy of milkvetch root for nourishing qi and alleviating water retention; when baical skullcap root is combined with rhubarb (dahuang), rhubarb can improve the efficacy of milkvetch root for clearing heat and purging fire.

3.1.4 Mutual restraint

It means that the toxicity or side effects of a medicinal can be eliminated and removed by another medicinal, such as, the toxicity of raw pinellia tuber (banxia) and raw dragon arum (nanxing) can be eliminated and removed by raw ginger (shengjiang), so raw pinellia tuber and raw dragon arum are restrained by raw ginger.

3.1.5 Mutual suppression

It means that one medicinal can eliminate or dissipate the toxicity or side effects of another medicinal. For example, raw ginger can eliminate or remove the toxicity or side effects of raw pinellia tuber and raw dragon arum, so raw ginger can suppress the toxicity of raw pinellia tuber and raw dragon arum.

3.1.6 Mutual Inhibition

It means the efficacy of one medicinal will be eliminated by another one, even lose totally. For example, ginseng (renshen) is inhibited by radish seed (laifuzi), because radish seed can eliminate the nourishing function of ginseng.

3.1.7 Mutual antagonism

When two medicinals are combined, they can produce

性反应或副作用,如"十八反"等。

3.2 用药禁忌

在临床应用中,为了安全起见,一些用药方面的禁忌需要重视,主要包括配伍禁忌、妊娠禁忌以及服药时的饮食禁忌。

3.2.1配伍禁忌,指某些药物在复方中禁止或不宜配伍运用。目前医药界共同认可的配伍禁忌,主要有"十八反"和"十九畏"。

十八反:甘草反甘遂、大戟、海藻、芫花;乌头反贝母、瓜蒌、半夏、白蔹、白及;藜芦反人参、沙参、丹参、玄参、苦参、细辛、芍药。

十九畏:硫黄畏朴硝,水银畏砒霜,狼毒畏密陀僧,巴豆畏牵牛,丁香畏郁金,川乌、草乌畏犀角,牙硝畏三棱,官桂畏石脂,人参畏五灵脂。

3.2.2 妊娠禁忌

妊娠禁忌药物,主要是根据其能引起堕胎或终止妊娠而提出来的,主要包括对孕妇和胎儿两方面:一方面对母体不利和产程不利;另一方面对胎儿发育影响

---

toxic effects or side effects, such as "the eighteen antagonisms".

3.2 Contraindication

In clinical applications, for the patients, safety, some medicinal contraindications need special attention, including prohibited combination, contradiction during pregnancy and dietary incompatibility.

3.2.1 Prohibited combination means medicinals in specific combinations should be avoided. At present, the commonly acknowledged prohibited combinations in TCM are "the eighteen antagonisms" and "the nineteen incompatibilities".

The eighteen antagonisms are: liquorice root (gancao) with gansui root (gansui), peking euphorbia (daji), seaweed (haizao) and lilac daphne flower bud (yuanhua); aconite (wutou) with fritillaria (beimu), snakegourd fruit (gualou), pinellia tuber (banxia), Japanese ampelopsis root (bailian) and common bletilla rubber (baiji); false hellebore (lilu) with ginseng (renshen), radix adenophorea (shashen), salvia (danshen), figwort root (xuanshen), light yellow sophora root (kushen), manchurian wildginger (xixin) and peony (shaoyao).

The nineteen incompatibilities are: sulfur (liuhuang) with mirabilite (puxiao), mercury (shuiyin) with arsenic (pishuang), euphorbia (langdu) with lithargyrum (mituoseng), croton fruit (badou) with pharbitis (qianniu), clove (dingxiang) with turmeric root tuber (yujin), common monkshood mother root (chuanwu) and kusnezoff monkshood root (caowu) with rhinoceros horn (xijiao), sodium sulfate (yaxiao) with common buried rubber (sanling), cassia bark (guangui) with stone ester (shizhi), ginseng (renshen) with flying squirrel's droppings (wulingzhi).

3.2.2 Contraindications during pregnancy

The contradicted medicinals during pregnancy are put forward based on the possibility of unintended abortion and stopping pregnancy, which include two aspects: for the mother and fetus. On the one hand, the negative effects are on the mother and labor; on the other hand, the negative effects are on the growth and development of the child.

中医理论 Basic Theory of Traditional Chinese Medicine

及小儿生长不利。根据其对妊娠危害程度的不同，一般分为禁用与慎用两类。属禁用的多系毒剧烈、药性峻猛及堕胎作用较强的药物；慎用药则主要是活血祛瘀、行气、攻下、温里等类药中的部分药物。

禁用药：水银、砒霜、雄黄、轻粉、斑蝥、马钱子、蟾酥、川乌、草乌、藜芦、胆矾、瓜蒂、巴豆、甘遂、大戟、芫花、牵牛子、商陆、麝香、干漆、水蛭、虻虫、三棱、莪术等。

慎用药：牛膝、川芎、红花、桃仁、姜黄、牡丹皮、枳实、枳壳、大黄、番泻叶、芦荟、芒硝、附子、肉桂等。

3.2.3　服食禁忌

是指服药期间对某些食物的禁忌，也就是通常所说的"禁口"或"忌口"。一般而言，在病人服药期间，均应忌食生冷、辛热、油腻、腥膻等不易消化的食物。根据患者病情的不同，饮食禁忌也有区别，如热性病应忌食辛辣、煎炸类等热性食物；寒性病应忌食寒凉食物；肝阳上亢、头晕目眩、烦躁易怒等应忌食胡椒、辣椒、大蒜、白酒等辛热助阳之品；

According to the different degrees of harm during pregnancy, it is generally divided into two categories: to be avoided completely or to be given cautiously. The medicinals to be avoided usually have severe toxicity and powerful efficacy on abortion; the medicinals to be given cautiously are mainly used for activating blood and dispelling stasis, moving qi, purging the offensive and warming the interior.

Medicinals to be avoided include mercury (shuiyin), arsenic (pishuang), realgar (xionghuang), calomel (qingfen), blister beetle (banmao), nux vomica (maqianzi), toad venom (chansu), common monkshood mother root (chuanwu), kusnezoff monkshood root (caowu), false hellebore (lilu), chalcanthite (danfan), pediculi melo (guadi), croton fruit (badou), gansui root (gansui), peking euphorbia (daji), lilac daphne flower bud (yuanhua), pharbitis seed (qianniuzi), pokeberry root (shanglu), musk (shexiang), dried lacquer (ganqi), leech (shuizhi), gadfly (mangchong), common buried rubber (sanling) and zedoary (ezhu) and so on.

Medicinals to be given cautiously include twotoothed achyranthes root (niuxi), sichuan lovage rhizome (chuanxiong), safflower (honghua), peach seed (taoren), turmeric (jianghuang), tree peony root bark (mudanpi), immature orange fruit (zhishi), orange fruit (zhike), rhubarb (dahuang), senna leaf (fanxieye), aloe (luhui), crystallized sodium sulfate (mangxiao), aconite (fuzi) and cassia bark (rougui) and so on.

3.2.3　Dietary incompatibility

It refers to incompatibility of some food during medication. In general, during medication, patients should not eat raw and cold, pungent and hot, greasy and fishy foods which are not easy to digest. According to the patient's condition, dietary incompatibility is also different. For example, in heat disease, spicy and fried foods should be forbidden; in cold disease, cold foods should be forbidden; patients with liver-yang hyperactivity, dizziness, irritability should not eat pepper, chili, garlic, liquor and other spicy and hot foods which may support yang; patients with weak

脾胃虚弱者应忌食油炸黏腻、不易消化的食物；疮疡、皮肤病患者，应忌食鱼、虾、蟹等腥膻及辛辣刺激性食品。

3.3 中药的用法

中药的服用法，由于中药临床应用以汤剂为主，故重点介绍中药的煎煮方法及服用方法。

3.3.1 给药途径

中药的传统给药途径，主要以内服和外用（口服和皮肤用药）为主。此外还有吸入、舌下给药、黏膜表面给药、直肠给药等多种途径。现代中药的给药途径又增添了皮下注射、肌内注射、穴位注射和静脉注射等。

临床用药时，具体应选择何种途径给药，应综合考虑药物的作用特点与症情的需要，如清热泻火时石膏生用，以内服为主；收湿敛疮时，必须是煅后外用。

3.3.2 煎煮方法

汤剂是中药临床最常用的剂型，因此，掌握正确的煎煮方法，也是保证临床用药疗效发挥的重要条件。

1）煎药器皿

最好先用陶瓷器皿，如砂锅、砂罐。因其化学性质稳定，不易与药物成分发生化学反应，并且导热均匀、保暖性能好；其次可用白色搪瓷器皿或不锈钢锅。煎药器皿切忌用铁、铜、铝等金属器具，因这些金属元素易与药液中的化学成分发生化学反应，致

spleen and stomach should not eat fried and greasy food which is not easy to digest; patients with ulcers and skin diseases should avoid eating fish, shrimp, crab and other fishy and spicy foods.

3.3 Administration

Since decoction plays a major role in clinical application, administration of Chinese medicinals focuses on the method of medicinal decocting and administration.

3.3.1 Route

The traditional route for administration mainly includes oral and skin administration. In addition, there are other routes including inhaling, sublingual, mucosal surface and rectal administration. Presently there are new routes including subcutaneous, intramuscular, acu-point and intravenous injections.

In clinical medication, the specific choice for administration should relate to medicinal characteristics and syndromes. Such as, raw gypsum (shigao) is taken orally for clearing heat and purging fire; calcining gypsum is used externally to astringe dampness and furuncle.

3.3.2 Method for decoction

Decoction is the most commonly used form in clinical application. Therefore, mastering the correct method of decoction is also an important element to ensure clinical therapeutic efficacy.

1) Decocting vessel

It is best to use ceramic utensils, such as casserole and sand tank. Because of its stable chemical properties, it is not easy to react with the chemical composition, and its thermal conductivity is well-distributed and thermal performance is excellent. The second choice is white enamel ware or stainless steel pot. Because of the chemical reaction between metal elements and chemical components in liquid medicinals, the curative effect is reduced and even toxicity

中医理论 Basic Theory of Traditional Chinese Medicine

使疗效降低,甚至还可产生毒副作用。

2）煎药用水

煎药用水:加水量原则上应根据饮片质地疏密、吸水性能及煎煮时间长短来确定。一般用水量为将饮片适当加压后,液面淹没过饮片约2厘米为宜。若质地坚硬、黏稠,或需久煎的药物,加水量可比一般药物略多;而质地疏松,或有效成分容易挥发,煎煮时间较短的药物,则加水量可比一般药物略少。为了有利于有效成分的充分溶出,缩短煎煮时间,避免因煎煮时间过长,导致部分有效成分耗损、破坏过多。煎煮之前多数药物宜用冷水浸泡,一般药物可浸泡20～30分钟,以种子、果实为主的药可浸泡1小时。夏天气温高,浸泡时间不宜过长,以免腐败变质。

3）煎煮火候

煎煮中药时,一般药物宜先武火后文火,即未沸时用大火,沸后用小火保持微沸状态。解表药及其他芳香性药物,一般用武火迅速煮沸,改用文火维持10～15分钟左右即可。有效成分不易煎出的矿物类、骨角类、贝壳类、甲壳类药及补益药,一般宜文火久煎,以使有效成分能充分溶出。

4）煎煮次数及药量

一般来说,一剂药可煎三次,最少应煎两次。每剂药煎取液量,成人约200～300ml,小儿减半。

5）特殊药物的煎煮方法

一般药物可以同时入煎,但

and side effects can be produced, iron, copper, aluminum and other metal utensils should be avoided.

2) The water for decoction

The principle of water volume for decoction should be based on medicinal texture density, water absorption and the length of decoction time. The general water volume should be 2 centimeters above the medicinals which are pressed into the utensil. If the medicinals are hard and sticky, or need a long time to decoct, the water volume should be larger than common medicinals; however, if the medicinals are loose, their active ingredients tend to volatilize, or need a short time to decoct, the water volume should be a little smaller than the common medicinals. In order to get the effective components fully dissolved, shorten the decocting time to avoid decocting too long, resulting in some loss, even excessive destruction of effective components. Most medicinals should be soaked with cold water. The common medicinals should be soaked for 20~30 minutes; seeds and fruits should be soaked for 1 hour. Because of the high temperature in summer, the soaking time should not be too long in order to avoid medicinal spoilage.

3) Decocting fire

When decocting medicinals, a strong fire is applied before a slow fire. That is to say, before boiling, use a strong fire and switch to a small fire after boiling. For diaphoretic and other aromatic medicinals, use a strong fire to bring the water to boil immediately, and then change into a slow fire for about 10~15 minutes. The effective component in minerals, bones, shells, crust and tonic is not easy to dissolve by decocting, so they need a slow fire to decoct for a long time to dissolve effective component thoroughly.

4) Decoction time and dosage

Generally, a dose of medicinals can be decocted three times, or at least twice. Each dose of liquid medicinal for adults is about 200 ~ 300 ml, and half of it for children.

5) Decocting method for special medicinals

The common medicinals can be decocted together.

部分药物因其性质、性能及临床用途不同，所需煎煮时间不同。有的还需作特殊处理。

先煎：如金石、矿物、贝壳类药物，因其有效成分不易煎出，应打碎先煎20～30分钟，然后与其他药物同煎；又如川乌、附子等药，应先煎半小时以上再入它药同煎，因经久煎可以降低其毒性烈性，以确保用药的安全。

后下：一些容易挥散或破坏而不耐煎者，如薄荷、白豆蔻、大黄、番泻叶等药，入药宜后下，待他药煎煮将成时投入，煎沸几分钟即可。

包煎：有些药物煎煮时易飘浮在药液面上，或成糊状，不便于煎煮及服用，如蒲黄、海金沙、车前子、葶苈子、辛夷、旋覆花等，宜用纱布包裹入水再煎。

另煎：一些贵重药物，如人参等宜另煎，以免煎出的有效成分被其他药渣所吸附，影响疗效，以致造成浪费。

烊化：胶类药物，如阿胶、龟板胶、鹿角胶等，容易黏附于其他药渣及锅底，既浪费药材，又容易熬焦，宜另行烊化，再与其他药汁兑服。

冲服：一些粉末状、或液状类药物，如芒硝、竹沥等药，宜用煎好的其他药液或用开水冲服。

However, because of the special properties, characteristics and clinical application of some medicinals, the decocting time is different, and some of them even need special treatment.

Decoct first   Since the effective component of stones, minerals and shells is not easy to dissolve, so they should be ground and decocted for 20~30 minutes, then decocted with other medicinals. Common monkshood mother root (chuanwu) and aconite (fuzi) should be decocted for more than half an hour, and then decocted with other medicinals in that long-time decoction can reduce toxicity of medicinals to ensure medication safety.

Decoct later   Medicinals with ingredients easy to volatilize and be destroyed, such as peppermint (bohe), cardamon fruit (baidoukou), rhubarb (dahuang), senna leaf (fanxieye), should be put in when the decoction is almost done, and then they are decocted for several minutes after boiling.

Wrap-decoct   Some medicinals tending to float on water or conglomerate into a paste are not easy to be decocted and taken, such as cattail pollen (puhuang), Japanese climbing fern spore (haijinsha), plantain seed (cheqianzi), pepperweed seed (tinglizi), biond magnolia flower-bud (xinyi) and inula flower (xuanfuhua), should be wrapped when decocted.

Decoct separately   Some expensive medicinals, such as ginseng (renshen), should be decocted separately lest that the effective ingredients being absorbed by dregs of other medicinals to cause efficacy loss and waste.

Melt   Glue-like medicinals, such as donkey hide gelatin (ejiao), glue of tortoise plastron (guibanjiao), deerhorn glue (lujiaojiao) are easy to stick to the dregs or pot, which is wasteful and easy to become carbonized. They should be melted and then mixed with other liquid medicinals.

Take infused   Some powder or liquid medicinals, such as crystallized sodium sulfate (mangxiao) and bamboo vinegar (zhuli) should be infused with a decoction or boiling water.

中医理论

Basic Theory of Traditional Chinese Medicine

3.4　服药方法

3.4.1　服药时间

一般中药汤剂，每日早晚二次分服。服药与进食都应间隔1小时左右，以免影响药物与食物的消化吸收及药效的发挥，具体服药时间应根据病情需要及药物特性来确定。

清晨空腹服：如峻下逐水药晨起空腹时服药，不仅有利于药物迅速入肠发挥作用，且可避免晚间频频起床影响睡眠。

饭前服：驱虫药、攻下药及其他治疗胃肠道疾病的药物宜饭前服用。因饭前服用，有利于药物的消化吸收，故多数药宜饭前服用。

饭后服：对胃肠道有刺激性的药物宜于饭后服用。消食药亦宜饭后及时服用，以利充分发挥药效。

特定时间服：如安神药用于治失眠，宜在睡前30分钟至1小时服药；缓下剂亦宜睡前服用，以便翌日清晨排便；涩精止遗药也应晚间服一次药；截疟药应在疟疾发作前两小时服药，急性病则不拘时服。

3.4.2　服药量

一般疾病服用汤剂，多为每日一剂，每剂分二服或三服。病情急重者，可每隔四小时左右服药一次，昼夜不停，使药力持续，利于控制病情。

应用发汗药、泻下药时，因

3.4　Administration Method

3.4.1　Administration time

Usually, a dose can be taken twice per day, one in the morning and the other in the night. There is about 1 hour interval between administration and taking food so as not to affect digestion and absorption of medicinals and food, and medicinal efficacy. Specific administration time should be determined by clinical needs and medicinal characteristics.

In the morning　Administration of drastic hydragogue in the morning when the stomach is empty can not only get the medicinal into intestines immediately to work, but also can avoid getting up frequently during night, which will interrupt sleep.

Before dinner　Vermifuge, purgative medicinals and other medicinals dealing with stomach and intestinal disease should be taken before dinner, which is conducive to medicinal digestion and absorption, so most of the medicinals should be taken before dinner.

After dinner　Medicinals which can irritate the stomach and intestines should be taken after dinner. Digestant medicinals should be taken immediately after dinner in order to utilize their full potential.

Particular time　The tranquilizer for treating insomnia should be taken 30 minutes to 1 hour before bedtime; a laxative should be taken before going to bed, which can promote defecation in the next morning; medicinals stopping seminal emissions should be taken one extra dosage during night; medicinals to check malaria should be taken two hours before the onset of malaria. For acute disease, medicinals should be taken at any time.

3.4.2　Administration dosage

Usually for common diseases, one dosage of decoction should be taken per day which is divided into two or three parts. For the acute illness, take once every four hours day and night so that the efficacy can continue and the illness can be controlled.

药力较强,服药应适可而止。一般以得汗、得下为度,不必尽剂,以免汗、下太过,损伤正气。呕吐病人服药宜小量频服。

3.4.3 服药冷热

一般汤剂,多宜温服,如热病,患者欲冷饮者所用寒药可凉服;特殊情况下,如用从治法时,中医也会有热药凉服,或凉药热服的医嘱。

至于丸、散等固体药剂,除特别规定外(黄酒、盐水等),一般都宜用温开水送服。

Sweat-inducing and purgative medicinals with powerful efficacy cannot be taken excessively, because too much sweating will damage the vital qi. Vomiting patients should take a small amount of dosage.

3.4.3 Administration temperature

The common decoction should be taken in a warm temperature. The patient with heat syndromes who prefers cold drink can take cold medicinals in a cool temperature. Under special circumstances, such as retrograde treatment, there will be the doctor's advice like taking hot medicinals in a cool temperature or taking cool medicinals in a warm temperature.

As for pills, powder and other solid drugs, except special provisions (rice wine and salty water etc.), they are generally taken with warm water.

中医理论

Basic Theory of Traditional Chinese Medicine

第八章　中医养生

Chapter 8　Health Preservation

养生是中华民族传统文化的一个有机组成部分，整个中医学说就是广义的养生学。

疾病的发生与病情发展，虽然和致病因素有直接关系，但中医学更强调正气在发病中的主导地位，正气是发病与不发病的内在根据。致病邪气是无处不在的，只要自身的正气充足，也是可以不发病的，此即"正气存内，邪不可干"。只有在正气不足、防御能力下降，或者邪气致病能力超过正气的抗御能力时，外邪才会乘虚侵袭而发病，因此说"邪之所凑，其气必虚"。顾护正气体现于中医临床诊疗的全过程，养生即增强正气的主要方法和手段。

中医养生流派有很多。比如静神（恬淡虚无以养神等）、动形（八段锦、五禽戏、易筋经等导引以练形）、固精（各种房中术等）、调气（包括各种门派、形式的气功）、食养（包括节食、辟谷等）以及药饵（丹药）等。

养生内容广泛、方法众多，而以调饮食、慎起居、适寒温、和

Health preservation is an organic component of traditional Chinese culture. The whole traditional Chinese medicine theory is, in a broad sense, health preservation.

Although the occurrence and development of the disease have a direct relationship with pathogenic factors, TCM emphasizes the leading role of the vital qi which is the internal basis of health or disease. Pathogenic evil is pervasive, but as long as the vital qi is sufficient, diseases will not occur, which is known as "the inside vital qi can keep the evil invasion away". The evil can attack and diseases will occur only when the vital qi is deficient leading to the decline of defensive ability or the pathogenecity of the evil is stronger than the defensive ability of the vital qi, so there is the saying "accumulated evil leads to qi deficiency". Protecting the vital qi is embodied in the whole process of clinical diagnosis and treatment. Health preservation is the main method to enhance the vital qi.

There are many schools of health preservation. For example, staying in a calm mood (keeping a peaceful and pure heart and limiting desires to nourish spirit), exercising (eight-section brocade, five-animal boxing, muscle-bone strengthening exercise and other Chinese physical and breathing exercises), preserving the kidney-essence (various instructions for sexual intercourse), regulating qi (qigong in various schools and forms), having a proper diet (dieting and refraining from eating) and taking tonics (drugs with cinnabar) and so on.

The content and methods of health preservation is various and wide, of which the basic concept lies in having

喜怒为其基本养生观点，其基本原则也不外乎以下几点：

1 顺应自然

人生活在自然界，其生命活动遵循自然界的客观规律而进行，人体的生理活动必须与自然界的变化规律相适应。《素问·四气调神大论篇》提出了"春夏养阳，秋冬养阴。"这种"顺时摄养"的原则，就是顺应四时阴阳消长节律进行养生，从而使人体生理活动与自然界变化的周期同步，保持机体内外环境的协调统一。顺应自然包括天时与地利。

2 精神调摄

中医学非常重视人的精神活动与身体健康的关系。七情太过，不仅可直接伤及脏腑，引起气机紊乱而发病，也可损伤人体正气，使人体的自我调节能力减退。所以，调神，或曰养性，是养生的一个重要方面。《素问·上古天真论》说："恬淡虚无，真气从之，精神内守，病安从来。"即言心的生理特征是喜宁静。心静则神安，神安则体内真气和顺，就不会生病。传统气功中的炼意调神，即含此原理。除此之外，通过养性调神，还可改善气质、优化性格，增强自身的心理调摄能力，起到

a proper diet, living a regular life, adapting to coldness and warmth and having moderate joy and anger. The following are the basic principles.

1 Complying with Nature

Human beings live in the natural environment, so their life activities should follow the objective laws of nature, and their bodies' physiological activities must be adapted to the laws of change in nature. *Plain Questions: Major Discussion of Regulation of Spirit According to the Changes of the Four Seasons* puts forward "nourishing yang in spring and summer and nourishing yin in autumn and winter". The principle of "health preservation according to seasons" is to follow the decreasing and increasing law of four seasons and yin and yang so that human physiological activities is synchronized with the cycle of natural changes to harmonize the internal and external environments of the body. Complying with the nature includes complying with the time and location.

2 Mental Adjustment

TCM attaches great importance to the relationship between people's mental activity and physical health. Excessive emotions can not only cause direct injury of viscera and diseases due to qi disorder, but also damage the vital qi, leading to the decline of body's self-regulating ability. Therefore, mental adjustment (also known as nature cultivation) is an important aspect of health. In *Plain Questions: Ancient Ideas on How to Preserve Natural Healthy Energy*, there is the saying "keeping a peaceful and pure heart and limiting desires to have a vigorous genuine qi". That is to say, the physiological characteristic of the heart is being fond of peace. Keeping a calm mood makes a peaceful mind which can smooth the genuine qi to prevent diseases. Mental adjustment and mood regulation in tradi-tional qigong contains the above principle. Besides, through nature cultivation and mood regulation, temperament can be improved, character can be optimized and psychological adjustment ability can be strengthened, which plays a role

中医理论 Basic Theory of Traditional Chinese Medicine

预防疾病、健康长寿的功用。

in disease prevention, health-keeping and longevity.

3　护肾保精

男女从青春发育期开始产生的性冲动是先天赋予的本能，是人类种族延续所必需的，是肾中精气充盈的表现。因精能化气，气能生神，神能御气、御形，故精是形气神的基础，所以中医历来强调肾精对人体生命活动的重要性。体现在养生上，即有护肾保精的主张。性生活要有节制，不可纵欲无度以耗竭其精。男女间正常的性生活，是生理所需，对身体是无害的。若性生活得不到满足，每易形成气机郁滞之症，但性生活要消耗肾精肾气，而肾精肾气关系到人体的生长、发育、生殖等功能及机体阴阳平衡的调节，性生活过度，必致肾精肾气亏损而使人易于衰老或患病，故中医学将房劳过度看作是疾病的主要病因之一。

护肾保精之法除房事有节外，尚有运动保健、按摩固肾、食疗保肾、针灸药物调治等，从而使人体精充气足、形健神旺，达到预防疾病、健康长寿的目的。

4　形体锻炼

古人养生，注重"形神合一"、动静结合。《吕氏春秋·尽数》以"流水不腐，户枢不蠹，动也"为例，阐释了"形气亦然，形不动则

3　Protecting Kidney to Nourish Essence

The sexual impulse is the innate instinct starting from the men and women's puberty. It is necessary for the continuation of human race and is the reflection of sufficient kidney-essence. The essence can be transformed into qi, qi can generate the spirit and the spirit can control qi and constitution, so the essence is the basis of constitution, qi and spirit. Therefore, TCM has always stressed the importance of kidney essence for human life activities. In health preservation, protecting the kidney to nourish the essence is proposed. Sexual life should be moderate, because indulging in carnal pleasure without restraint will deplete the essence. Normal sexual life between men and women is a harmless physical need to the body. If sexual desire cannot be satisfied, qi stagnation syndrome will be formed gradually. However, sexual life can consume the kidney-essence and qi which are related to the body's growth, development and reproductive function and balance regulation of yin and yang. Excessive sexual life will surely cause loss of kidney-qi and essence to make a person subject to aging and illness, so TCM regards excessive sexual life as one of the main causes of illnesses.

Besides restraining sexual life to protect the kidney and nourish the essence, there are other methods, such as exercise and massage to strengthen the kidney, food therapy to nourish the kidney, acupuncture and drug treatment and so on to make the essence and qi abundant, body strong and spirit vigorous to achieve the goal of illness prevention, health and longevity.

4　Exercising

For health preservation, the ancient people laid emphasis on "harmonization between soma and spirit" and "association of activity and inertia". *Master Lü's Spring and Autumn Annals* takes "the running water does not stink

精不流,精不流则气郁"的道理。中医学认为锻炼形体可以促进气血流畅,使人体肌肉筋骨强健,脏腑功能旺盛,并可借形动以济神,从而使身体健康,益寿延年,同时也能预防疾病。传统的健身术如太极拳、易筋经、八段锦以及一些偏于健身的武术等,即具此特色。形体锻炼的要点有三:一是运动量要适度,要因人而异,做到"形劳而不倦";二是要循序渐进,运动量由小到大;三是要持之以恒,方能收效。

5 调摄饮食

调摄饮食主要包括注意饮食宜忌及药膳保健两个方面。

5.1 注意饮食宜忌

食物有偏性。一般说来,食性最好寒温适宜,或据体质而调配:体质偏热之人,宜食寒凉而忌温热之品;体质偏寒者,进食宜温而忌凉;平体之人,宜进平衡饮食而忌偏。

各种食物含有不同的营养成分,要调配适宜,不可偏食。正如《素问•藏气法时论》说:"五谷为养,五果为助,五畜为益,五菜为充。气味合而服之,以补益精气。"

此外,从预防的角度看,某些易使旧病复发或加重的"发物"亦不宜食。

and the spinning door-hinge does not rust" as an example to interpret the lesson "motionlessness leads to stagnant essence, while the stagnant essence leads to qi stagnation". TCM advocates that exercising can promote qi and blood to flow smoothly, strengthen muscles, tendons and bones, enhance the function of viscera and nourish the spirit in order to get a good health and a long life. The traditional exercising, such as taiji, muscle-bone strengthening exercise, eight-section brocade and some other body building martial arts, has the health preserving characteristics. Three points should be adhered for exercising: firstly, taking exercise should be appropriate in amount for different people; secondly, exercise should be taken regularly; thirdly, taking exercise is effective only with perseverance.

5 Having a Proper Diet

A proper diet includes two aspects: compatibility of diet and medicated diet.

5.1 Compatibility and incompatibility of diet

Each kind of food has its nature. Generally speaking, the best diet should be moderate in the food's nature and suitable for the person's constitution. For example, the person with a warm constitution had better take the food of cold nature but not of warm or hot nature; the person with a cold constitution had better take the food of warm nature but not of cold nature; the person with a moderate constitution had better keep a balanced diet.

Different food boasts of different nutrients. People should keep a balanced diet but not a biased one. As *Plain Questions: Discussion on the Association of the Zang-qi with Four Seasons* says, "Five grains are taken for growth; five fruits are to assist; five animals for benefit and five vegetables for supplement. Delicious food is taken to nourish and supplement the essence and qi."

In addition, from the perspective of prevention, some food having a trend to irritate the recurrence of an old illness or aggravate the illness is not suitable for eating.

中医理论 Basic Theory of Traditional Chinese Medicine

中医理论 Basic Theory of Traditional Chinese Medicine

5.2 药膳保健

药食同源。药膳是在中医学理论指导下,将食物与中药,以及食物的辅料、调料等相配合,通过加工调制而成的膳食。这些食品具有防治疾病和保健强身的作用。药膳常用的中药如人参、枸杞子、黄芪、黄精、莲子、百合、苡仁、芡实、菊花等,药性平和,可以长期服用,适应面较广。

正确的食用方法还应做到因时制宜、药食结合、辨证施膳等。

药膳兼有药、食二者之长,这是中医养生颇具特色的一种方法。

6 针灸、推拿、药物调养

药物调养是长期服食一些对身体有益的药物以扶助正气,平调体内阴阳,从而达到健身防病益寿的目的。其对象多为体质偏差较大或体弱多病者,前者则应根据患者的阴阳气血的偏颇而选用有针对性的药物,后者则以补益脾胃、肝肾为主。药物调养,往往长期服食才能见效。

推拿,是通过各种手法,作用于体表的特定部位,以调节机体生理病理状况,达到治疗效果和保健强身的一种方法。其原理有三:一是纠正解剖位置异常,二是调整体内生物信息,三是改变系统功能。

针灸包括针法和灸法,即通

5.2 Medicated Diet

Medicine and food are homologous. Medicated diet in the guidance of the theory of TCM is the allocated combination of food, food accessories and seasoning in a proper percentage, which have the function of preventing and controlling diseases and keeping fit. The herb used in the medicated diet contains ginseng, medlar, astragalus, polygonatum, lotus seeds, lily, coix seed, gorgon fruit and chrysanthemum which are mild in nature and can be taken for a long time and used widely.

The proper diet should be combined with season, medicine and syndrome differentiation.

Medicated diet possessing the advantages of drug and food is a distinctive method of health preservation.

6 Acupuncture, Massage, Medicinal Maintenance

Medicinal maintenance refers to taking some beneficial drugs on a long term basis to assist the vital qi and balance yin and yang inside the body in order to achieve the aim of fitness, disease prevention and longevity. Persons with a largely deviated constitution and are weak in physique and constantly ill usually follow this way. The former should be treated with the targeted drug according to his or her physical deviation of yin and yang, qi and blood; the latter should be treated by replenishing spleen and stomach, liver and kidney.

Massage, through a variety of techniques, works on specific parts of the body surface to regulate the body's physiological and pathological conditions in order to achieve the effect of treatment and health care. Three principles should be followed in massage: the first is to correct the abnormal anatomical position; the second is to adjust the biological information of the body; the third is to change the system function.

Acupuncture includes needling and moxibustion.

过针刺手法或艾灸的物理热效应及艾绒的药性对穴位的特异刺激作用,通过经络系统的感应传导及调节机能,而使人身气血阴阳得到调整而恢复平衡,从而发挥其治疗保健及防病效能。

Through the needling therapy or the physical thermal effect of moxibustion and the drug effect of moxa on the acupoint, specific stimulating effect can be achieved. Through the conduction, induction and regulation function of the meridian system, the balance of qi and blood, yin and yang can be regulated and restored, so as to exert the effect of treatment, health care and disease prevention.

中医理论

Basic Theory of Traditional Chinese Medicine

附录1 常见中医典籍名中文、拼音、英文对照表

中医理论

Basic Theory of Traditional Chinese Medicine

书名	拼音	英文译名
周礼	Zhou Li	The Rites of Zhou
黄帝内经	Huangdi Neijing	Huangdi's Internal Classic
伤寒杂病论	Shanghan Zabing Lun	Treatise on Cold Damage and Miscellaneous Diseases
神农本草经	Shennong Bencao Jing	Shennong's Classic of Materia Medica
难经	Nan Jing	Classic of Difficult Issues
素问	Su Wen	Plain Questions
尚书正义	Shangshu Zhengyi	Revelation to the Book of History
难经	Nan Jing	Classic of Difficult Issues
灵枢	Ling Shu	Miraculous Pivot
伤寒论	Shanghan Lun	Treatise on Cold Damage Diseases
礼记	Li Ji	The Book of Rites
脉经	Mai Jing	Pulse Classic
濒湖脉诀	Binhu Maijue	Binhu's Sphygmology
诊家正眼	Zhenjia Zhengyan	Key to Physicians
本草纲目	Bencao Gangmu	Compendium of Materia Medica
吕氏春秋	Lüshi Chunqiu	Master Lü's Spring and Autumn Annals

附录 2　常用中药名中文、拼音、拉丁文、英文对照表
（按拼音顺序）

汉语	拼音	拉丁文	英文
A			
艾叶	aiye	Artemisiae Argyi	argy wormwood leaf
B			
巴豆	badou	Fructus Crotonis	croton fruit
巴豆霜	badoushuang	——*	defatted croton seed powder
巴戟天	bajitian	Radix Morindae Officinalis	morinda root
白豆蔻	baidoukou	Fructus Ammomi Rotundus	cardamon fruit
白附子	baifuzi	Rhizoma Typhonii	giant typhonium rhizome
白及	baiji	Rhizoma Bletillae	common bletilla rubber
白芥子	baijiezi	Sinapis Alba	white mustard seed
白菊花	baijuhua	Dendranthema morifolium	chrysanthemum
白蔹	bailian	Ampelopsis japonica	Japanese ampelopsis root
白芍	baishao	Radix Paeoniae Alba	debark peony root
白术	baizhu	Rhizoma Atractylodis Macrocephalae	largehead atractylodes rhizome
白芷	baizhi	Radix Angelicae Dahuricae	dahurian angelica root
败酱草	baijiangcao	Herba Patriniae	atrina glass
斑蝥	banmao	Mylabris	blister beetle
板蓝根	banlangen	Radix Isatidis	isatis root
半边莲	banbianlian	Herba Lobeliae Chinensis	Chinese lobelia herb
半夏	banxia	Rhizoma Pinelliae	pinellia tuber
薄荷	bohe	Herba Menthae	peppermint
北口芪	beikouqi	——	stilbene of Northeast China
北细辛	beixixin	Asarum heterotropoides	manchurian wildginger
贝母	beimu	Bulbus Fritillaria	fritillaria
鳖甲	biejia	Carapax Trionycis	turtle shell

*——表示没有相应的拉丁文名称。

汉语	拼音	拉丁文	英文
C			
苍耳	canger	Fructus Xanthii	siberian cocklebur fruit
苍术	cangzhu	Rhizoma Atractylodis	atractylodes rhizome
草乌	caowu	Radix Aconiti Kusnezoffii	kusnezoff monkshood root
侧柏叶	cebaiye	Cacumen Platycladi	Chinese arborvitae twig and leaf
柴胡	chaihu	Radix Bupleuri	Chinese thorowax root
蝉衣	chanyi	Periostracum Cicadae	cicada slough
蟾酥	chansu	Venenum Bufonis	toad venom
车前子	cheqianzi	Semen Plantaginis	plantain seed
沉香	chenxiang	Lignum Aquilariae Resinatum	Chinese eaglewood
陈皮	chenpi	Pericarpium Citri Reticulatae	dried tangerine peel
陈棕	chenzong	——	petiolo-nervus trachycarpi
川贝母	chuanbeimu	Bulbus Fritillariae Cirrhosae	tendrilleaf fritillary bulb
川楝子	chuanlianzi	Fructus Meliae Toosendan	szechwan chinaberry fruit
川牛膝	chuanniuxi	Radix Cyathulae	medicinal cyathula root
川乌	chuanwu	Radix Aconiti	common monkshood mother root
川芎	chuanxiong	Rhizoma Ligustici Chuanxiong	sichuan lovage rhizome
垂盆草	chuipencao	Herba Sedi	stringy stonecrop herb
磁石	cishi	Magnetitum	magnetite
D			
大枫子	dafengzi	Hydnocarpus anthelmintica	chaulmoogra seed
大腹皮	dafupi	Pericarpium Arecae	areca peel
大黄	dahuang	Radix et Rhizoma Rhei	rhubarb
大戟	daji	Euphorbia pekinensis	peking euphorbia
大青叶	daqingye	Folium Isatidis	dyers woad leaf
大枣	dazao	Fructus Jujubae	Chinese date
代赭石	daizheshi	——	haematitum
丹参	danshen	Radix Salviae Miltiorrhizae	salvia
胆矾	danfan	——	chalcanthite
淡豆豉	dandouchi	Semen Sojae Preparatum	fermented soybean

汉语	拼音	拉丁文	英文
淡竹叶	danzhuye	Herba Lophatheri	lophatherum herb
当归	danggui	Radix Angelicae Sinensis	Chinese angelica
灯心草	dengxincao	Medulla Junci	common rush
地鳖虫	dibiechong	Eupolyphaga Seu Steleophaga	eupolyphaga sinensis walker
地骨皮	digupi	Cortex Lycii	Chinese wolfberry root-bark
地黄	dihuang	Rehmannia glutinosa	radix rehmanniae
丁香	dingxiang	Flos Caryophylli	clove
冬虫夏草	dongchongxiacao	Cordyceps	Chinese caterpillar fungus
兜铃	douling	Aristolochia contorta	dutchmanspipe fruit
独活	duhuo	Radix Angelicae Pubescentis	pubescent angelica
杜仲	duzhong	Cortex Eucommiae	eucommia bark
E			
莪术	ezhu	Curcuma zedoaria (Christm.) Rosc	zedoary
阿胶	ejiao	——	donkey hide gelatin
F			
番红花	fanhonghua	Crocus sativus L	saffron
番木鳖	fanmubie	——	nux vomica
番泻叶	fanxieye	Folium Sennae	senna leaf
防风	fangfeng	Radix Saposhnikoviae	divaricate saposhnikovia root
凤仙花子	fengxianhuazi	——	impatiens balsamina seed
茯苓	fuling	Poria cocos	Indian buead
附子	fuzi	Aconitum carmichaeli Debx	aconite
G			
甘草	gancao	Radix Glycyrrhizae	liquorice root
甘遂	gansui	Radix Euphorbiae Kansui	gansui root
干姜	ganjiang	Rhizoma Zingiberis	dried ginger
干漆	ganqi	Resina Toxicodendri	dried lacquer
葛根	gegen	Radix Puerariae	kudzuvine root

中医理论 Basic Theory of Traditional Chinese Medicine

汉语	拼音	拉丁文	英文
钩藤	gouteng	Ramulus Uncariae Cum Uncis	gambir plant nod
谷芽	guya	Fructus Setariae Germinatus	millet sprout
骨碎补	gusuibu	Rhizoma Drynariae	fortune's drynaria rhizome
瓜蒂	guadi	——	pediculi melo
瓜蒌	gualou	Fructus Trichosanthis	snakegourd fruit
官桂	guangui	Cortex Cinnamomi	Cassia bark
龟板	guiban	Carapax et Plastrum Testudinis	tortoise carapace and plastron
龟板胶	guibanjiao	——	glue of tortoise plastron
桂皮	guipi	Cinnamomum tamala	cinnamon bark
桂枝	guizhi	Ramulus Cinnamomi	cassia twig
H			
孩儿参	haiershen	Pseudostellaria heterophylla	radix pseudostell
海风藤	haifengteng	Caulis Piperis Kadsurae	kadsura pepper stem
海浮石	haifushi	——	pumice stone
海狗肾	haigoushen	——	urine seal testes and penis
海金沙	haijinsha	Spora Lygodii	Japanese climbing fern spore
海藻	haizao	Sargassum	seaweed
寒水石	hanshuishi	——	glauberitum
诃黎勒	helilie	haritaki	terminalia
何首乌	heshouwu	Radix Polygoni Multiflori	fleeceflower root
荷叶	heye	Folium Nelumbinis	lotus leaf
鹤草芽	hecaoya	Agrimonia pilosa	agrimony
红花	honghua	Flos Carthami	safflower
红藤	hongteng	Sargentodoxa cuneata	sargentgloryvine stem
厚朴	houpo	Cortex Magnoliae Officinalis	officinal magnolia bark
胡黄连	huhuanglian	Rhizoma Picrorhizae	figwortflower picrorhiza rhizome
胡椒	hujiao	Fructus Piperis Nigri	pepper fruit
胡麻仁	humaren	Sesamum indicum	sesame seed
胡桃仁	hutaoren	Juglans regia	walnut meat

汉语	拼音	拉丁文	英文
花蕊石	huaruishi	——	ophicalcitum
滑石	huashi	Talcum	talc
黄柏	huangbai	Cortex Phellodendri	amur cork-tree
黄狗肾	huanggoushen	——	dog penis
黄连	huanglian	Rhizoma Coptidis	golden thread
黄芪	huangqi	Radix Astragali seu Hedysari	milkvetch root
黄芩	huangqin	Radix Scutellariae	baical skullcap root
J			
鸡内金	jineijin	Endothelium Corneum Gigeriae Galli	inner membrane of chicken gizzard
鸡血藤	jixueteng	Caulis Spatholobi	suberect spatholobus stem
急性子	jixingzi	Semen Impatientis	garden balsam seed
姜	jiang	Zingiber officinale Roscoe	ginger
姜黄	jianghuang	Rhizoma Curcumae Longae	turmeric
金银花	jinyinshua	Flos Lonicerae	honeysuckle bud and flower
桔梗	jiegeng	Radix Platycodonis	platycodon root
菊花	juhua	Flos Chrysanthemi	chrysanthemum
决明子	juemingzi	Semen Cassiae	cassia seed
K			
苦参	Kushen	Radix Sophorae Flavescentis	light yellow sophora root
苦楝皮	Kulianpi	Cortex Meliae	Sichuan chinaberry bark
款冬花	Kuandonghua	Flos Farfarae	common coltsfoot flower
昆布	Kunbu	Thallus Laminariae	kelp
L			
莱菔子	laifuzi	Semen Raphani	radish seed
狼毒	langdu	Euphorbia ebracteolata	euphorbia
藜芦	lilu	Veratrum nigrum	false hellebore
连翘	lianqiao	Fructus Forsythiae	weeping forsythia capsule
莲子	lianzi	Semen Nelumbinis	lotus seed
辽五味	liaowuwei	Schisandra sphenanthera	schisandra chinensis
灵磁石	lingcishi	——	magnetite

汉语	拼音	拉丁文	英文
刘寄奴	liujinu	Artemisia; anomala	diverse wormwood herb
硫黄	liuhuang	——	sulfur
龙胆草	longdancao	Radix Gentianae	Chinese gentian
芦根	lugen	Rhizoma Phragmitis	reed rhizome
芦荟	luhui	Aloe	aloe
炉甘石	luganshi	Galamina	calamine
鹿角	lujiao	Cornu Cervi	antler
鹿角胶	lujiaojiao	Colla Corni Cervi	deerhorn glue
鹿茸	lurong	Cornu Cervi Pantotrichum	pilose antler
络石藤	luoshiteng	Caulis Trachelospermi	Chinese starjasmine stem
M			
麻黄	mahuang	Herba Ephedrae	ephedra
马钱子	maqianzi	Semen Strychni	nux vomica
麦芽	maiya	Fructus Hordei Germinatus	germinated barley
曼陀罗	mantuoluo	Datura stramonium	datura stramonium
芒硝	mangxiao	Natrii Sulfas	crystallized sodium sulfate
猫爪草	maozhuacao	Radix Ranunculi Ternati	catclaw buttercup root
虻虫	mengchong	Tabanus	gadfly
密陀僧	mituoseng	——	lithargyrum
牡丹皮	mudanpi	Cortex Moutan Radicis	tree peony root bark
牡蛎	muli	Concha Ostreae	oyster shell
木蝴蝶	muhudie	Semen Oroxyli	Indian trumpet flower seed
木香	muxiang	Radix Aucklandiae	common aucklandia root
木通	mutong	Caulis Akebiae	akebia stem
木贼草	muzeicao	Herba Equiseti Hiemalis	common scouring rush herb
N			
南星	nanxing	Arisaema heterophyllum Blume	dragon arum
牛膝	niuxi	Radix Achyranthis Bidentatae	twotoothed achyranthes root
女贞子	nüzhenzi	Fructus Ligustri Lucidi	glossy privet fruit
P			
佩兰	peilan	Herba Eupatorii	fortune eupatorium herb

汉语	拼音	拉丁文	英文
硼砂	pengsha	——	borax
砒霜	pishuang	——	arsenic
枇杷叶	pipaye	Folium Eriobotryae	loquat leaf
蒲公英	pugongying	Herba Taraxaci	dandelion
蒲黄	puhuang	Pollen Typhae	cattail pollen
朴硝	puxiao	——	mirabilite
Q			
七叶一枝花	qiyeyizhihua	Paris chinensis	Paris polyphylla
蕲蛇	qishe	——	agkistrodon
牵牛	qianniu	Pharbitidis	pharbitis
牵牛子	qianniuzi	Semen Pharbitidis	pharbitis seed
前胡	qianhu	Radix Peucedani	hogfennel root
羌活	qianghuo	Rhizoma et Radix Notopterygii	incised notopterygium rhizome and root
秦艽	qinjiao	Radix Gentianae Macrophyllae	largeleaf gentian root
秦椒	qinjiao	Zanthoxylum bungeanum	xanthoxylum piperitum
青黛	qingdai	Indigo Naturalis	natural indigo
青风藤	qingfengteng	Caulis Sinomenii	orientvine vine
青蒿	qinghao	Herba Artemisiae Annuae	sweet wormwood herb
青皮	qingpi	Pericarpium Citri Reticulatae Viride	immature tangerine peel
轻粉	qingfen	Calomelas	calomel
R			
人参	renshen	Radix Ginseng	ginseng
人发	renfa	——	human hair
忍冬藤	rendongteng	Caulis Lonicerae	honeysuckle stem
肉桂	rougui	Cortex Cinnamomi	cassia bark
乳香	ruxiang	Olibanum	frankincense
S			
三棱	sanleng	Rhizoma Sparganii	common buried rubber
桑白皮	sangbaipi	Cortex Mori	white mulberry root-bark

汉语	拼音	拉丁文	英文
桑槐	sanghuai	——	mulberry and sophora japonica
桑寄生	sangjisheng	Herba Taxilli	Chinese taxillus herb
桑叶	sangye	Folium Mori	mulberry leaf
沙参	shashen	Adenophora stricta	radix adenophorea
山豆根	shandougen	Radix Sophorae Tonkinensis	vietnamese sophora root
山甲片	shanjiapian	Manis pentadactyla Linnaeus	pangolin scales
山药	shanyao	Rhizoma Dioscoreae	common yam rhizome
山楂	shanzha	Fructus Crataegi	hawthorn fruit
山茱萸	shanzhuyu	Fructus Corni	asiatic cornelian cherry fruit
商陆	shanglu	Radix Phytolaccae	pokeberry root
芍药	shaoyao	Paeonia lactiflora	peony
麝香	shexiang	Moschus	musk
伸筋草	shenjincao	Herba Lycopodii	common clubmoss herb
神曲	Shenqu	Massa Medicata Fermentata	medicated leaven
升麻	Shengma	Rhizoma Cimicifugae	largetrifoliolious bugbane rhizome
生地黄	Shengdihuang	Rehmannia glutinosa Libosch	rehmanniae radix
石膏	shigao	Gypsum Fibrosum	gypsum
石决明	shijueming	Concha Haliotidis	abalone shell
石榴皮	shiliupi	Pericarpium Granati	pomegranate rind
石楠藤	shinanteng	Piper puberulum	piper wallichii
石脂	shizhi	——	stone ester
使君子	shijunzi	Fructus Quisqualis	rangooncreeper fruit
首乌藤	shouwuteng	Caulis Polygoni Multiflori	tuber fleece flower stem
熟大黄	shudahuang	——	prepared rhubarb
熟地黄	shudihuang	Radix Rehmanniae Preparata	prepared rehmannia root
水银	shuiyin	——	mercury
水蛭	shuizhi	Hirudo	leech
松香	songxiang	Pinus massoniana	rosin
苏合香	suhexiang	Styrax	storax

Basic Theory of Traditional Chinese Medicine

汉语	拼音	拉丁文	英文
苏叶	suye	Perilla frutescens	perilla leaf
苏子	suzi	Perilla frutescens (L.) Britt. var. acuta (Thunb.) kudo	perilla
T			
胎盘	taipan	——	placenta
檀香	tanxiang	Lignum Santali Albi	sandalwood
桃仁	taoren	Semen Persicae	peach seed
天麻	tianma	Rhizoma Gastrodiae	tall gastrodia tuber
甜杏仁	tianxingren	Amygdalus Communis Vas	dessert almond
葶苈子	tinglizi	Semen Lepidii	pepperweed seed
通草	tongcao	Medulla Tetrapanacis	ricepaperplant pith
土鳖虫	tubiechong	Eupolyphaga Seu Steleophaga	ground beetle
W			
乌梢蛇	wushaoshe	Zaocys	black-tail snake
乌头	wutou	Aconitum carmichaeli Debx.	aconite
乌贼骨	wuzeigu	Cleistocactus sepium	cuttlefish bone
吴茱萸	wuzhuyu	Fructus Evodiae	medicinal evodia fruit
蜈蚣	wugong	Scolopendra	centipede
五灵脂	wulingzhi	Faeces Togopteri	flying squirrel's droppings
五味子	wuweizi	Fructus Schisandrae Chinensis	Chinese magnoliavine fruit
X			
西瓜霜	xiguashuang	——	watermelon frost
西红花	xihonghua	Stigma Croci	saffron
犀角	xijiao	Rhinoceros unicornis L	rhinoceros horn
细辛	xixin	Herba Asari	manchurian wildginger
夏枯草	xiakucao	Spica Prunellae	common selfheal fruit-spike
香附	xiangfu	Rhizoma Cyperi	nutgrass galingale rhizome
辛夷	xinyi	Flos Magnoliae	biond magnolia flower-bud
杏仁	xingren	Semen Armeniacae Amarum	bitter apricot seed
雄黄	xionghuang	——	realgar
熊胆汁	xiongdanzhi	——	bear bile

中医理论

Basic Theory of Traditional Chinese Medicine

汉语	拼音	拉丁文	英文
徐长卿	xuchangqing	Radix Cynanchi Paniculati	paniculate swallowwort root
续断	xuduan	Radix Dipsaci	himalayan teasel root
玄参	xuanshen	Radix Scrophulariae	figwort root
旋覆	xuanfu	Inula japonica Thunb	inula
旋覆花	xuanfuhua	Flos Inulae	inula flower
Y			
牙硝	yaxiao	——	sodium sulfate
延胡索	yanhusuo	Corydalis yanhusuo	rhizoma corydalis
阳起石	yangqishi		actinolite
益母草	yimucao	Herba Leonuri	motherwort herb
茵陈	yinchen	Herba Artemisiae Scopariae	virgate wormwood herb
迎春花	yingchunhua	Jasminum nudiflorum Lindl.	winter jasmine
鱼腥草	yuxingcao	Herba Houttuyniae	heartleaf houttuynia herb
禹余粮	yuyuliang	Limonitum	limonite
郁金	yujin	Radix Curcumae	turmeric root tuber
芫花	yuanhua	Flos Genkwa	lilac daphne flower bud
远志	yuanzhi	Radix Polygalae	milkwort root
月季花	yuejihua	Flos Rosae Chinensis	Chinese rose flower
Z			
藏红花	zanghonghua	Crocus sativus L.	Saffron
蚤休	zaoxiu	Paris chinensis	Paris polyphylla
泽泻	zexie	Rhizoma Alismatis	oriental waterplantain rhizome
知母	zhimu	Rhizoma Anemarrhenae	common anemarrhena rhizome
枳壳	zhike	Fructus Aurantii	orange fruit
枳实	zhishi	Fructus Aurantii Immaturus	immature orange fruit
朱砂	zhusha	——	cinnabar
猪胆汁	zhudanzhi	——	pig bile
猪苓	zhuling	Polyporus Umbellatus	polyporus
竹沥	zhuli		bamboo vinegar

续表

汉语	拼音	拉丁文	英文
紫草	zicao	Radix Arnebiae	arnebia root
紫河车	ziheche	Placenta Hominis	human placenta
紫花地丁	zihuadiding	Herba Violae	Tokyo violet herb
紫苏叶	zisuye	Folium Perillae	perilla leaf
紫苏子	zisuzi	Fructus Perillae	perilla fruit
紫菀	ziwan	Radix Asteris	tatarian aster root

中 医 理 论

Basic Theory of Traditional Chinese Medicine